T0198260

COVID 19: How the Pandemic Changed Psychiatry for Good

Editors

ROBERT L. TRESTMAN
ARPAN WAGHRAY

PSYCHIATRIC CLINICS OF NORTH AMERICA

www.psych.theclinics.com

Consulting Editor
HARSH K. TRIVEDI

March 2022 • Volume 45 • Number 1

ELSEVIER

1600 John F. Kennedy Boulevard • Suite 1800 • Philadelphia, Pennsylvania, 19103-2899

http://www.theclinics.com

PSYCHIATRIC CLINICS OF NORTH AMERICA Volume 45, Number 1
March 2022 ISSN 0193-953X, ISBN-13: 978-0-323-84858-9

Editor: Megan Ashdown
Developmental Editor: Diana Grace Ang

Psychiatric Clinics of North America (ISSN 0193-953X) is published quarterly by Elsevier Inc., 360 Park Avenue South, New York, NY 10010-1710. Months of issue are March, June, September, and December. Business and Editorial Offices: 1600 John F. Kennedy Blvd., Suite 1800, Philadelphia, PA 19103-2899. Periodicals postage paid at New York, NY and additional mailing offices. Subscription prices are $345.00 per year (US individuals), $985.00 per year (US institutions), $100.00 per year (US students/residents), $414.00 per year (Canadian individuals), $509.00 per year (international individuals), $1005.00 per year (Canadian & international institutions), and $220.00 per year (international students/residents), $100.00 per year (Canadian & students/residents). Foreign air speed delivery is included in all *Clinics*' subscription prices. All prices are subject to change without notice. **POSTMASTER:** Send address changes to *Psychiatric Clinics of North America*, Elsevier Health Sciences Division, Subscription Customer Service, 3251 Riverport Lane, Maryland Heights, MO 63043. **Customer Service: 1-800-654-2452 (US). From outside the United States, call 1-314-447-8871. Fax: 1-314-447-8029. E-mail: journalscustomerservice-usa@elsevier.com (for print support)** and **journalsonlinesupport-usa@elsevier.com (for online support)**.

Reprints. For copies of 100 or more, of articles in this publication, please contact the Commercial Reprints Department, Elsevier Inc., 360 Park Avenue South, New York, New York 10010-1710. Tel.: 212-633-3874, Fax: 212-633-3820, E-mail: reprints@elsevier.com.

Psychiatric Clinics of North America is covered in *MEDLINE/PubMed (Index Medicus), Current Contents/Social and Behavioral Sciences, Social Science Citation Index, Embase/Excerpta Medica,* and PsycINFO.

Contributors

CONSULTING EDITOR

HARSH K. TRIVEDI, MD, MBA
President and Chief Executive Officer, Sheppard Pratt, Clinical Professor of Psychiatry, University of Maryland School of Medicine, Baltimore, Maryland, USA

EDITORS

ROBERT L. TRESTMAN, PhD, MD
Professor and Chair of Psychiatry and Behavioral Medicine, Virginia Tech/Carilion School of Medicine and Carilion Clinic, Carilion Clinic Department of Psychiatry and Behavioral Medicine, Roanoke, Virginia, USA

ARPAN WAGHRAY, MD
Chief Medical Officer, Behavioral Medicine, Providence Health and Services, CMO, Well Being Trust, Executive Medical Director, Behavioral Medicine, Issaquah, Washington, USA

AUTHORS

KELLY B. AHERN, BS
Department of Psychiatry, Washington University School of Medicine, St Louis, Missouri, USA

MANUEL G. ALVAREZ ROMERO, BA
Research Coordinator, Department of Emergency Medicine, University of Arkansas for Medical Sciences, Little Rock, Arkansas, USA

AZZIZA BANKOLE, MD
Virginia Tech Carilion School of Medicine, Carilion Center for Healthy Aging, Roanoke, Virginia, USA

JOSHUA BEREZIN, MD, MS
New York State Office of Mental Health, New York, New York, USA

LESLIE BUCKLEY, MD, MPH
Addictions Division, Centre for Addiction and Mental Health, Department of Psychiatry, University of Toronto, Toronto, Ontario, Canada

MATTHEW BUTLER, MD
Maudsley BRC Preparatory Clinical Research Training Fellow, Institute of Psychiatry, Psychology and Neuroscience, King's College, London

SHIREEN F. CAMA, MD
Program Director in Child and Adolescent Psychiatry, Cambridge Health Alliance, Instructor, Harvard Medical School, Cambridge, Massachusetts, USA

FLAVIO CASOY, MD
New York State Office of Mental Health, New York, New York, USA

DENISE CHANG, MD
Assistant Professor, Department of Psychiatry and Behavioral Sciences, University of Washington, Seattle, Washington, USA

WAI TAT CHIU, AM
Department of Health Care Policy, Harvard Medical School, Boston, Massachusetts, USA

BENJAMIN CROSS, MD
Foundation Year One Doctor, East Lancashire Hospitals NHS Trust, Burnley, United Kingdom

MARA DE MAIO, PhD
Director, Child and Adolescent Services, Institute of Living, Hartford, Connecticut, USA

SANDRA M. DEJONG, MD, MSc
Senior Consultant to Child and Adolescent Psychiatry Training, Cambridge Health Alliance, Assistant Professor, Harvard Medical School, Cambridge, Massachusetts, USA

WAYNE K. DERUITER, PhD
Nicotine Dependence Service, Centre for Addiction and Mental Health, Toronto, Ontario, Canada

MARK H. DUNCAN, MD
Assistant Professor, Department of Psychiatry and Behavioral Sciences, University of Washington, Seattle, Washington, USA

JENNIFER M. ERICKSON, DO
Assistant Professor, Department of Psychiatry and Behavioral Sciences, University of Washington, Seattle, Washington, USA

MATTHEW D. ERLICH, MD
New York State Office of Mental Health, New York, New York, USA

DANISH HAFEEZ
School of Medical Sciences, The University of Manchester, Manchester, United Kingdom

YAMILETTE HERNANDEZ, BS
New York State Office of Mental Health, New York, New York, USA

IRVING H. HWANG, MA
Department of Health Care Policy, Harvard Medical School, Boston, Massachusetts, USA

MICHAEL JUSTIN COFFEY, MD, FAPA, FANPA
Professor of Psychiatry, Chair of Psychiatry and Behavioral Health, Geisinger, Danville, Pennsylvania, USA

SUZANNE KERNS, MBBS
Assistant Professor of Psychiatry, Medical University of South Carolina, Charleston, South Carolina, USA

RONALD C. KESSLER, PhD
Department of Health Care Policy, Harvard Medical School, Boston, Massachusetts, USA

ERIC J. LENZE, MD
Department of Psychiatry, Washington University School of Medicine, St Louis, Missouri, USA

MAO FONG LIM, MD
Foundation Year Two Doctor, Cambridge University Hospitals NHS Foundation Trust, Cambridge, United Kingdom

OSNAT C. MELAMED, MD, MSc
Nicotine Dependence Service, Centre for Addiction and Mental Health, Department of Family and Community Medicine, University of Toronto, Toronto, Ontario, Canada

LAURENCE H. MILLER, MD
Senior Psychiatrist, Division of Medical Services, Arkansas Department of Human Services, Clinical Professor, Department of Psychiatry, University of Arkansas for Medical Sciences, Little Rock, Arkansas, USA

BRIGITTA E. MIYAMOTO, MD
Fellow in Child and Adolescent Psychiatry, Cambridge Health Alliance, Cambridge, Massachusetts, USA

JOSHUA C. MORGANSTEIN, MD
Associate Professor and Vice Chair, Department of Psychiatry, Deputy Director, Center for the Study of Traumatic Stress, School of Medicine, Uniformed Services University, Bethesda, Maryland, USA

HAMILTON MORRIN, MD
Foundation Year Two Doctor, Maidstone & Tunbridge Wells NHS Trust, Maidstone, United Kingdom

TIMOTHY R. NICHOLSON, PhD
Senior Clinical Lecturer, Institute of Psychiatry, Psychology and Neuroscience, King's College, London

JOSEPH PARKS, MD
Vice President, Practice Improvement and Medical Director, Practice Improvement and Consulting, National Council for Mental Wellbeing, Washington, DC, USA

CHANDRA PENTHALA, BA
Research Associate, Department of Emergency Medicine, University of Arkansas for Medical Sciences, Little Rock, Arkansas, USA

TOM POLLAK, PhD
NIHR Clinical Lecturer, Institute of Psychiatry, Psychology and Neuroscience, King's College, London

VICTOR PUAC-POLANCO, MD, DrPH
Department of Health Care Policy, Harvard Medical School, Boston, Massachusetts, USA

ANNA D.H. RATZLIFF, MD, PhD
Professor, Depression Therapy Research Endowed Professorship, Director, UW Psychiatry Residency Training Program, Co-Director, AIMS Center, Director, UW Integrated Care Training Program, Department of Psychiatry and Behavioral Sciences, University of Washington, Seattle, Washington, USA

EMMA RACHEL RENGASAMY, MD
Academic Foundation Year Two Doctor, Cwm Taf Morgannwg University Health Board, Wales, United Kingdom

NANCY A. SAMPSON, BA
Department of Health Care Policy, Harvard Medical School, Boston, Massachusetts, USA

SOHAG SANGHANI, MD
Assistant Professor of Psychiatry, Donald and Barbara Zucker School of Medicine at Hofstra/Northwell, Hempstead, New York, USA

JOHN SANTOPIETRO, MD
Assistant Professor of Psychiatry, University of Connecticut School of Medicine, Senior Vice President, Hartford HealthCare, Physician-in-Chief, Behavioral Health Network, Hartford, Connecticut, USA; Assistant Clinical Professor of Psychiatry, Yale School of Medicine, New Haven, Connecticut, USA

PETER SELBY, MBBS, MHSc
Nicotine Dependence Service, Centre for Addiction and Mental Health, Departments of Family and Community Medicine, and Psychiatry, Dalla Lana School of Public Health, University of Toronto, Toronto, Ontario, Canada

MANU S. SHARMA, MD
Assitant Professor of Psychiatry, Yale School of Medicine, New Haven, Connecticut, USA

THOMAS E. SMITH, MD
New York State Office of Mental Health, New York, New York, USA

RAMANPREET TOOR, MD
Assistant Professor, Department of Psychiatry and Behavioral Sciences, University of Washington, Seattle, Washington, USA

HARSH K. TRIVEDI, MD, MBA
President and Chief Executive Officer, Sheppard Pratt, Clinical Professor of Psychiatry, University of Maryland School of Medicine, Baltimore, Maryland, USA

LEE WACHTEL, MD
Associate Professor of Psychiatry, Kennedy Krieger Institute, Baltimore, Maryland, USA

MICHAEL P. WILSON, MD, PhD
Assistant Professor, Departments of Emergency Medicine and Psychiatry, University of Arkansas for Medical Sciences, Little Rock, Arkansas, USA

PETER YELLOWLEES, MBBS, MD
Allen Stoudemire Endowed Distinguished Professor of Psychiatry, Department of Psychiatry and Behavioral Sciences, University of California, Davis, Sacramento, California, USA

KEVIN YOUNG, PhD
Program Director, Psychology Training, Institute of Living, Hartford, Connecticut, USA; Assistant Professor, Psychiatry, University of Connecticut School of Medicine

REBECCA YOWELL, BS
Director, Reimbursement Policy and Quality, American Psychiatric Association, Washington, DC, USA

ALAN M. ZASLAVSKY, PhD
Department of Health Care Policy, Harvard Medical School, Boston, Massachusetts, USA

SCOTT L. ZELLER, MD
Assistant Clinical Professor, Department of Psychiatry, University of California, Riverside, Riverside, California, USA; Vice President, Acute Psychiatry, Vituity, Emeryville, California, USA

HANNAH N. ZIOBROWSKI, PhD, MPH
Department of Health Care Policy, Harvard Medical School, Boston, Massachusetts, USA

Contents

PSYCHIATRIC CLINICS OF NORTH AMERICA

FORTHCOMING ISSUES

June 2022
Workforce and Professional Diversity in Psychiatry
Altha J. Stewart and Howard Y. Liu, *Editors*

September 2022
Addiction Psychiatry: Challenges and Recent Advances
George Kolodner, Sunil Khushalani, and Christopher Welsh, *Editors*

RECENT ISSUES

December 2021
Ethics in Psychiatry
Rebecca Weintraub Brendel and Michelle Hume, *Editors*

September 2021
Sport Psychiatry: Maximizing Performance
Andy Jagoda and Silvana Riggio, *Editors*

June 2021
Medical Education in Psychiatry
Robert J. Boland and Hermioni L. Amonoo, *Editors*

SERIES OF RELATED INTEREST

Child and Adolescent Psychiatric Clinics of North America
https://www.childpsych.theclinics.com/

Neurologic Clinics
https://www.neurologic.theclinics.com/

THE CLINICS ARE AVAILABLE ONLINE!
Access your subscription at:
www.theclinics.com

Preface

There's No Going Back: The Transformation of Psychiatry and Psychiatric Care Postpandemic

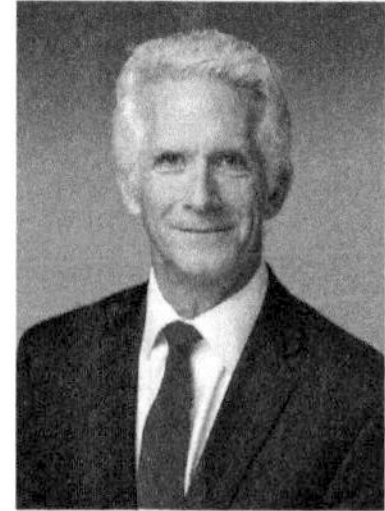

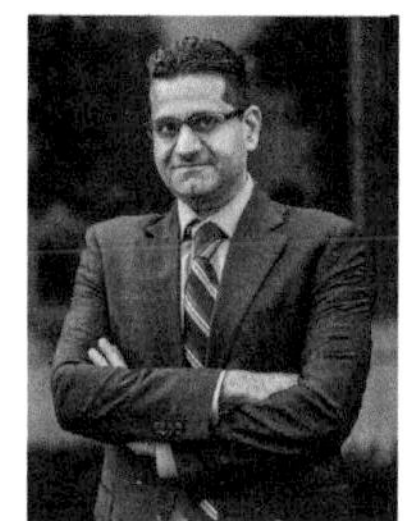

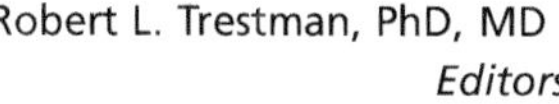

Robert L. Trestman, PhD, MD   Arpan Waghray, MD
Editors

The COVID-19 pandemic is not the first, nor sadly the last, crisis we will face as a country. Mental illness and addiction were at crisis levels long before COVID-19. During and postpandemic, the isolation, uncertainty, economic hardships, and social dislocation led to what has been described as the "Second Pandemic" of despair, substance misuse, and mental illness. Nor did the impact of the pandemic fall on each of us equally. The longstanding inequities in health and health care became accentuated during the pandemic, placing disproportionate burdens on those already marginalized or underresourced.

The COVID-19 pandemic created additional barriers for people already suffering from mental illness and substance use disorders, requiring psychiatrists and other mental health providers to rapidly adapt the way psychiatric care is delivered. Some of these changes have been very positive, enhancing the patient experience, improving access to care, and transforming the work life of psychiatric providers.

There are many lessons learned and promising practices that will persist beyond the pandemic. In this issue of *Psychiatric Clinics of North America*, we take a comprehensive look at the impact of the pandemic on psychiatric practice in a variety of care settings and for different populations. In each, we incorporate some of the ways in which health inequity played a part: through social or structural determinants, financial constraints, and other extant biases.

We begin with a piece authored by Dr Ron Kessler and colleagues examining changes in prevalence of mental illness and substance use disorders consequent to the pandemic and the social upheavals that followed. The increases that are found result from multiple previously known factors: genetic risks and preexisting illness;

Psychiatr Clin N Am 45 (2022) xv–xvii
https://doi.org/10.1016/j.psc.2021.11.016

isolation and loss of social support; financial and housing instability; increased family distress; and so forth.

The potential of a new causative factor may also be in play: the fact that the SARS-CoV-2 virus and its many variants may have inflammatory effects on the brain. Dr Mathew Butler and colleagues thoughtfully address the evolving knowledge base of the viral neuropathology and potential pathways that may lead to psychiatric illness.

We then transition to domains of clinical care during the pandemic. Dr Thomas Smith and colleagues describe the adaptations of a major state's health care system to deal with inpatient psychiatric care across the various stages of the pandemic. In parallel to inpatient changes, Dr Manu Sharma and colleagues reflect on the experience of transforming outpatient psychiatric care. For many practices, clinics, and systems, this was an almost overnight phenomenon: converting from in-person to virtual care with a speed unimaginable even 1 year earlier.

Many of us in psychiatry have worked to integrate our work into primary care for many years. Dr Ratzliff and colleagues address some of the opportunities utilized during the pandemic to accelerate that work, as well as discuss some of the ongoing pragmatic challenges. As we all know, the emergency departments of every hospital were hard hit. In emergency psychiatry, though, the pattern was by no means linear. Dr Scott Zeller takes a close look into the patterns and disruptions that occurred in psychiatric care in emergency departments, along with the innovations that allowed our patients to continue to receive that critical level of triage, evaluation, and treatment.

While mental illness per se was a major and growing concern, so too was substance use. The isolation and stressors all contributed to a dramatic surge in substance use disorders and overdose deaths during the pandemic. Dr Peter Selby and colleagues examine the ways in which the treatment of substance use disorders was transformed during the pandemic, and how what we learned may shape the future of addiction treatment.

While the pandemic had a broad impact on society, it had a profound impact on those of us charged to care for the sick. Dr Peter Yellowlees takes a detailed look into the impact of the pandemic on health care workers in general and psychiatric personnel in particular. The lessons learned in providing comprehensive support will likely serve to sustain and enhance the profession and change the culture to one that recognizes the importance of seeking and accepting help for ourselves.

Interventional psychiatry has evolved into a complex field over the past years, including not only electroconvulsive therapy, but also transcranial magnetic stimulation, vagal nerve stimulation, and ketamine and related treatments, among others. Administering such treatment during the pandemic created multiple challenges. Dr Justin Coffey describes the impact of the pandemic on interventional psychiatry and the adaptations developed to allow for ongoing access to these critical services.

Children and the elderly are psychiatric populations that are among the most vulnerable. Each have long required unique treatment adaptations and skills to assess and to provide appropriate care. Dr Sandra DeJong and colleagues discuss the challenges and adaptations to care delivery for children and adolescents during the pandemic, and Dr Azziza Bankole reviews the multiple adaptations required to deliver care to the elderly, whether at home or in institutional settings.

Among the many changes that were required during the pandemic, some of the most extensive were the ways in which care was financed. The federal government, individual states, and commercial insurers each modified regulations and funding mechanisms to support transformed service delivery in a complex and sometimes inconsistent fashion. Dr Laurence Miller and colleagues help us understand the changes in detail and look at the impact these changes had on care and care delivery.

The largest freestanding nongovernmental psychiatric care system in the United States is Sheppard Pratt, based in Maryland. Dr Harsh Trivedi, President and CEO of Sheppard Pratt, utilizes the changes made in that system to speak to lessons learned that may have significant application for the future of psychiatric care.

Psychiatric care has improved dramatically over the past few decades, largely driven by research findings and the implementation of those findings. The pandemic created profound challenges to ongoing clinical research, in some cases halting it completely. Dr Eric Lenze and colleagues describe some of those impacts and some of the remarkable adaptations researchers made to pursue clinical research despite the restrictions of a pandemic.

Each disaster, whether flood, draught, tornado, or violent disruption, has anticipated psychiatric consequences. The pandemic, which brought together a confluence of lethal disease, social unrest, and political instability, is an extreme and lengthy disaster. Dr Joshua Morganstein, whose career has focused on the psychiatric consequences of disaster, addressed our inadequate preparedness for this event and what we have learned to better position us for any future pandemic.

In conceiving this wide-ranging issue of *Psychiatric Clinics of North America*, whose title is "COVID-19: How the Pandemic Changed Psychiatry for Good," we attempted to bring together the spectrum of experiences and knowledge that span the impact of the pandemic on clinical psychiatry. We hope that the many lessons learned and shared throughout this issue help the readers better understand the impact of the pandemic on psychiatric practice and reimagine excellence in the delivery of care.

Robert L. Trestman, PhD, MD
Virginia Tech/Carilion School of Medicine
Carilion Clinic
Department of Psychiatry and
Behavioral Medicine
2017 South Jefferson Street
1st Floor Administrative Suite
Roanoke, VA 24014, USA

Arpan Waghray, MD
Behavioral Medicine
Providence Health and Services
Well Being Trust
Behavioral Medicine
Swedish Health Services
751 NE Blakely Drive, IS 4475
Issaquah, WA 98029, USA

E-mail addresses:
rltrestman@carilionclinic.org (R.L. Trestman)
arpan.waghray@swedish.org (A. Waghray)

Changes in Prevalence of Mental Illness Among US Adults During Compared with Before the COVID-19 Pandemic

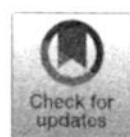

Ronald C. Kessler, PhD*, Wai Tat Chiu, AM, Irving H. Hwang, MA, Victor Puac-Polanco, MD, DrPH, Nancy A. Sampson, BA, Hannah N. Ziobrowski, PhD, MPH, Alan M. Zaslavsky, PhD

KEYWORDS

• Cohort study • COVID-19 • Health disparities • Mental disorders • Trend study

KEY POINTS

- Although thousands of articles have been published over the past 18 months on the mental health effects of COVID-19, only a few describing US samples were based on research designs that support valid inferences about changes in prevalence or disparities in common mental disorders either during the pandemic or before the pandemic or over the course of the pandemic.
- Reports based on nonprobability general population surveys carried out early in the pandemic estimated that point prevalence of clinically significant anxiety-depression increased by relative risk (RR) = 5.0 to 8.0 during the pandemic compared with before the pandemic. A more focused analysis of available evidence suggests that the true change was probably in the range RR = 1.3 to 1.5, although the increase could have been greater in persistent anxiety-depression or in some segments of the population.
- Disparities in prevalence of anxiety-depression during the pandemic compared with before the pandemic appear to have increased among people younger than 60 years of age, members of racial/ethnic minorities, and people with education levels less than a 4-year college degree.
- Changes in prevalence over the course of the pandemic have occurred (both up and down at different times), but health disparities have not changed substantially overall based on sex, age, education, or race/ethnicity.

 **Video content accompanies this article at http://www.psych.theclinics.com.**

Department of Health Care Policy, Harvard Medical School, 180 Longwood Ave, Ste 215, Boston, MA 02115-5899, USA
* Corresponding author.
E-mail address: kessler@hcp.med.harvard.edu

Psychiatr Clin N Am 45 (2022) 1–28
https://doi.org/10.1016/j.psc.2021.11.013

As of August 2021, COVID-19 infection has caused more than 637,000 US deaths,[1] and the pandemic has caused many more deaths owing to external causes (most notably drug overdose)[2] beyond those projected from previous years. Mitigation measures have resulted in massive changes in day-to-day life and an unemployment rate early in the pandemic that was higher than any other time since the Great Depression.[3] Unemployment remains high even now, 18 months after the pandemic began. Even more importantly, the *long-term* unemployment rate, an indicator of severe financial distress,[4,5] is currently more than double the prepandemic rate.[5] In addition, many more people are living on reduced incomes and are experiencing uncertainties about their financial futures.[6] Adding to these stresses, the pandemic occurred during a time of civic polarization that highlighted inequalities exacerbated by the pandemic,[7] leading to wide variation in responses to government mitigation efforts and consequent variations in pandemic spread.[8]

In the context of this enormous complexity, we were asked by the editors to review the literature on evolving changes in prevalence of mental disorders in the US adult general population during compared with those measured before the pandemic. Concerns about such changes have been raised since the beginning of the pandemic[9,10] based partly on evidence from past infectious disease outbreaks[11–13] and other natural disasters[14] documenting adverse mental health effects of these events owing to exposure to component stressors, such as job loss,[15] death of a loved one,[16] social isolation,[17] and multiple accumulated stressors that often occur during major disasters.[18]

TRENDS IN MENTAL DISORDER PREVALENCE SINCE BEFORE THE COVID-19 PANDEMIC

A search of American Psychological Association PsycINFO, OVID Medline, Embase, Scopus, and Web of Science for published English language articles on COVID-19 and mental health in July 2021 found 14,094 articles, including 49 reviews of research on the pandemic's effects on general population mental health.[19] Most of these reviews were not quantitative and concluded merely that the pandemic had the potential to increase psychopathology (eg, Ref.[20]) and that certain segments of the population are likely to be at especially high risk (eg, Refs.[21,22]). Most of the underlying studies in the reviews were based on nonprobability samples without established prepandemic baselines.

Accurate trend estimates require before and after comparisons based either on true trend studies (ie, sampling and field procedures that are the same before and after) or cohort studies (ie, the same individuals are assessed before and after). Trend studies are more common. Caution is needed in interpreting their results, though, as the pandemic might have changed response rates and field survey procedures. In the case of administrative trend data (eg, emergency department [ED] visits), there may have been new barriers to health care access during the pandemic. Cohort surveys are less subject to these biases but suffer from attrition bias. The remainder of this section reviews trend and cohort studies that attempted to make before and after comparisons of mental health in the COVID-19 pandemic.

Noncomparable Trend Surveys

Twenge and Joiner[23] carried out a national survey of n = 19,330 adults in April 2020 from an online consumer panel sample that was designed to be representative of the US population on broad geographic and sociodemographic characteristics.[24] The same short self-report screening scale of serious mental illness (SMI)[25] used in the US government's 2018 National Health Interview Survey (NHIS)[26] was administered in that online survey. The investigators estimated that SMI prevalence increased 8-fold in the United States since the 2018 NHIS. However, the NHIS was a face-to-face household survey carried out by the Census Bureau with a response rate of 61%, whereas the online survey was based on a nonprobability sample with an unknown response rate. That sample, although balanced to the population on basic geographic-demographic characteristics, might have been quite different from the population on psychological characteristics.[27] Other widely cited studies that used similar noncomparable trend designs (ie, comparing the prevalence of mental illness in prepandemic benchmark government surveys to estimates in online nonprobability surveys carried out during the pandemic) came to a similar conclusion: that there were massive increases in the prevalence of common mental disorders (CMD) during the pandemic, with relative risk (RR) ranging from 3.0 to 5.0.[23,28–31] These comparisons all had the same fundamental design flaw as the Twenge and Joiner study. Although methods exist to improve estimates of population prevalence in such nonprobability surveys,[32] particularly when other surveys with the same instruments and more systematic sampling are available, these methods were not used in any of these noncomparable trend studies.

Several other studies compared prevalence estimates in baseline prepandemic benchmark government surveys with estimates in the Centers for Disease Control and Prevention (CDC) Household Pulse Survey (HPS), a major ongoing US government trend survey initiated in April 2020 to track mental health, health insurance coverage, and problems accessing care during the pandemic.[33] The HPS has so far collected self-report survey data from more than 2.7 million respondents. The HPS includes the 4-item Patient Health Questionnaire (PHQ-4) screening scale of current anxiety-depression,[34] which was the same scale used in the benchmark NHIS and in subsamples of another important national benchmark government survey, the CDC Behavioral Risk Factor Surveillance Survey (BRFSS).[35] The studies that used the HPS as the follow-up survey during the pandemic and made comparisons with prepandemic estimates based on the 2018 or 2019 NHIS or BRFSS drew similar conclusions to those of the studies that used commercial noncomparable trend surveys: that the prevalence of clinically significant PHQ-4 scores increased during the pandemic with RR of 3.0 to 5.0.[23,28,36]

However, none of these HPS trend study reports noted that the HPS, unlike the NHIS or BRFSS, is one of the Census Bureau's "Experimental Data Products,"[37] which the Bureau uses to provide rapid response to time-sensitive questions before more definitive results can be generated from benchmark surveys. The HPS achieves this rapid response by using an online self-report questionnaire administered to large samples of people residing in households across the country recruited via e-mail and text invitations either weekly (in the first 12 HPS waves) or biweekly (in subsequent HPS waves). As in online consumer surveys, the HPS uses weights to match sample distributions to Census population distributions on the cross-classification of age, sex, race/ethnicity, education, and geography (the 50 states, the District of Columbia, and the 15 largest metropolitan statistical areas). However, unlike benchmark government surveys like the NHIS, the weekly phase 1 HPS (April 14 to July 23, 2020) had a response rate of only 1.3% to 2.9%. The response rate increased in subsequent HPS phases to 6.3% to 10.3% based on important design changes, including shifting to a 2-week rather than 1-week field period.[38] The Census Bureau documentation is clear that these low response rates make it hazardous to compare prevalence estimates in the HPS with those in earlier benchmark government surveys,[39] but this caution did not deter researchers from making such comparisons and declaring that COVID-19 had a dramatic effect on US mental health.

COHORT SURVEYS

A living systematic review of high-quality cohort studies is being carried out by a Canadian research group to assess pandemic effects on population mental health.[40]

Study inclusion requires the same participants to be assessed both before and during the pandemic with either a high follow-up response rate or usage of a statistical adjustment for follow-up survey nonresponse bias. A first report by this research group posted in May 2021 based on 33 cohorts[41] concluded, in striking contrast to the results of the noncomparable trend studies described above, that "mental health in the general population has not worsened compared to pre-COVID-19 levels."

To begin reconciling the striking inconsistency between this conclusion and the conclusion of the noncomparable trend surveys, it is important to note that the cohort studies in the review were international, covered diverse population segments, and varied enormously in size. Focusing only on the large national probability-based samples in the review shows clearly that pandemic impact differed significantly both within and across countries and over time. A national UK cohort study in the review, which was made up of more than 40,000 households studied since 2009,[42] found that the prevalence (95% confidence interval [CI]) of current clinically significant CMD[43] was significantly higher in April 2020 than the average across the 19 prepandemic waves (29.5% [28.0–31.0] vs 20.8% [19.4–22.2]),[44] but that current prevalence decreased to the prepandemic level (20.8% [19.5–22.1]) in a follow-up survey 5 months later.[45] In comparison, a large Norwegian cohort study based on a panel of more than 230,000 people studied since 1984[42] initiated a new wave of data collection shortly before the start of the pandemic to assess 30-day prevalence of CMD using the World Health Organization Composite International Diagnostic Interview.[46] That survey was carried out in random replicates to test the new instrument. The prevalence (95% CI) was significantly higher in the first random replicate (15.3% [12.4–18.8]) implemented just before the pandemic started (January 28 to March 11, 2020), than in the replicate carried out during the first 3 months of the pandemic (March 12 to May 31; 8.7% [6.8–11.0]). The prevalence then increased back to the prepandemic level in the next 2 random replicates (June 1 to July 21; 14.2% [11.4–17.5] and August 1 to September 18; 11.9% [9.0–15.6]).[47] These large studies demonstrate clearly that pandemic effects on mental health varied both by country and by time of assessment during the pandemic.

With those results in mind, it is noteworthy that only 3 of the 33 studies in the cohort study review[40] came from the United States. These all involved small population segments: a convenience sample of n = 2288 sex- and gender-minority adults and 2 even smaller (n = 178–205) samples of students from single universities. Significant increases in screening scales of current anxiety-depression were found in all 3 studies. Although each study reported results in terms of means rather than proportions with clinically significant disorders, standardized mean differences can be converted into estimates of RR if we make assumptions about prepandemic prevalence and distributions.[48] When we did this using the assumption that prepandemic anxiety-depression prevalence was in the plausible range of 5% to 10%, the RR equivalents were 1.3 to 2.8, which are below the lower end of the 3.0 to 8.0 range estimated in the noncomparable trend surveys.

All 3 US cohort studies in the review were carried out in small population segments, whereas the trend surveys were based on samples of the general population. We are aware of only one US cohort study that was carried out in a national general population sample shortly before and then again during the pandemic. This study was not included in the systematic review because it did not meet the requirement for a high follow-up response rate or nonresponse adjustment. Based on the RAND American Life Panel (ALP),[49] this cohort study included an online survey of n = 2555 adults ages 20+ in February 2019, n = 2020 of whom also completed a follow-up survey in May 2020. SMI was assessed using the same screening scale as in the 2018 NHIS.[25] However, the 2019 survey used the "worst month" version of that scale, which asks respondents to think of the 1 month in the past 12 when they had the most persistent and severe psychological distress when answering the questions, whereas the 2020 survey used the past-month version of the scale, which asks respondents to think of the month before the survey in answering the questions. The recommended approach is to administer both versions in a single survey,[50] with the past-month version administered first to obtain information that approximates point prevalence and then only administering the worst month questions to the subset of respondents who report having a worse month than the current one. The latter estimate is needed in some jurisdictions for policy planning purposes.

SMI prevalence (95% CI) in these ALP cohort surveys was 10.9% (7.6–14.0) 12-month prevalence in 2019 and 10.1% (6.9–13.3) 1-month prevalence in 2020.[51] Based on previous surveys that administered both versions of the scale to the same samples of respondents,[50] the ratio of 1-month to 12-month prevalence in high-income countries is estimated to have a median (interquartile range) of 73.8% (50.4–80.2; Appendix Table 1). This would put the prepandemic 1-month SMI prevalence estimate in the ALP sample at 8.0% and RR during the pandemic versus before at approximately RR = 1.3. The latter is at the lower end of the RR = 1.3 to 2.8 range across the 3 true US cohort studies in the systematic review and well below the RR = 3.0 to 8.0 range in the US noncomparable trend surveys.

Taken together, these results suggest that the noncomparable trend surveys substantially overestimated the effect of the pandemic on population mental health. A central reason for this is likely to be selection bias owing to very high nonresponse in the nonprobability online surveys used to assess mental disorders during the pandemic. As mentioned earlier, although these nonprobability surveys were balanced to the population on basic geographic-demographic characteristics, it is likely that they were different in psychological characteristics from the population in ways that were not corrected by adjustments for geographic-demographic variables. To that point, it is noteworthy that the 8.0% best estimate of SMI prevalence in the prepandemic ALP survey, which had a similar sample design as the other online surveys used in the noncomparable trend comparisons, was more than 2 times the 3.4% estimate in the 2018 NHIS.[23] Although the ALP is described as a "nationally representative, probability-based panel,"[49] it is "representative" only in the sense that weights were used to make the joint distribution of the weighted sample on basic sociodemographic and geographic variables comparable to the distribution of the Census population. There is no reason to assume that the mental health of people in the ALP sample represents the mental health of the US population. The ALP response rate is likely less than 5%[52] compared with the 61% response rate of the 2018 NHIS.

TRUE TREND SURVEYS

True trend studies can provide equally, if not more, accurate information about change in disorder prevalence than cohort studies but with lower statistical power. Three relevant large-scale US government benchmark trend surveys exist to do this. Two of them, the NHIS and the BRFSS, were already mentioned. The third is the National Health and Nutrition Examination Survey (NHANES), a face-to-face household survey that combines physical examinations with self-reports in a sample of about 5000 respondents per year.[53] The 2020 to 2021 NHIS and NHANES are both face-to-face surveys that were disrupted by the pandemic. The BRFSS, in comparison, is a telephone survey that continued without interruption during the pandemic in monthly replicates interviewing more than 400,000 respondents each year.[35] At the time of writing this article, the 2020 BRFSS were only recently posted. We are not aware of any reports that have analyzed BRFSS trends into 2020.

We are aware of only one other true US national trend survey that has reported relevant data as of now: the annual November Gallup Poll Health and Healthcare survey. This is a national telephone survey carried out since 2001 in a random digit dial telephone sample with demographic weighting targets comparable to those in online surveys carried out during the pandemic.[54] However, unlike the latter, the same design and field procedures used for many years in the annual Gallup survey were repeated in its November 2020 survey. One of the survey questions is "*How would you describe your own mental health or emotional well-being at this time? Would you say it is excellent, good, only fair, or poor?*" The proportion of respondents who answered "fair" or "poor" was higher in the 2020 survey than in any year since the survey began 2 decades ago: 23% compared with a median (interquartile range) in previous years of 13% (13–15). RR in 2020 versus 2019 was 1.5.[55] Responses to this type of general excellent-to-poor mental health question are known to be strongly correlated with prevalence of CMDs (Appendix Table 2). Thus, although the Gallup survey does not provide direct estimates of depression anxiety, it does indirectly support the finding in cohort studies of more modest elevations in prevalence.

Administrative Trend Data

Emergency department visits

As noted above, changes in factors other than true prevalence can influence trends in administrative data, making it important to be cautious in interpreting such data. These extraneous influences are perhaps not clearer than in trend data on ED visits, which dropped by 42% nationwide in the first 2 months of the COVID-19 pandemic compared with the same months in 2019,[56] increased subsequently up until August 2020 to become about 15% lower than in the prior year, and then decreased again to become about 25% lower than the prior year in the first months of 2021.[57] The disorder-specific patterns in these ED visit trends are inconsistent with changes in true prevalence.[58,59] The trends more likely occurred because people who would otherwise have come to the ED failed to do so because of fear of COVID-19 exposure, minimizing nonurgent care, or reduced access to care because of loss of insurance in conjunction with job loss.

Based on this complex set of possibilities, some researchers have focused on *proportional* changes in presenting problems in ED visits rather than *absolute* changes.[57,60] These studies show that even though absolute volume of ED visits for mental health problems decreased since the beginning of the pandemic, the proportional decrease has been lower than that for many other presenting problems. This finding has sometimes been interpreted to mean that a higher proportion of mental disorders that would otherwise be seen at an ED exceed the severity threshold that led people to seek ED treatment even during the pandemic.[60] However, this interpretation is difficult to accept given that substantial reductions in ED visits occurred for many life-threatening illnesses during the pandemic, resulting in the proportion of deaths from natural causes occurring at home increasing substantially since the beginning of the pandemic.[61]

Another possibility is that alternatives to ED treatment decreased more for mental disorders than physical disorders during the pandemic.[62] A related possibility is that changes in relative severity of ED presentations within conditions changed during than before the pandemic in ways that led to differences in overall visits across conditions because of delays in typical help-seeking patterns. For example, the number of patients presenting at EDs with complicated appendicitis increased significantly during the pandemic, whereas the number with uncomplicated appendicitis decreased, indicating that people with appendicitis were waiting longer before going to the ED during the pandemic than before.[63] We are aware of no attempts to compare changes in severity of ED mental disorder presentations during versus before the pandemic.

Although these complexities make it impossible to draw firm conclusions from ED trend data about changes in true prevalence of mental disorders during the pandemic, there are 2 exceptions: ED visits for suicide attempts among adolescents and Emergency Medical Services (EMS) activations for drug overdoses both increased in *absolute* numbers during the pandemic. The most plausible interpretation of these increases is that they were caused by true increases in prevalence, as the ED would normally be the first-line treatment for both these presentations. The number of adolescent (ages 12–17) ED visits for suspected suicide attempts was 22.3% higher in the summer of 2020 than the summer of 2019 and 39.1% higher in the winter of 2021 than the winter of 2019.[64] No comparable absolute increase occurred among adults. In the case of drug overdoses, although an absolute increase in number of ED visits reported by the CDC[60] appears to have been an artifact of the ED sample in that study increasing in size over time,[62] data from the National Emergency Medical Services Information System documents a 42.1% increase in EMS activations for overdose-related cardiac arrests in 2020 compared with 2019.[65] This appears to be another example of delays in help-seeking resulting in a higher proportion of comparatively severe cases presenting for care during than before the pandemic. The fact that this dramatic increase in EMS activations was not reflected in ED visits suggests that many of the overdoses resulted in death before reaching the ED. As we see in the next subsection, mortality trend data are consistent with this interpretation.

Mortality

Total number of deaths in the United States increased by 503,976 in 2020 compared with 2019.[66] An estimated 345,323 of these excess deaths were classified by CDC as directly owing to COVID-19,[67] making COVID-19 the third leading cause of death in 2020 behind only heart disease and cancer. However, there were also substantial increases in death from several other leading causes, including cardiometabolic disorders: heart disease (20% of the total excess not owing directly to COVID-19), diabetes (8%), and stroke (6%).[68] These increases presumably occurred because of disrupted treatments and incorrect classification of some such deaths as due to chronic conditions when they were in fact due to COVID-19.[69]

Suicide deaths did not increase in 2020. Indeed, the US suicide rate was slightly lower in 2020 than 2019,[68] consistent with evidence from other countries in the early months of the pandemic.[70] However, initial declines in suicides during other infectious disease outbreaks have sometimes been followed by increases,[71] so it might be that increased suicides will occur as a late consequence of the COVID-19 pandemic. Preliminary evidence for such a scenario has already been reported in Japan.[72]

Deaths owing to 3 other external causes increased significantly during the pandemic: homicides, drug overdoses, and unintentional injury deaths.[73] The most recent CDC quarterly provisional mortality data found that there were 30% more homicides in both the second and the third quarters of 2020 compared with the same quarters in 2019.[74] An important factor in this trend is that close to 80% of all US homicides are committed with firearms,[75] and firearm sales skyrocketed during the early part of the pandemic in conjunction with the social and political unrest and violent protests that surrounded the last year of the Trump presidency.[76] A recent report found that between-state variation in increased firearm purchases during the COVID-19 pandemic was correlated with between-state increases in both fatal and nonfatal firearm-related interpersonal violence during the early months of the pandemic.[77] Importantly, this significant pattern was only for domestic violence (RR = 1.8–2.6), not for nondomestic violence (RR = 0.8–1.0).

Although the increased RR in firearm-related domestic violence was higher than that for increased drug overdose deaths (RR = 1.5 in Q2 2020), overdoses accounted for a much larger absolute number of excess deaths.[74] Indeed, the CDC estimated that drug overdose deaths increased by 22,473 in 2020 compared with 2019 (14% of the total excess deaths not owing directly to COVID-19),[78] which was a worsening of a trend that began in 2019.[79] As a result, the United States saw the highest number of overdose deaths, 95,230 total in 2020, ever recorded in a single year.[78] The pandemic also saw an increased proportion of overdose deaths owing to synthetic opioids other than methadone, with the greatest increases observed in the West and among racial/ethnic minorities and people living in socioeconomically disadvantaged communities.[80]

Although drug overdoses accounted for most increased unintentional injury deaths so far during the pandemic, an increase in unintentional firearm deaths also occurred. We noted above that firearm sales spiked early in the pandemic. It is noteworthy that a similar spike in firearm purchasing in the aftermath of the Sandy Hook school shooting was found to be associated with a time-lagged spike in unintentional firearm deaths that covaried with between-state variation in increased firearm purchasing.[81] A similar increase during the COVID-19 pandemic can be inferred from the observation that the absolute increase in firearm deaths in the second and third quarters (Q2–Q3) of 2020 increased more than firearm-related homicides.[74] Although we are aware of no direct study of such deaths among adults, unintentional firearm-related injuries increased among children by RR = 1.9 during 2020 Q2–Q3 and were especially pronounced in states with high increases during the pandemic in firearms purchases.[82]

Surprisingly, road traffic fatalities were another significant contributor to the increase in unintentional injury deaths during the first year of the pandemic. The National Safety Council (NSC) estimated that 42,060 people died in motor vehicle crashes in 2020, which represented an 8% increase compared with 2019. This happened despite the number of miles driven in 2020 dropping 13% compared with 2019.[83] The 2020 increase in rate of traffic deaths was the largest single-year jump documented by the NSC in the last 96 years. Similar findings were described by the National Highway Traffic Safety Administration.[84]

Crisis Line Calls

Numerous mass media stories early in the pandemic reported that suicide and mental health crisis lines were being overwhelmed with increased calls[85] and that increased crisis line calls from teenagers continued as school closings went into the next fall.[86] We are aware of only one large-scale study on this trend. That study examined trends in calls to the National Suicide Prevention Lifeline (NSCL)[87] and found that call volume increased in 2020 Q2 compared with 2019 Q2 in 28 states by RR = 1.01 to 1.3 but decreased in the remaining 22 states.[88] No association was found between state-level COVID-19 infection and change in NSCL call volume. We subsequently examined associations of the state-level call volume data in this report with (i) state-level prevalence of anxiety-depression in the 2 years before the beginning of the pandemic (as assessed in the BRFSS), (ii) increase in state-level anxiety-depression over 2020 Q2 compared with 2018 to 2019 (as assessed in the HPS compared with predicted values based on the BRFSS), and (iii) increases in the state-level unemployment rate in 2020 Q2 compared with 2019 Q2. None of these associations was significant either statistically or substantively ($R^2 = -0.020$–0.011).

A more focused study of 911 calls for mental health issues in Detroit during the early months of the pandemic found that call volume declined relative to the same months in the prior 3 years.[89] This finding is broadly consistent with 2 surveys carried out in April 2020 and April 2021 by the National Association of Emergency Medical Technicians with leaders of EMS agencies throughout the country.[90] Of agencies, 61% reported decreases in call volume in the 2020 and 43% in 2021. In comparison, several reports showed that 911 calls for domestic violence increased RR = 1.1 to 1.3 during the early months of the pandemic (reviewed by Refs.[91–93]). However, more recent evidence suggests that call volume might have subsequently returned to prepandemic levels.[94]

SUMMARY OF THE EVIDENCE ON TRENDS IN MENTAL DISORDER PREVALENCE SINCE BEFORE THE PANDEMIC

Taken together, the above evidence suggests that COVID-19 has so far had a significant impact on point prevalence of anxiety-depression spectrum disorders and serious drug use disorders in the US adult population, albeit substantially less than that posited by early reviews. The point prevalence of anxiety-depression likely increased by about 30% to 50%, although the impact on more persistent anxiety-depression was not assessed in any of these studies. It is also noteworthy that data collected in within-pandemic cohort and trend surveys reviewed later in the article show that the numerator for these ratios (ie, prevalence within the pandemic) changed rather substantially over the course of the pandemic. In particular, the during-pandemic waves in the ALP national cohort survey and the Gallup national trend survey both occurred at times during the pandemic estimated to have comparatively high prevalence. Effects in this range RR = 1.3 to 1.5 are important, but not nearly as high as the RR = 3.0 to 8.0 estimates obtained in the noncomparable trend studies that have been the major focus of media attention.

CHANGES IN MENTAL HEALTH DISPARITIES SINCE BEFORE THE PANDEMIC

Another important question concerns disparities in the effects of the pandemic on population mental health. We know from previous research that the component stressors caused by the pandemic, including job loss,[95] death of a loved one,[96] social isolation,[97] and a combination of multiple such stressors,[98] have negative effects on mental health. Given that exposure to these experiences during the pandemic has been significantly higher in some already disadvantaged segments of the population[99,100] and that the psychological impact of pandemic-related stressors might have been greater among already disadvantaged segments of the population,[101] we might expect that prepandemic health disparities would be magnified by the pandemic.

Research on this possibility can be carried out most directly by making comparisons within cohorts. The one true cohort study we described above, the RAND ALP, did this and found that individual-level increases in psychological distress during compared with before the pandemic were significantly more common among women than men (odds ratio [OR] = 1.9), respondents younger than 60 compared with those 60+ years old (OR = 2.4–1.7), and Hispanic compared with non-Hispanic white individuals (OR = 1.9).[51]

Trend data can also be used to make such comparisons, but less powerfully so than in cohort studies because trend studies require evidence of variation in the associations of social disadvantage with mental disorder over time (ie, statistical interactions). However, as only one of the large government benchmark trend surveys with relevant information has been reported for 2020 (the BRFSS reported these data in August 2021, after this article was completed), data from noncomparable trend surveys are the only ones available to provide preliminary information, albeit with the recognition that the differences in sample frames, field procedures, and response rates could introduce bias into these comparisons.

The noncomparable trend survey reports all presented data on the sociodemographic correlates of anxiety-depression during the pandemic, but in most cases did not comment on the possibility that these associations predated the pandemic. The few studies that made such comparisons found consistently that anxiety-depression increased most dramatically among young adults and least among black individuals,[23,36] but these were weak comparisons because the surveys carried out during the pandemic were relatively small.

We carried out a more thorough analysis of such differences by comparing associations of core sociodemographic variables (age, sex, race-ethnicity, education) with anxiety-depression in the publicly available 2018 to 2019 BRFSS (n = 839,366) and 2020 to 2021 CDC HPS (n = 2,373,044) data sets. The outcome was a dichotomous measure representing a clinically significant score for anxiety-depression on the PHQ-4 screening scale (6+ on the 0–12 response scale).[34] Some preprocessing was needed before the comparisons could be made, though, as the PHQ-4 was administered only to a subsample of BRFSS respondents. We consequently imputed predicted probabilities of clinically significant PHQ-4 scores to the remainder of the BRFSS sample based on a logistic regression model estimated in the subsample where the PHQ-4 was administered. Predictors in the model included all the sociodemographic variables in the substantive analysis reported below plus scores on the screening scales of mental disorder included in all BRFSS interviews (questions about number of days in poor mental health and number of days of role impairment owing to poor mental or physical health). The model had strong cross-validated accuracy in a holdout test sample (area under the receiver operating characteristic curve [AUC = 0.90]). The associations of the sociodemographic variables with predicted scores were also comparable in cross-validation to those with the observed scores (Appendix Table 3). To make associations comparable in the 2 surveys, we coarsened the observed PHQ-4 score in the HPS to generate a predicted score similar to the predicted score in the BRFSS. That predicted score had a comparable association with the observed dichotomy for PHQ-4 = 6+ as in the BRFSS (AUC = .88, Appendix Fig. 1).

As expected, comparisons across the 2 surveys found that estimated prevalence of PHQ-4 = 6+ scores was substantially higher in the HPS (26.4%) than the BRFSS (10.9%; **Table 1**). However, the RR among women compared with men was the same in the 2 surveys (RR = 1.2), resulting in the HPS:BRFSS interaction with sex being $RR_{H:B}$ = 1.0. This suggests that prevalence increased by similar proportions among women and men. On the other hand, the prevalence of PHQ-4 = 6+ increased substantially more for respondents younger than 60 than those 60+ years of age. in the HPS (29.9%–41.8%) compared with before the pandemic (ie, 2018–2019 BRFSS, resulting in $RR_{H:B}$ = 1.6–1.7 for 18–59 compared with 60+). Unlike some previous reports suggesting that prevalence increased less among blacks than other individuals, we found that proportional prevalence was slightly higher among non-Hispanic black individuals than non-Hispanic white individuals in HPS than BRFSS ($RR_{H:B}$ = 1.2) and much higher among Hispanic individuals ($RR_{H:B}$ = 1.8) and other races ($RR_{H:B}$ = 1.8) than non-Hispanic white individuals. Finally, we found that individuals with lower education levels had higher PHQ-4 scores both before and during the pandemic, but that these differences became more pronounced during the pandemic, resulting in $RR_{H:B}$ being relatively comparable across the 3 lower levels of education relative to the highest level (1.5–1.7).

CHANGES IN MENTAL DISORDER PREVALENCE OVER THE COURSE OF THE PANDEMIC

Although the HPS is by far the largest trend survey carried out during the pandemic, several nongovernment multiwave trend surveys were initiated shortly after the onset of the pandemic to track the prevalence and correlates of diverse policy-related issues

Table 1
Change in the univariate and multivariate associations of sociodemographic variables with clinically significant anxiety-depression (PHQ-4 = 6+) between the 2018-2019 CDC Behavioral Risk Factors Surveillance Survey (n = 839,366) and April 2020 to July 2021 CDC Household Pulse Survey (n = 2,373,044)[a]

	Behavioral Risk Factors Surveillance Survey (BRFSS)						Household Pulse Survey (HPS)						HPS: BRFSS			
	Prevalence		Univariate		Multivariate		Prevalence		Univariate		Multivariate		Univariate		Multivariate	
	%	(SE)	RR	(95% CI)	RR	(95% CI)	%	(SE)	RR	(95% CI)	RR	(95% CI)	RR	(95% CI)	RR	(95% CI)
Sex																
Female	12.0	(0.1)	1.2[b]	(1.2–1.3)	1.3[b]	(1.3–1.3)	28.8	(0.0)	1.2[b]	(1.2–1.2)	1.3[b]	(1.3–1.3)	1.0[b]	(0.9–1.0)	1.0	(1.0–1.0)
Male	9.8	(0.1)	1.0		1.0		24.2	(0.0)	1.0		1.0		1.0		1.0	
χ^2_1			229.7[b]		387.2[b]				310.3[b]		748.2[b]		3.9[b]		0.5	
Age																
18–29	14.4	(0.1)	1.8[b]	(1.8–1.9)	2.0[b]	(1.9–2.0)	41.8	(0.1)	3.1[b]	(3.0–3.2)	2.9[b]	(2.8–3.0)	1.7[b]	(1.6–1.8)	1.5[b]	(1.4–1.6)
30–44	11.2	(0.1)	1.4[b]	(1.4–1.5)	1.7[b]	(1.6–1.7)	29.9	(0.1)	2.2[b]	(2.1–2.3)	2.3[b]	(2.2–2.4)	1.6[b]	(1.5–1.6)	1.4[b]	(1.3–1.5)
45–59	11.5	(0.1)	1.5[b]	(1.4–1.5)	1.6[b]	(1.5–1.6)	31.4	(0.1)	2.3[b]	(2.3–2.4)	2.3[b]	(2.2–2.4)	1.6[b]	(1.5–1.7)	1.5[b]	(1.4–1.5)
60+	7.9	(0.0)	1.0		1.0		13.5	(0.0)	1.0		1.0		1.0			
χ^2_3			1029.0[b]		1345.9[b]				4231.6[b]		4135.6[b]		507.3[b]		311.0[b]	
Education																
Less than high school	19.5	(0.2)	4.2[b]	(4.0–4.3)	5.0[b]	(4.8–5.2)	59.5	(0.2)	6.8[b]	(6.6–7.0)	6.5[b]	(6.3–6.7)	1.6[b]	(1.5–1.7)	1.3[b]	(1.2–1.4)
High school graduate	13.4	(0.1)	2.9[b]	(2.8–3.0)	2.9[b]	(2.8–3.0)	37.3	(0.1)	4.3[b]	(4.2–4.4)	4.4[b]	(4.3–4.5)	1.5[b]	(1.4–1.6)	1.5[b]	(1.5–1.6)
Some college	10.7	(0.1)	2.3[b]	(2.2–2.4)	2.3[b]	(2.2–2.3)	34.2	(0.1)	3.9[b]	(3.8–4.0)	3.8[b]	(3.8–3.9)	1.7[b]	(1.6–1.8)	1.7[b]	(1.6–1.8)
College graduate/more	4.7	(0.0)	1.0		1.0		8.8	(0.0)	1.0		1.0		1.0			
χ^2_3			4706.8[b]		5395.0[b]				22,755.0[b]		21,496.2[b]		625.1[b]		623.3[b]	
Race																
Non-Hispanic black	15.8	(0.1)	1.5[b]	(1.4–1.5)	1.2[b]	(1.2–1.3)	39.9	(0.1)	1.8[b]	(1.8–1.9)	1.3[b]	(1.3–1.3)	1.2[b]	(1.2–1.3)	1.1[b]	(1.0–1.1)
Hispanic	9.5	(0.1)	0.9[b]	(0.8–0.9)	0.6[b]	(0.5–0.6)	34.1	(0.1)	1.6[b]	(1.5–1.6)	1.0	(1.0–1.0)	1.8[b]	(1.7–1.9)	1.7[b]	(1.6–1.8)
Other race	8.9	(0.1)	0.8[b]	(0.8–0.9)	0.8[b]	(0.7–0.8)	32.5	(0.1)	1.5[b]	(1.4–1.6)	1.3[b]	(1.2–1.3)	1.8[b]	(1.7–1.9)	1.6[b]	(1.5–1.7)

(continued on next page)

Table 1
(continued)

	Behavioral Risk Factors Surveillance Survey (BRFSS)						Household Pulse Survey (HPS)						HPS: BRFSS			
	Prevalence		Univariate		Multivariate		Prevalence		Univariate		Multivariate		Univariate		Multivariate	
	%	(SE)	RR	(95% CI)	RR	(95% CI)	%	(SE)	RR	(95% CI)	RR	(95% CI)	RR	(95% CI)	RR	(95% CI)
Non-Hispanic white	10.7	(0.0)	1.0		1.0		21.7	(0.0)	1.0		1.0		1.0			
χ^2_3			578.7[b]		744.0[b]				2838.6[b]		533.1[b]		722.6[b]		517.1[b]	
Total	10.9	(0.0)					26.4	(0.0)								

[a] Estimated using robust Poisson regression models.[102] The dependent variable was a random 0/1 draw from a Bernoulli distribution with a fixed random seed from a separate predicted probability assigned to each respondent from an imputed predicted probability generated by a separate internally cross-validated logistic regression in each sample. These models are described in Appendix Tables 3 (BRFSS) and 4 (HPS). The imputation was necessary in BRFSS because the PHQ-4 was administered only in 3 stated in 2018, although, as detailed in Appendix Table 3, other measures assessed in the entre sample were strongly associated with PHQ 4 = 6+ (AUC = .90). The imputation was not necessary in HPS because the PHQ-4 was administered in the entire sample. However, for purposes of making a fair comparison of predictors with the outcome across the 2 surveys, we coarsened the PHQ score (Appendix Table 4) to make the association between true scores and predicted probabilities comparable across surveys. In addition, a propensity score 1/p weight was imposed on the HPS data to adjust for the fact that the 12% of respondents missing the PHQ-4 questions were not random with respect to sociodemographic characteristics, geography, or time. Logistic regression with the same predictors as in the substantive model as well as dummy variables for state and survey wave was used to estimate predicted probability of answering the PHQ-4 questions for purposes of generating the 1/p weight.

[b] Significant at the 0.05 level.

(eg, Refs.[103–106]). The 2 largest and with the most waves among these are as follows: (i) *The COVID States Project (CSP)*, a series of Internet trend surveys carried out roughly monthly in samples mostly of n = 20,000 to 25,000 respondents from nonprobability consumer panels[107]; and (ii) *The University of Southern California Understanding America Study (UAS) Panel*, a panel of approximately n = 9500 people assembled by the USC Center for Economic and Social Research beginning in 2014 to carry out diverse surveys on a wide range of topics,[108] but carrying out an ongoing tracking survey on COVID-related topics beginning at the very onset of the pandemic. Each UAS panel member was invited to respond on one assigned day every 2 weeks beginning in early March 2020, with the rotation changing to 1 day every month since mid-March 2021.[109] This design allows for aggregation of trend data over weekly, biweekly, or other designated time intervals and allows analysis of cohort (ie, within-person) changes.

The HPS, CSP, and UAS all use either the PHQ-4, which includes separate 2-item subscales of anxiety (Generalized Anxiety Disorder (GAD)-2) and depression (PHQ-2), or, in the case of the CSP, the full PHQ-9 depression scale in addition to the GAD-2, to track anxiety-depression during the pandemic. We aggregated prevalence estimates by month within surveys using standard thresholds of clinically significant anxiety (GAD-2 = 3+) and depression (PHQ-2 = 3+ or PHQ-9 = 10+) and plotted trends (**Fig. 1**). These trends are quite different across surveys, with Pearson correlations of month-by-month variation in the range $r = 0.39$ (UAS anxiety and CSP depression) to $r = -0.13$ (UAS depression and CPS anxiety; **Table 2**). Overall, correlations (mean [range]) are highest between HPS and CSP ($r = 0.26$ [0.15–0.38]) and lower between these surveys and UAS ($r = 0.08$ [−0.13–0.39]). It is noteworthy in this regard that HPS and CSP are both trend surveys in which only a subset of respondents participate in more than one wave, whereas the UAS is a rolling panel trend survey in which the n = 9500 UAS panel members were surveyed many times both before and since the onset of the pandemic. This repeated surveying might have led to panel fatigue, which could account for why prevalence estimates are substantially lower in UAS than the other 2 surveys even though all 3 surveys were weighted to be nationally representative on the cross-classification of demographic-geographic variables.[110]

Several other patterns in the trend figure are noteworthy. First, the UAS panel was already active before the pandemic, allowing the first COVID-19 survey to be fielded more quickly, 1 month after the United States declared COVID-19 a public health emergency[111] than the HPS and CSP surveys. This allowed UAS to pick up an acute upswing in both anxiety-depression associated with the statewide stay-at-home orders that began in late March (eg, California, 19 March 2020; New York and Illinois, 20 March 2020; New Jersey, 21 March 2020; Ohio, 22 March 2020; and many other states. 23 March 2020). However, UAS prevalence estimates dropped precipitously after the April spike and showed only attenuated evidence of subsequent spikes that were picked up in the other surveys.

HPS, in comparison, picked up a 1-month spike in prevalence in July 2020, the month the United States surpassed 3 million COVID-19 cases. CSP did not field a wave that month. An increase in prevalence between August 2020 and November 2020 (the first time 100,000 COVID-19 cases were reported in a single day[112]) was then detected by all 3 surveys, with the increase continuing in December for depression in HPS (CSP did not have a December 2020 wave), although this trend was weak and only for anxiety in UAS. The time between August and November coincided with the most dramatic increase to date in COVID-19 deaths, with a peak at the end of December (4169 COVID-19 deaths, January 13, 2021).[113] Anxiety-depression prevalence declined after that time period in conjunction with a precipitous decline in COVID-19 cases through mid-June (8463 cases, June 14, 2021 compared with a high of 292,713 cases, January 6, 2021) and

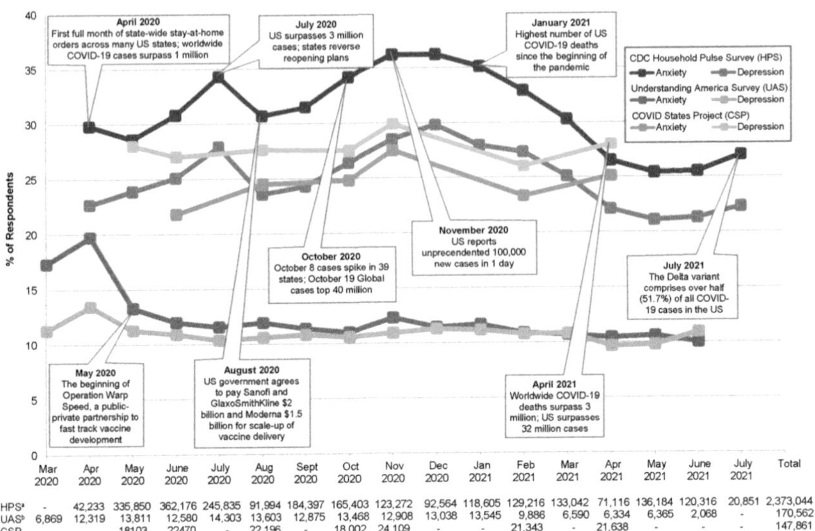

	Mar 2020	Apr 2020	May 2020	June 2020	July 2020	Aug 2020	Sept 2020	Oct 2020	Nov 2020	Dec 2020	Jan 2021	Feb 2021	Mar 2021	Apr 2021	May 2021	June 2021	July 2021	Total
HPS[a]	-	42,233	335,850	362,176	245,835	91,994	184,397	165,403	123,272	92,564	118,605	129,216	133,042	71,116	136,184	120,316	20,851	2,373,044
UAS[b]	6,869	12,319	13,811	12,580	14,303	13,603	12,875	13,468	12,908	13,038	13,545	9,886	6,590	6,334	6,365	2,068	-	170,562
CSP	-	-	18103	22470	-	22,196	-	18,002	24,109	-	-	21,343	-	21,638	-	-	-	147,861

Fig. 1. Comparing trends in anxiety and depression during the pandemic across studies: HPS, CSP, UAS. [a]There were 2,745,185 observations in the HPS from April 2020 to July 2021. In this figure, the authors excluded any observations that were missing values for questions on anxiety or depression from the PHQ-4 for a total sample size of 2,373,044 observations. In instances when multiple waves of the survey were carried out in a single month, equal weight was given to the surveys as a function of number of days in the month covered rather than comparative sample size. In instances when a single wave was carried out across 2 months, the overall prevalence in that wave to both months was attributed based on number of days covered. For example, if a single wave was carried out in the last 5 days of 1 month and the first 2 days of the next month, the prevalence in the survey was counted as applying to 5 days in the first month and 2 days in the second month. If one additional wave was carried out over in the first month for a total of 14 days, for example, the prevalence in the overlapping wave would contribute 5/19 to the estimated prevalence in the month (and the first wave would contribute 14/19 to the estimated prevalence). [b]There were 173,823 observations in the UAS. In this figure, the authors excluded 3261 observations that were missing values for questions on anxiety or depression from the PHQ-4 or who had an incomplete survey date for a total sample size of 170,562 observations. It is noteworthy in this regard that HPS and CSP are both trend surveys in which only a tiny proportion of respondents participate in more than one wave, whereas the UAS is a rolling panel trend survey in which the n = 9500 UAS panel members are surveyed repeatedly over time. This might have led to panel fatigue, which could account for why prevalence estimates are substantially lower in UAS than the other 2 surveys even though all 3 surveys were weighted to be nationally representative on the cross-classification of demographic-geographic characteristics.

COVID-19 deaths through early July (140 deaths, July 11, 2021). A slight upswing in HPS anxiety-depression and UAS depression occurred near the end of the time series, which coincided with the emergence of the Delta variant[114] and subsequent increases in cases and deaths. The last CSP wave was in April but showed an upswing in anxiety-depression prevalence before the other surveys.

CHANGES IN MENTAL HEALTH DISPARITIES OVER THE COURSE OF THE PANDEMIC

The bulk of research on mental health disparities during the pandemic has focused on comparative cross-sectional analyses. These show clearly that socially

Table 2
Pearson correlations between monthly trends in clinically significant anxiety-depression prevalence across major within-pandemic tracking surveys between March 2020 and July 2021

	HPS		UAS		CSP	
	Anx	**Dep**	**Anx**	**Dep**	**Anx**	**Dep**
Household Pulse Survey (HPS)						
Anxiety (Anx)	1.0					
Anxiety (Anx) and Depression (Dep) should be slightly indented under Household Pulse Survey (HPS)						
Depression (Dep)	1.0[a]	1.0				
Understanding America Survey (UAS)						
Anxiety (Anx)	0.0	−0.1	1.0			
Anxiety (Anx) and Depression (Dep) should be slightly indented under Understanding America Survey (UAS)						
Depression (Dep)	0.2	0.1	0.8[a]	1.0		
COVID States Project (CSP)						
Anxiety (Anx)	0.4	0.3	0.2	−0.1	1.0	
Anxiety (Anx) and Depression (Dep) should be slightly indented under COVID States Project (CSP)						
Depression (Dep)	0.2	0.2	0.4	0.0	0.9[a]	1.0

[a] Significant at the 0.05 level, 2-sided test based on a sample of between 6 and 16 mo. See **Fig. 1** for the number of common monthly data points for each pair of surveys.

disadvantaged segments of the population are at increased risk of exposure to pandemic-related stressors, including personal infection, death of a loved one, and financial loss.[99,100,115,116] These analyses also document significant over-time associations between aggregate changes in pandemic-related stressors and changes in anxiety-depression.[117–122] We are not aware of studies investigating the possibility that the associations of individual-level exposure to pandemic-related stressors with subsequent onset-worsening of anxiety-depression are different among disadvantaged than other segments of the population. The latter studies would require the use of cohort data, as it would be necessary to control for baseline anxiety-depression owing to the existence of reciprocal relationships between prior mental disorders and some types of stressor exposure.[123,124] Nonetheless, the existing evidence on stressor exposure is sufficient to think that mental health disparities might have increased over the course of the pandemic.

We are not aware of any attempt to determine whether systematic changes have occurred in these disparities over the course of the pandemic. We expanded our earlier analysis of sociodemographic correlates in the HPS to do this. We began by disaggregating the HPS data over 6 time periods within the pandemic, indicating corresponding to changes in anxiety-depression prevalence. We then estimated the same model as in **Table 1** separately within each of these time periods and compared results. To facilitate these comparisons, the RR estimates were centered within each of the 6 time periods so that they multiplied to 1.0 across categories of each predictor.

Women had an elevated risk of clinically significant PHQ-4 scores compared with men over the full HPS series (29.6% vs 23.5%, $\chi^2_1 = 650.8$, $P<.001$) with an unadjusted

RR of 1.3 that varied only modestly) across the time periods defined here and were not changed meaningfully by multivariate controls for other sociodemographics (**Table 3**). A similar consistency over time can be seen in the association between age and PHQ-4 scores. The univariate association is significant in the total sample (χ^2_3 = 3582.5, *P*<.001) based on a monotonically decreasing prevalence with age from a high of 38.7% among respondents ages 18 to 29 to a low of 17.6% among those 60+ years and intermediate prevalence among those ages 30 to 44 years (30.8%) and 45 to 59 years (27.0%). Centered RR among the youngest respondents varies monotonically but modestly with time in the range RR = 1.3 to 1.6. Similarly small but nonmonotonic changes in centered RR can be seen in the other age groups.

An even stronger consistency over time can be seen in the association between education and PHQ-4 scores. The total sample association is significant (χ^2_3 = 1900.8, *P*<.001) based on a monotonically decreasing prevalence from 34.2% at the lowest level (less than high school) to a low of 22.2% at the highest level (college graduate) and intermediate prevalence of 28.3% to 29.7% in the 2 middle categories (high school graduate, some college). In the adjusted model, centered RR was 1.2 to 1.3 among those with lowest education, RR = 0.7 to 0.8 among those with highest education, and RR = 1.0 to 1.1 among those with intermediate education. A significant association of race ethnicity with PHQ-4 scores, finally, was found in the total sample (χ^2_3 = 331.3, *P*<.001), with highest prevalence among Hispanic individuals (30.3%), lowest among non-Hispanic white individuals (24.8%), and intermediate among non-Hispanic black individuals (29.3%) and other races (28.8%). However, this association decreased dramatically in magnitude in the multivariate model that adjusted for age, sex, and education model (χ^2_3 = 11.6, *P* = .009) resulting in the centered RR becoming nonsignificantly different from the total sample average in only 1 of the 6 intervals each among Hispanic individuals (RR = 0.95) and other races (RR = 1.1), none of the 6 among non-Hispanic black individuals, and 2 of the 6 among non-Hispanic white individuals (RR = 0.95–0.97).

Taken as a whole, these results suggest that mental health disparities based on sex, age, education, and race ethnicity have not changed substantially as of this stage in the pandemic despite the clear evidence that disadvantaged segments of society have been more highly exposed than others to pandemic-related stressors. Whether this is due to a greater resilience among disadvantaged segments of the population is unclear from the simple analyses reported here. More nuanced analysis would be needed to investigate this issue directly by estimating interactions between individual-level exposure to pandemic-related stressors and disadvantaged social status to predict subsequent onset of worsening of anxiety-depression. This kind of analysis is beyond the scope of the current review but could be carried out in the UAS cohort, although the much lower estimated prevalence of anxiety-depression in the UAS than the other 2 major tracking surveys might undercut the persuasiveness of the results.

Another possibility is that the associations of disadvantaged social status with anxiety-depression are more complex than in the simple additive model considered here. For example, there might be important interactions among the indicators of disadvantage, or there might be important geographic variation in these associations. Consistent with the latter, a study carried out in the early months of the pandemic with HPS data showed that the associations of COVID-19-related financial stressors with anxiety-depression were dampened in states with supportive policies for dealing with reduced income (Medicaid, unemployment insurance, restrictions on landlord and utility company responses to nonpayment).[125] Based on this result, it is plausible to think that more disaggregated analyses might show evidence of significant time-space variation in health disparities throughout the pandemic.

Table 3
Variation in the multivariate associations of sociodemographic variables with clinically significant anxiety-depression (PHQ-4 = 6+) across weeks of the CDC Household Pulse Survey, April 2020 to July 2021 (n = 2,373,044)[b,c]

	April–June 2020 (n = 650,000)				Late June–July 2020 (n = 336,084)				August–October 2020 (n = 426,584)			
	Prevalence				Prevalence				Prevalence			
	%	(SE)	RR	(95% CI)	%	(SE)	RR	(95% CI)	%	(SE)	RR	(95% CI)
Sex												
Female	28.7	(0.1)	1.1[a]	(1.1–1.2)	31.8	(0.1)	1.1[a]	(1.1–1.1)	29.3	(0.1)	1.1[a]	(1.1–1.2)
Male	22.3	(0.1)	0.9[a]	(0.9–0.9)	26.5	(0.1)	0.9[a]	(0.9–0.9)	22.6	(0.1)	0.9[a]	(0.9–0.9)
χ^2_1			244.5[a]				101.9[a]				441.6[a]	
Age												
18–29	36.5	(0.2)	1.4[a]	(1.3–1.4)	40.5	(0.3)	1.3[a]	(1.3–1.4)	37.8	(0.3)	1.4[a]	(1.3–1.4)
30–44	28.7	(0.1)	1.1[a]	(1.1–1.2)	34.5	(0.1)	1.2[a]	(1.1–1.2)	31.4	(0.1)	1.2[a]	(1.1–1.2)
45–59	26.2	(0.1)	1.0	(1.0–1.0)	30.0	(0.1)	1.0	(1.0–1.0)	26.2	(0.1)	1.0[a]	(0.9–1.0)
60+	16.3	(0.1)	0.6[a]	(0.6–0.7)	19.3	(0.1)	0.6[a]	(0.6–0.7)	18.3	(0.1)	0.7[a]	(0.6–0.7)
χ^2_3			806.4[a]				633.7[a]				1276.5[a]	
Education												
Less than high school	31.9	(0.4)	1.2[a]	(1.1–1.2)	37.7	(0.6)	1.2[a]	(1.1–1.3)	32.6	(0.5)	1.2[a]	(1.1–1.3)
High school graduate	27.8	(0.2)	1.1[a]	(1.0–1.1)	30.3	(0.2)	1.0	(1.0–1.1)	26.3	(0.2)	1.0	(0.9–1.0)
Some college	27.9	(0.1)	1.0	(1.0–1.1)	32.6	(0.2)	1.0[a]	(1.0–1.1)	29.7	(0.1)	1.0[a]	(1.0–1.1)
College graduate/more	20.9	(0.1)	0.8[a]	(0.8–0.8)	24.6	(0.1)	0.8[a]	(0.8–0.8)	23.0	(0.1)	0.8[a]	(0.8–0.8)
χ^2_3			457.8[a]				328.5[a]				627.2[a]	
Race												
Non-Hispanic black	29.2	(0.2)	1.0	(1.0–1.1)	30.3	(0.3)	0.9	(0.9–1.0)	27.0	(0.3)	1.0	(0.9–1.0)
Hispanic	29.0	(0.2)	1.0	(1.0–1.0)	32.3	(0.3)	0.9[a]	(0.9–1.0)	30.3	(0.2)	1.0	(1.0–1.1)
Other race	26.9	(0.2)	1.0	(1.0–1.1)	34.5	(0.3)	1.1[a]	(1.1–1.2)	27.0	(0.2)	1.0	(0.9–1.0)
Non-Hispanic white	23.6	(0.1)	1.0[a]	(0.9–1.0)	27.2	(0.1)	1.0	(1.0–1.0)	24.9	(0.1)	1.0	(1.0–1.0)

(continued on next page)

Table 3
(continued)

	April–June 2020 (n = 650,000)				Late June–July 2020 (n = 336,084)				August–October 2020 (n = 426,584)			
	Prevalence				Prevalence				Prevalence			
	%	(SE)	RR	(95% CI)	%	(SE)	RR	(95% CI)	%	(SE)	RR	(95% CI)
χ^2_3			5.7				17.5[a]				3.2	
Total	25.4	(0.0)			29.0	(0.1)			26.0	(0.1)		

	November–February 2021 (n = 354,843)				February–March 2021 (n = 257,066)				April–July 2021 (n = 348,467)			
	Prevalence				Prevalence				Prevalence			
	%	(SE)	RR	(95% CI)	%	(SE)	RR	(95% CI)	%	(SE)	RR	(95% CI)
Sex												
Female	33.9	(0.1)	1.1[a]	(1.1–1.2)	30.0	(0.1)	1.1[a]	(1.1–1.1)	23.9	(0.1)	1.1[a]	(1.1–1.2)
Male	26.5	(0.1)	0.9[a]	(0.9–0.9)	24.2	(0.1)	0.9[a]	(0.9–0.9)	18.9	(0.1)	0.9[a]	(0.9–0.9)
χ^2_1			328.8[a]				202.5[a]				230.7[a]	
Age												
18–29	44.7	(0.3)	1.4[a]	(1.3–1.4)	41.4	(0.4)	1.4[a]	(1.4–1.5)	36.2	(0.3)	1.6[a]	(1.5–1.6)
30–44	35.7	(0.1)	1.1[a]	(1.1–1.2)	31.8	(0.2)	1.1[a]	(1.1–1.2)	26.2	(0.1)	1.2[a]	(1.1–1.2)
45–59	30.6	(0.1)	1.0[a]	(0.9–1.0)	26.3	(0.2)	0.9[a]	(0.9–1.0)	21.3	(0.1)	0.9[a]	(0.9–1.0)
60+	21.4	(0.1)	0.7[a]	(0.6–0.7)	18.4	(0.1)	0.6[a]	(0.6–0.7)	13.0	(0.1)	0.6[a]	(0.5–0.6)
χ^2_3			993.5[a]				1010.5[a]				1377.0[a]	
Education												
Less than high school	40.1	(0.6)	1.2[a]	(1.1–1.3)	35.3	(0.7)	1.2[a]	(1.1–1.3)	29.9	(0.6)	1.3[a]	(1.2–1.3)
High school graduate	32.0	(0.2)	1.0	(1.0–1.0)	28.5	(0.3)	1.0	(1.0–1.0)	23.5	(0.2)	1.0[a]	(1.0–1.1)
Some college	33.9	(0.2)	1.0[a]	(1.0–1.0)	31.4	(0.2)	1.0[a]	(1.0–1.1)	25.3	(0.2)	1.1[a]	(1.0–1.1)
College graduate/more	26.0	(0.1)	0.8[a]	(0.8–0.8)	22.9	(0.1)	0.8[a]	(0.8–0.8)	16.9	(0.1)	0.7[a]	(0.7–0.7)
χ^2_3			765.5[a]				586.2[a]				1055.2[a]	

Race												
Non-Hispanic black	34.4	(0.3)	1.1	(1.0–1.1)	30.3	(0.3)	1.0	(1.0–1.1)	24.0	(0.3)	1.0	(0.9–1.1)
Hispanic	34.6	(0.3)	1.0	(0.9–1.0)	30.6	(0.3)	1.0	(0.9–1.0)	26.5	(0.2)	1.0	(1.0–1.1)
Other race	31.3	(0.3)	1.0	(0.9–1.0)	29.2	(0.3)	1.0	(1.0–1.1)	23.7	(0.2)	1.0	(1.0–1.1)
Non-Hispanic white	28.7	(0.1)	1.0	(0.9–1.0)	25.7	(0.1)	1.0	(1.0–1.0)	19.7	(0.1)	0.9[a]	(0.9–1.0)
χ^2_3			4.5				4.8				11.7[a]	
Total	30.3	(0.1)			27.1	(0.1)			21.4	(0.1)		

[a] Significant at the 0.05 level.
[b] Estimated in multivariate robust Poisson regression models[102] with dummy variable controls for the separate waves within the time intervals. The time intervals were as follows: (1) 8 waves between April 23 and June 23, 2020; (2) 4 waves between June 25 and July 21; (3) 5 waves between August 19 and October 26; (4) 5 waves between October 28 and February 1,2021; (5) 4 waves between February 3 and March 29; (6) 6 waves between April 14 and July 5,2021. Time intervals were selected by inspection of consistency and changes in prevalence across waves.
[c] Controlled by weeks 1.0 within variables within time period.

Finally, it is important to recognize that we examined RR rather than absolute-risk difference. This means that prevalence of clinically significant anxiety-depression across the segments of the population considered here has not changed *proportionally* over the pandemic, but absolute differences would increase as overall prevalence increased if overall prevalence increased during the pandemic. The same observation was made by Swaziek and Wozniak[122] in an analysis comparing early waves of the HPS data with the BRFSS data.

PREDICTING FUTURE CHANGES IN MENTAL DISORDER PREVALENCE AND DISPARITIES

If anything about the data reviewed here is clear, it is that the impact of COVID-19 on mental disorders is challenging to document. This is even truer for forecasting future effects of the pandemic on population mental health. There are some promising signs in the expansion of tele-mental health care to reach hard-to-reach people in need of care and the increased use of scalable interventions to address the rising demand for treatment of emotional problems during the pandemic. However, there are also enormous uncertainties. We noted in the previous section that the effects of some pandemic-related stressors have so far been buffered by government policies, but uncertainties exist about the long-term sustainability of these policies.[126] Indeed, the Supreme Court recently ended the Biden administration's eviction moratorium in the same week that the government announced the US inflation rate hit a 30-year high.[127]

In addition, uncertainties exist about the duration of the pandemic, with its ever-increasing number of variants, the long-term prognosis of the 10% to 30% of COVID-19 survivors[128] who experience the post-COVID-19 syndrome now referred to as PASC (postacute sequelae of COVID),[129] and the extent to which COVID-19 infection will have long-term neuropsychiatric effects.[130] We know from research on prior infectious disease outbreaks and other natural disasters that prolongation of the physical threat phase,[131] as is occurring in the evolving COVID-19 pandemic, along with the proliferation of secondary financial stressors we are experiencing can create what has been referred to as a "second disaster" with more severe negative effects on mental health than the original disaster.[132] That these events are occurring in the fractious political environment in which we are now living only compounds the problem. The implications of this confluence of factors for population mental health are likely to be substantial, at least in the short term, and especially so for the more economically disadvantaged segment of society.

ACKNOWLEDGMENTS

The authors appreciate the helpful comments of Alan Kazdin, Roy Perlis, Michael Schoenbaum, and Jose Zubizarreta on an earlier version of the paper. We appreciate being given access to data from surveys administered by the Understanding America Study, which is maintained by the Center for Economic and Social Research (CESR) at the University of Southern California and is supported in part by the Bill & Melinda Gates Foundation and by grant U01AG054580 from the National Institute on Aging. The authors also appreciate access to public use microdata files from the CDC Household Pulse Survey and CDC Behavioral Risk Factor Surveillance Survey. We thank Roy Perlis for providing us with summary data from the COVID States Project for use in **Fig. 1**. The COVID States Project is a joint project of Northeastern University, Harvard University, Rutgers University, and Northwestern University and is supported by the National Science Foundation under grants SES-2029292 and SES-2029792 and is also supported by a grant from the Knight Foundation, the Russell Sage Foundation, and the Peter G. Peterson Foundation. Their data collection was also supported in part by Amazon. Any opinions, findings, and conclusions or recommendations expressed herein are those of the authors and do not necessarily reflect the views of the principals or funders of these surveys.

DISCLOSURE

In the past 3 years, Dr R.C. Kessler was a consultant for Datastat, Inc, Holmusk, RallyPoint Networks, Inc, and Sage Therapeutics. He has stock options in Mirah, PYM, and Roga Sciences. The other authors report no conflicts.

SUPPLEMENTARY DATA

Supplementary data related to this article can be found online at https://doi.org/10.1016/j.psc.2021.11.013.

REFERENCES

1. Center for Disease Control and Prevention. COVID data tracker. Available at: https://covid.cdc.gov/covid-data-tracker/#datatracker-home. Accessed August 6, 2021.
2. David KB, Aborode AT, Olaoye DQ, et al. Increased risk of death triggered by domestic violence, hunger, suicide, exhausted health system during COVID-19 pandemic: why, how and solutions. Front Sociol 2021;6:648395.
3. Falk G, Romero PD, Carter JA, et al. Unemployment rates during the COVID-19 pandemic. Available at: https://fas.org/sgp/crs/misc/R46554.pdf. Accessed August 7, 2021.
4. Amadeo K. What is long-term unemployment?. Available at: https://www.thebalance.com/long-term-unemployment-what-it-is-causes-and-effects-3305518. Accessed August 11, 2021.
5. U.S. Bureau of Labor Statistics. Unemployed 27 weeks or longer as a percent of total unemployed. Available at: https://www.bls.gov/charts/employment-situation/unemployed-27-weeks-or-longer-as-a-percent-of-total-unemployed.htm. Accessed August 7, 2021.
6. Center on Budget and Policy Priorities. Tracking the COVID-19 economy's effects on food, housing, and employment hardships. Available at: https://www.cbpp.org/sites/default/files/atoms/files/8-13-20pov.pdf. Accessed August 5, 2021.
7. Dimock M, Gramlich J. How America changed during Donald Trump's presidency. Available at: https://www.pewresearch.org/2021/01/29/how-america-changed-during-donald-trumps-presidency/. Accessed August 5, 2021.
8. Iacoella F, Justino P, Martorano B. Do pandemics lead to rebellion? Policy responses to COVID-19, inequality, and protests in the USA. Available at: https://www.wider.unu.edu/sites/default/files/Publications/Working-paper/PDF/wp2021-57-pandemics-rebellion-policy-responses-COVID-19-inequality-protests-USA.pdf. Accessed August 6, 2021.
9. Galea S, Merchant RM, Lurie N. The mental health consequences of COVID-19 and physical distancing: the need for prevention and early intervention. JAMA Intern Med 2020;180(6):817–8.
10. Pfefferbaum B, North CS. Mental health and the Covid-19 pandemic. N Engl J Med 2020;383(6):510–2.
11. Cavicchioli M, Ferrucci R, Guidetti M, et al. What will be the impact of the Covid-19 quarantine on psychological distress? Considerations based on a systematic

review of pandemic outbreaks. Healthcare (Basel). 2021;9(1). https://doi.org/10.3390/healthcare9010101.
12. Chu IY, Alam P, Larson HJ, et al. Social consequences of mass quarantine during epidemics: a systematic review with implications for the COVID-19 response. J Trav Med 2020;27(7). https://doi.org/10.1093/jtm/taaa192.
13. Shah K, Kamrai D, Mekala H, et al. Focus on mental health during the coronavirus (COVID-19) pandemic: applying learnings from the past outbreaks. Cureus 2020;12(3):e7405.
14. Goldmann E, Galea S. Mental health consequences of disasters. Annu Rev Public Health 2014;35(1):169–83.
15. Paul K, Moser K. Unemployment impairs mental health: meta-analysis. J Vocat Behav 2009;74:264–82.
16. Thimm JC, Kristoffersen AE, Ringberg U. The prevalence of severe grief reactions after bereavement and their associations with mental health, physical health, and health service utilization: a population-based study. Eur J Psychotraumatol 2020;11(1):1844440.
17. Wang J, Lloyd-Evans B, Giacco D, et al. Social isolation in mental health: a conceptual and methodological review. Soc Psychiatry Psychiatr Epidemiol 2017;52(12):1451–61.
18. Galea S, Brewin CR, Gruber M, et al. Exposure to hurricane-related stressors and mental illness after Hurricane Katrina. Arch Gen Psychiatry 2007;64(12):1427–34.
19. Majid U, Hussain SAS, Wasim A, et al. A systematic map of non-clinical evidence syntheses published globally on COVID-19. Disaster Med Public Health Prep 2021;1–19. https://doi.org/10.1017/dmp.2021.236.
20. Chen PJ, Pusica Y, Sohaei D, et al. An overview of mental health during the COVID-19 pandemic. Diagnosis (Berl) 2021;8(4):403–12. https://doi.org/10.1515/dx-2021-0046.
21. Phiri P, Ramakrishnan R, Rathod S, et al. An evaluation of the mental health impact of SARS-CoV-2 on patients, general public and healthcare professionals: a systematic review and meta-analysis. EClinicalMedicine 2021;34:100806.
22. Rodríguez-Fernández P, González-Santos J, Santamaría-Peláez M, et al. Psychological effects of home confinement and social distancing derived from COVID-19 in the general population–a systematic review. Int J Environ Res Public Health 2021;18(12). https://doi.org/10.3390/ijerph18126528.
23. Twenge JM, Joiner TE. Mental distress among U.S. adults during the COVID-19 pandemic. J Clin Psychol 2020;76(12):2170–82.
24. Lucid Holdings LLC. Academic research with Lucid. Available at: https://luc.id/academic-solutions/. Accessed August 6, 2021.
25. Kessler RC, Barker PR, Colpe LJ, et al. Screening for serious mental illness in the general population. Arch Gen Psychiatry 2003;60(2):184–9.
26. National Center for Health Statistics. National health interview survey. Available at: https://www.cdc.gov/nchs/nhis/index.htm. Accessed August 6, 2021.
27. American Association for Public Opinion Research. AAPOR report on online panels. Available at: https://www.aapor.org/Education-Resources/Reports/Report-on-Online-Panels. Accessed August 8, 2021.
28. Czeisler M, Lane RI, Petrosky E, et al. Mental health, substance use, and suicidal ideation during the COVID-19 pandemic - United States, June 24-30, 2020. MMWR Morb Mortal Wkly Rep 2020;69(32):1049–57.
29. Daly M, Sutin AR, Robinson E. Depression reported by US adults in 2017-2018 and March and April 2020. J Affect Disord 2021;278:131–5.

30. Ettman CK, Abdalla SM, Cohen GH, et al. Prevalence of depression symptoms in US adults before and during the COVID-19 pandemic. JAMA Netw Open 2020;3(9):e2019686.
31. McGinty EE, Presskreischer R, Han H, et al. Psychological distress and loneliness reported by US adults in 2018 and april 2020. JAMA 2020;324(1):93–4.
32. Yang S, Kim JK, Song R. Doubly robust inference when combining probability and non-probability samples with high dimensional data. J R Stat Soc Ser B Stat Methodol 2020;82(2):445–65.
33. United States Census Bureau. Measuring household experiences during the Coronavirus pandemic. Available at: https://www.census.gov/data/experimental-data-products/household-pulse-survey.html. Accessed August 8, 2021.
34. Kroenke K, Spitzer RL, Williams JB, et al. An ultra-brief screening scale for anxiety and depression: the PHQ-4. Psychosomatics 2009;50(6):613–21.
35. National Center for Chronic Disease Prevention and Health Promotion DoPH. Behavioral risk factor surveillance system. Available at: https://www.cdc.gov/brfss/index.html. Accessed August 8, 2021.
36. Twenge JM, McAllister C, Joiner TE. Anxiety and depressive symptoms in U.S. Census Bureau assessments of adults: trends from 2019 to fall 2020 across demographic groups. J Anxiety Disord 2021;83:102455.
37. United States Census Bureau. Experimental data products. Available at: https://www.census.gov/data/experimental-data-products.html. Accessed August 7, 2021.
38. United States Census Bureau. Household pulse survey technical documentation. Available at: https://www.census.gov/programs-surveys/household-pulse-survey/technical-documentation.html. Accessed August 8, 2021.
39. Peterson S, Toribio N, Farber J, et al. Nonresponse bias report for the 2020 Household Pulse Survey. Available at: https://www2.census.gov/programs-surveys/demo/technical-documentation/hhp/2020_HPS_NR_Bias_Report-final.pdf. Accessed August 8, 2021.
40. He C. The Depressd project: changes in mental health symptoms. Available at: https://www.depressd.ca/research-question-1-symptom-changes. Accessed August 8, 2021.
41. Sun Y, Wu Y, Bonardi O, et al. Comparison of mental health symptoms prior to and during COVID-19: evidence from a living systematic review and meta-analysis. medRxiv 2021;21256920. https://doi.org/10.1101/2021.05.10.21256920.
42. Institute for Social and Economic Research (ISER). Understanding society: the UK household longitudinal study. Available at: https://www.understandingsociety.ac.uk/. Accessed August 7, 2021.
43. Pevalin DJ. Multiple applications of the GHQ-12 in a general population sample: an investigation of long-term retest effects. Soc Psychiatry Psychiatr Epidemiol 2000;35(11):508–12. https://doi.org/10.1007/s001270050272.
44. Pierce M, Hope H, Ford T, et al. Mental health before and during the COVID-19 pandemic: a longitudinal probability sample survey of the UK population. Lancet Psychiatry 2020;7(10):883–92. https://doi.org/10.1016/s2215-0366(20)30308-4.
45. Daly M, Robinson E. Longitudinal changes in psychological distress in the UK from 2019 to September 2020 during the COVID-19 pandemic: evidence from a large nationally representative study. Psychiatry Res 2021;300:113920. https://doi.org/10.1016/j.psychres.2021.113920.
46. Kessler RC, Ustün TB. The World Mental Health (WMH) survey initiative version of the World Health Organization (WHO) composite international diagnostic interview (CIDI). Int J Methods Psychiatr Res 2004;13(2):93–121. https://doi.org/10.1002/mpr.168.

47. Knudsen AKS, Stene-Larsen K, Gustavson K, et al. Prevalence of mental disorders, suicidal ideation and suicides in the general population before and during the COVID-19 pandemic in Norway: a population-based repeated cross-sectional analysis. Lancet Reg Health - Europe 2021;4:100071. https://doi.org/10.1016/j.lanepe.2021.100071.
48. Murad MH, Wang Z, Chu H, et al. When continuous outcomes are measured using different scales: guide for meta-analysis and interpretation. BMJ 2019;364:k4817.
49. RAND Corporation. RAND American Life Panel (ALP). Available at: https://www.rand.org/research/data/alp.html. Accessed August 8, 2021.
50. Kessler RC, Green JG, Gruber MJ, et al. Screening for serious mental illness in the general population with the K6 screening scale: results from the WHO World Mental Health (WMH) survey initiative. Int J Methods Psychiatr Res 2010; 19(Suppl 1):4–22.
51. Breslau J, Finucane ML, Locker AR, et al. A longitudinal study of psychological distress in the United States before and during the COVID-19 pandemic. Prev Med 2021;143:106362.
52. Gutsche TL, Kapteyn A, Meijer E, et al. The RAND continuous 2012 presidential election poll. Public Opin Q 2014;78:233–54.
53. National Center for Health Statistics. National Health and Nutrition Examination Survey. Available at: https://www.cdc.gov/nchs/nhanes/about_nhanes.htm. Accessed August 8, 2021.
54. Gallup News Service. Gallup Poll social series: health and healthcare. Available at: https://news.gallup.com/poll/327311/americans-mental-health-ratings-sink-new-low.aspx. Accessed August 10, 2021.
55. Brenan M. Americans' mental health ratings sink to new low. Available at: https://news.gallup.com/poll/327311/americans-mental-health-ratings-sink-new-low.aspx. Accessed August 8, 2021.
56. Hartnett KP, Kite-Powell A, DeVies J, et al. Impact of the COVID-19 pandemic on emergency department visits - United States, January 1, 2019-May 30, 2020. MMWR Morb Mortal Wkly Rep 2020;69(23):699–704.
57. Adjemian J, Hartnett KP, Kite-Powell A, et al. Update: COVID-19 pandemic-associated changes in emergency department visits - United States, December 2020-January 2021. MMWR Morb Mortal Wkly Rep 2021;70(15):552–6.
58. Bhambhvani HP, Rodrigues AJ, Yu JS, et al. Hospital volumes of 5 medical emergencies in the COVID-19 pandemic in 2 US medical centers. JAMA Intern Med 2021;181(2):272–4.
59. Lange SJ, Ritchey MD, Goodman AB, et al. Potential indirect effects of the COVID-19 pandemic on use of emergency departments for acute life-threatening conditions - United States, January-May 2020. MMWR Morb Mortal Wkly Rep 2020;69(25):795–800.
60. Holland KM, Jones C, Vivolo-Kantor AM, et al. Trends in US emergency department visits for mental health, overdose, and violence outcomes before and during the COVID-19 pandemic. JAMA Psychiatry 2021;78(4):372–9.
61. Pathak EB, Garcia RB, Menard JM, et al. Out-of-hospital COVID-19 deaths: consequences for quality of medical care and accuracy of cause of death coding. Am J Public Health 2021;111(S2):S101–6.
62. Schoenbaum M, Colpe L. Challenges to behavioral health and injury surveillance during the COVID-19 pandemic. JAMA Psychiatry 2021;78(8):924–5.
63. Orthopoulos G, Santone E, Izzo F, et al. Increasing incidence of complicated appendicitis during COVID-19 pandemic. Am J Surg 2021;221(5):1056–60.

64. Yard E, Radhakrishnan L, Ballesteros MF, et al. Emergency department visits for suspected suicide attempts among persons aged 12-25 years before and during the COVID-19 pandemic - United States, January 2019-May 2021. MMWR Morb Mortal Wkly Rep 2021;70(24):888–94.
65. Friedman J, Mann NC, Hansen H, et al. Racial/ethnic, social, and geographic trends in overdose-associated cardiac arrests observed by US Emergency Medical Services during the COVID-19 pandemic. JAMA Psychiatry 2021;78(8):886–95.
66. Ahmad FB, Cisewski JA, Miniño A, et al. Provisional mortality data - United States, 2020. MMWR Morb Mortal Wkly Rep 2021;70(14):519–22.
67. National Center for Health Statistics. Instructions for classification of underlying and multiple causes of death. Available at: https://www.cdc.gov/nchs/nvss/manuals/2a-2021.htm. Accessed August 19, 2021.
68. Ahmad FB, Anderson RN. The leading causes of death in the US for 2020. JAMA 2021;325(18):1829–30.
69. Gupta S, Hayek SS, Wang W, et al. Factors associated with death in critically ill patients with coronavirus disease 2019 in the US. JAMA Intern Med 2020;180(11):1436–47.
70. Pirkis J, John A, Shin S, et al. Suicide trends in the early months of the COVID-19 pandemic: an interrupted time-series analysis of preliminary data from 21 countries. Lancet Psychiatry 2021;8(7):579–88.
71. Leaune E, Samuel M, Oh H, et al. Suicidal behaviors and ideation during emerging viral disease outbreaks before the COVID-19 pandemic: a systematic rapid review. Prev Med 2020;141:106264.
72. Tanaka T, Okamoto S. Increase in suicide following an initial decline during the COVID-19 pandemic in Japan. Nat Hum Behav 2021;5(2):229–38.
73. Faust JS, Du C, Mayes KD, et al. Mortality from drug overdoses, homicides, unintentional injuries, motor vehicle crashes, and suicides during the pandemic, march-august 2020. JAMA 2021;326(1):84–6.
74. Ahmad FB, Cisewski JA. Quarterly provisional estimates for selected indicators of mortality, 2019-Quarter 1, 2021. Available at: Available at: https://www.cdc.gov/nchs/nvss/vsrr/mortality-dashboard.htm. Accessed August 10, 2021.
75. Statista. Percentage of homicides by firearm in the United States from 2006 to 2019. Available at: https://www.statista.com/statistics/249783/percentage-of-homicides-by-firearm-in-the-united-states/. Accessed August 8, 2021.
76. Levine P, McKnight R. Three million more guns: the Spring 2020 spike in firearm sales. Available at: https://www.brookings.edu/blog/up-front/2020/07/13/three-million-more-guns-the-spring-2020-spike-in-firearm-sales/. Accessed August 20, 2021.
77. Schleimer JP, McCort CD, Shev AB, et al. Firearm purchasing and firearm violence during the coronavirus pandemic in the United States: a cross-sectional study. Inj Epidemiol 2021;8(1):43.
78. Ahmad FB, Rossen L, Sutton P. Provisional drug overdose death counts. National Center for Health Statistics; 2021.
79. Wilson N, Kariisa M, Seth P, et al. Drug and opioid-involved overdose deaths — United States, 2017–2018. MMWR Morb Mortal Wkly Rep 2020;69:290–7. https://doi.org/10.15585/mmwr.mm6911a4.
80. CDC Health Alert Network. Emergency preparedness and response. Available at: https://emergency.cdc.gov/han/2020/han00438.asp. Accessed August 19, 2021.
81. Levine PB, McKnight R. Firearms and accidental deaths: evidence from the aftermath of the Sandy Hook school shooting. Science 2017;358(6368):1324–8.

82. Cohen JS, Donnelly K, Patel SJ, et al. Firearms injuries involving young children in the United States during the COVID-19 pandemic. Pediatrics 2021;148(1). e2020042697.
83. National Safety Council. Motor vehicle deaths in 2020 estimated to be highest in 13 years, despite dramatic drops in miles driven. Available at: https://www.nsc.org/newsroom/motor-vehicle-deaths-2020-estimated-to-be-highest. Accessed October 2, 2021.
84. National Highway Traffic Safety Administration's National Center for Statistics and Analysis. Early estimate of motor vehicle traffic fatalities in 2020. Available at: https://crashstats.nhtsa.dot.gov/Api/Public/ViewPublication/813115. Accessed October 2, 2021.
85. Hirt S. As calls to crisis hotlines spike amid the coronavirus, those who respond feel the strain. Available at: https://www.usatoday.com/story/news/2020/06/15/crisis-hotline-call-volume-spikes-straining-social-workers/5266072002/. Accessed August 20, 2021.
86. Cooke K, Pell M, Lesser B. As school activity shut down amid COVID, 911 drug calls for youth skyrocketed. Available at: https://www.reuters.com/investigates/special-report/health-coronavirus-trauma/. Accessed August 19, 2020.
87. The National Suicide Prevention Lifeline. About the Lifeline. Available at: https://suicidepreventionlifeline.org/about/. Accessed August 20, 2021.
88. Tjeltveit A. COVID-19 and the National Suicide Prevention Lifeline. Available at: https://storymaps.arcgis.com/stories/063fbdbfb7c743b78e56abf79fc284b9.
89. Lersch KM. COVID-19 and mental health: an examination of 911 calls for service. Policing: A J Policy Pract 2020. https://doi.org/10.1093/police/paaa049. paaa049.
90. National Association of Emergency Medical Technicians. How COVID-19 has impacted our nation's EMS agencies. Available at: https://www.naemt.org/docs/default-source/covid-19/covid-impact-survey-06-03-2021.pdf?sfvrsn=c62fea93_4. Accessed August 20, 2021.
91. Boserup B, McKenney M, Elkbuli A. Alarming trends in US domestic violence during the COVID-19 pandemic. Am J Emerg Med 2020;38(12):2753–5.
92. McCrary J, Sanga S. The impact of the coronavirus lockdown on domestic violence. Am L Econ Rev 2021;23(1):137–63.
93. National Domestic Violence Hotline. A snapshot of domestic violence during COVID-19. Available at: https://www.thehotline.org/resources/a-snapshot-of-domestic-violence-during-covid-19/. Accessed August 20, 2021.
94. Ta M, Collins H, Neal S, et al. Domestic violence patterns in King County, WA: March – August 2020. Available at: https://kingcounty.gov/depts/health/covid-19/~/media/depts/health/communicable-diseases/documents/C19/domestic-violence-patterns-in-king-county.ashx. Accessed August 19, 2020.
95. Krueger AB, Mueller AI. The lot of the unemployed: a time use perspective. J Eur Econ Assoc 2012;10(4):765–94.
96. Fernández-Alcántara M, Kokou-Kpolou CK, Cruz-Quintana F, et al. Editorial: New perspectives in bereavement and loss: complicated and disenfranchised grief along the life cycle. Front Psychol 2021;12:691464.
97. Erzen E, Ö Çikrikci. The effect of loneliness on depression: a meta-analysis. Int J Soc Psychiatry 2018;64(5):427–35.
98. Mortazavi SS, Assari S, Alimohamadi A, et al. Fear, loss, social isolation, and incomplete grief due to COVID-19: a recipe for a psychiatric pandemic. Basic Clin Neurosci 2020;11(2):225–32.

99. Center on Budget and Policy Priorities. Tracking the COVID-19 recession's effects on food, housing, and employment hardships. Available at: https://www.cbpp.org/research/poverty-and-inequality/tracking-the-covid-19-recessions-effects-on-food-housing-and. Accessed August 20, 2021.
100. Gould E, Kassa M. Young workers hit hard by the COVID-19 economy: workers ages 16–24 face high unemployment and an uncertain future. Available at: https://files.epi.org/pdf/203139.pdf. Accessed August 19, 2020.
101. Saban M, Myers V, Luxenburg O, et al. Tipping the scales: a theoretical model to describe the differential effects of the COVID-19 pandemic on mortality. Int J Equity Health 2021;20(1):140.
102. Chen W, Qian L, Shi J, et al. Comparing performance between log-binomial and robust Poisson regression models for estimating risk ratios under model misspecification. BMC Med Res Methodol 2018;18(1):63.
103. Han H, Anderson K, Barry CL, et al. The Johns Hopkins COVID-19 Civic Life and Public Health Survey. Available at: https://snfagora.jhu.edu/project/the-johns-hopkins-covid-19-civic-life-and-public-health-survey/. Accessed August 19, 2021.
104. The Data Foundation. Improving government and society by using data to inform public policymaking. Available at: https://www.datafoundation.org/. Accessed August 19, 2021.
105. Pew Research Center. About Pew Research center. Available at: https://www.pewresearch.org/about/. Accessed August 22, 2021.
106. Czeisler MÉ, Howard ME, Czeisler CA, et al. The COPE Initiative: findings. Available at: https://www.thecopeinitiative.org/findings. Accessed August 20, 2021.
107. Lazer D, Baum MA, Ognyanova K, et al. The state of the nation: a 50-state COVID-19 survey. Available at: https://covidstates.org/. Accessed August 20, 2021.
108. The University of Southern California. Welcome to the Understanding America Study. Available at: https://uasdata.usc.edu/index.php. Accessed August 19, 2020.
109. The University of Southern California. Understanding Coronavirus in America. Available at: https://covid19pulse.usc.edu/. Accessed August 19, 2020.
110. Czeisler MÉ, Wiley JF, Czeisler CA, et al. Tempering optimism from repeated longitudinal mental health surveys. Lancet Psychiatry 2021;8(4):274–5.
111. Staff AJMC. What we're reading: U.S. declares coronavirus a public health emergency; FDA approves peanut allergy drug; California healthcare tax rejected. Available at: https://www.ajmc.com/view/what-were-reading-us-declares-coronavirus-a-public-health-emergency-fda-approves-peanut-allergy-drug-california-healthcare-tax-rejected. Accessed August 22, 2021.
112. Staff AJMC. What we're reading: U.S. records 100,000 COVID-19 cases; FDA staff support Alzheimer drug; CDC director urges asymptomatic testing. Available at: https://www.ajmc.com/view/what-we-re-reading-us-records-100-000-covid-19-cases-fda-staff-support-alzheimer-drug-cdc-director-urges-asymptomatic-testing. Accessed August 22, 2021.
113. Center for Disease Control and Prevention. Trends in number of COVID-19 cases and deaths in the U.S. reported to CDC, by state/territory. Available at: https://covid.cdc.gov/covid-data-tracker/#trends_dailycases. Accessed August 22, 2021.
114. Center for Disease Control and Prevention. Variant proportions. Available at: https://covid.cdc.gov/covid-data-tracker/#monitoring-varaint-heading. Accessed August 21, 2021.
115. Chakrabarti S, Hamlet LC, Kaminsky J, et al. Association of human mobility restrictions and race/ethnicity-based, sex-based, and income-based factors with

inequities in well-being during the COVID-19 pandemic in the United States. JAMA Netw Open 2021;4(4):e217373.
116. Thomas K, Darling J, Cassil A. U.S. pandemic Misery Index tracks COVID-19 hardships no. 3, May 2021. Available at: https://uasdata.usc.edu/index.php. Accessed August 20, 2021.
117. Daly M, Robinson E. Acute and longer-term psychological distress associated with testing positive for COVID-19: longitudinal evidence from a population-based study of US adults. Psychol Med 2021;1–8.
118. Holman EA, Thompson RR, Garfin DR, et al. The unfolding COVID-19 pandemic: a probability-based, nationally representative study of mental health in the United States. Sci Adv 2020;6(42). https://doi.org/10.1126/sciadv.abd5390.
119. Pai N, Vella SL. COVID-19 and loneliness: a rapid systematic review. Aust N Z J Psychiatry 2021. https://doi.org/10.1177/00048674211031489. 48674211031489.
120. Perlis RH, Ognyanova K, Santillana M, et al. Association of acute symptoms of COVID-19 and symptoms of depression in adults. JAMA Netw Open 2021;4(3):e213223.
121. Robinson E, Daly M. Explaining the rise and fall of psychological distress during the COVID-19 crisis in the United States: longitudinal evidence from the Understanding America Study. Br J Health Psychol 2021;26(2):570–87. https://doi.org/10.1111/bjhp.12493.
122. Swaziek Z, Wozniak A. Disparities old and new in US mental health during the COVID-19 pandemic. Fisc Stud 2020;41(3):709–32.
123. Kessler RC, Heeringa S, Lakoma MD, et al. Individual and societal effects of mental disorders on earnings in the United States: results from the national comorbidity survey replication. Am J Psychiatry 2008;165(6):703–11.
124. Taquet M, Luciano S, Geddes JR, et al. Bidirectional associations between COVID-19 and psychiatric disorder: retrospective cohort studies of 62354 COVID-19 cases in the USA. Lancet Psychiatry 2021;8(2):130–40.
125. Donnelly R, Farina MP. How do state policies shape experiences of household income shocks and mental health during the COVID-19 pandemic? Soc Sci Med 2021;269:113557.
126. Rigby E. The COVID-19 economy, unemployment insurance, and population health. JAMA Netw Open 2021;4(1):e2035955.
127. Bartash J. Inflation rate hits 30-year high, PCE shows, as U.S. confronts major shortages. Available at: https://www.marketwatch.com/story/inflation-rate-hits-30-year-high-pce-shows-as-u-s-confronts-major-shortages-11630068319. Accessed August 22, 2021.
128. Moghimi N, Di Napoli M, Biller J, et al. The neurological manifestations of post-acute sequelae of SARS-CoV-2 infection. Curr Neurol Neurosci Rep 2021;21(9):44.
129. Lerner AM, Robinson DA, Yang L, et al. Toward understanding COVID-19 recovery: National Institutes of Health workshop on postacute COVID-19. Ann Intern Med 2021;174(7):999–1003.
130. Kumar S, Veldhuis A, Malhotra T. Neuropsychiatric and cognitive sequelae of COVID-19. Front Psychol 2021;12(553). https://doi.org/10.3389/fpsyg.2021.577529.
131. Raphael B. When disaster strikes: how individuals and communities cope with catastrophe. New York: Basic Books; 1986.
132. Gersons BPR, Smid GE, Smit AS, et al. Can a 'second disaster' during and after the COVID-19 pandemic be mitigated? Eur J Psychotraumatol 2020;11(1):1815283.

Emerging Knowledge of the Neurobiology of COVID-19

Matthew Butler, MD[a,*], Benjamin Cross, MD[b], Danish Hafeez[c], Mao Fong Lim, MD[d], Hamilton Morrin, MD[e], Emma Rachel Rengasamy, MD[f], Tom Pollak, PhD[a], Timothy R. Nicholson, PhD[a]

KEYWORDS

• COVID-19 • SARS-CoV-2 • Neurobiology • Delirium • Long COVID
• Neuropsychiatry

KEY POINTS

- COVID-19 causes a wide range of neuropsychiatric complications in both the acute and postacute phases.
- Acute neuropsychiatric complications are likely due to factors such as systemic inflammation and parainfectious immune mechanisms as opposed to direct viral neurotropism.
- Prolonged neuropsychiatric symptoms may result as sequalae from severe (hospitalized) COVID-19 illness.
- As well as this, debilitating neuropsychiatric symptoms may arise in relatively minor (nonhospitalized) COVID-19 cases.
- Studies on the *in utero* effects of SARS-CoV-2 infection are urgently required in order to qualify or refute a potential predisposition that a minority of children of infected mothers may have for increased risk of neurodevelopmental and neuropsychiatric disorders.

INTRODUCTION

COVID-19, the syndrome caused by infection with the novel coronavirus SARS-CoV-2, has, at the time of writing, affected more than 200 million people worldwide.[1] In mild COVID-19 illnesses, which constitute the large majority, viral replication tends to be confined to the upper respiratory tract, although in severe cases COVID-19 may affect

Conflict of interest: The authors declare no commercial or financial conflicts of interest.
[a] Institute of Psychiatry, Psychology and Neuroscience, King's College, 16 De Crespigny Park, SE5 8AF London; [b] East Lancashire Hospitals NHS Trust, Casterton Ave, Burnley, BB10 2PQ; [c] School of Medical Sciences, The University of Manchester, Oxford Rd, Manchester, M13 9PL, UK; [d] Cambridge University Hospitals NHS Foundation Trust, Hills Rd, Cambridge, CB2 0QQ, UK; [e] Maidstone & Tunbridge Wells NHS Trust, Tonbridge Rd, Royal Tunbridge Wells, TN2 4QJ, UK; [f] Cwm Taf Morgannwg University Health Board, Ynysmeurig House, Navigation Park, Abercynon, CF45 4SN, UK
* Corresponding author. Neuropsychiatry Research and Education Group, Institute of Psychiatry, Psychology & Neuroscience, 16 De Crespigny Park, London, SE5 8AF
E-mail address: Matthew.butler@kcl.ac.uk

Psychiatr Clin N Am 45 (2022) 29–43
https://doi.org/10.1016/j.psc.2021.11.001

multiple organs, including the central nervous system.[2] Indeed, high rates of neuropsychiatric complications in COVID-19 were expected based on data from previous coronavirus epidemics.[3]

Large studies have indicated high rates of neurologic and neuropsychiatric complications of COVID-19, which in the majority are nonspecific and include fatigue, myalgia, depression, anxiety, and headache.[4] As well as these common neuropsychiatric complications, there are rarer central nervous system complications, such as encephalitis and, possibly, psychosis.[5,6] In the acute phase of COVID-19, delirium is the most common neuropsychiatric manifestation and is thought to arise secondary to the inflammatory response to SARS-CoV-2 replication.[7] Furthermore, cerebral vasculopathy secondary to the inflammatory response likely predisposes to complications ranging from acute infarctions (ie, stroke) to subtle microvascular alterations.[8]

Toward the beginning of the pandemic it was hypothesized that SARS-CoV-2 may be neurotropic: that is, able to directly invade and replicate inside neuronal cells.[9] The scientific community had good reason to suspect this, as SARS-CoV-2 was found to enter human host cells via the angiotensin-converting enzyme 2, a transmembrane protein expressed by multiple tissue types across the body, including in the nasal neuroepithelium, where it is found in high levels.[10] Many patients with acute COVID-19 were found to experience anosmia, which in some cases is long-lasting, suggesting possible viral interference with the olfactory neurons, which may have represented a possible route of entry into the proximal central nervous system.[11] This hypothesis has been supported by preclinical data, which have suggested that the virus is able to replicate inside laboratory simulations of central nervous system tissue, such as brain organoids,[12] as well as suggestions from some neuroimaging data.[13] There are, however, limits to the conclusions that can be drawn from these in vitro studies, and there has been very scant evidence of neurotropism from clinical and postmortem studies.[9]

Over the roughly 18 months of the pandemic, the neurotropic hypothesis has gradually fallen out of favor, and there have been other, more nuanced, neurobiological hypotheses posited to explain the high rates of neuropsychiatric complications of COVID-19.[9] Many of these hypotheses implicate the immune response to the virus, which is likely to be responsible for many of the acute neuropsychiatric complications of the disorder but is also a potential contributing factor to longer term neuropsychiatric sequelae of COVID-19, many of which are currently known as "long COVID."[14] Indeed, large numbers of patients with long COVID symptoms, ranging from persistent anosmia, to neurocognitive abnormalities, to persistent and disabling fatigue, will continue to suffer as a longer term result of the pandemic.[2,14]

What follows is a broad discussion of the current neurobiological hypotheses on the cause and pathophysiology of both the acute and longer-term neuropsychiatric complications of COVID-19. These mechanistic factors are discussed in relation to the commonest neuropsychiatric syndromes that arise in the context of COVID-19.

DISCUSSION

What are the Mechanisms Behind Acute Neuropsychiatric Complications of COVID-19?

Delirium

Delirium is a syndrome defined as an acute disturbance in attention and awareness, as well as impairment in other aspects of cognition such as memory or perception, which tends to fluctuate in severity over days or hours. In this article the authors use delirium as the default term for such patients, reserving the term acute encephalopathy for clinical syndromes that incorporate rapidly developing pathobiological brain processes with additional neurologic signs or symptoms (for a consensus recommendation on this issue please see Ref.[15]).

Delirium is common, and the incidence in elderly hospital inpatients has been estimated to be up to 35%.[16] Although the cause is often multifactorial, it is well established that infections and the resultant systemic inflammatory response may lead to delirium in predisposed individuals, perhaps through cytokine-induced cholinergic neurotransmitter deficiencies.[17] Data have indicated that many patients with COVID-19 experience delirium in the acute phase—in some populations up to half of all cases—and in some delirium can be the sole presenting feature.[18] There is evidence demonstrating a higher prevalence of delirium in those with severe infection,[19] especially in those admitted to intensive care (ICU)[20] and in the elderly or those with dementia.[7] Despite this, delirium in COVID-19 has also affected those without typical risk factors, including younger patients.[21]

Some authors have suggested that patients with COVID-19 may be at risk of a dysfunctional immune response mediated by massive cytokine release, known as a "cytokine storm."[22] Massive cytokine release is postulated as being responsible for multiorgan pathology in severe COVID-19, for example, acute respiratory distress syndrome. Some patients have shown cytokine storm immune responses to other epidemic viruses, such as H1N1 influenza[23] and other coronaviruses.[24] Despite the theoretic risk of a cytokine storm, the data have not been consistently supportive of its common presence in COVID-19.[25] Whether or not patients with COVID-19 experience cytokine storms, high levels of circulating inflammatory markers, as is seen in any immune response to an infectious pathogen, may lead to central nervous system complications such as delirium.

Patients with COVID-19 have also been shown to have high levels of circulating serum cytokines, such as interferon-gamma (IFN-γ) and interleukin-17 (IL-17), which suggest a proinflammatory T-helper type I (Th1) and Th17 immune response.[26] Proinflammatory cytokines, such as IL-6, IL-8, and tumor necrosis factor alpha, seen in severe COVID-19,[27] can interfere with blood-brain barrier (BBB) permeability via upregulation of cyclooxygenase-2 and activation of matrix metalloproteases.[28] This COVID-19–related BBB breakdown has been shown in both preclinical[29] and clinical research.[30] Disruption of the BBB may facilitate entry of inflammatory or immune mediators, which induce or mediate neuroinflammation via microglial activation and T-cell invasion.[31] If severe enough, this may lead to lasting neuronal damage and subsequent cognitive impairment.[32]

Affective disorders

Depression has been reported at high levels in patients with acute COVID-19, although most studies to date have used basic screening tools in hospitalized patients, both of which are factors that may misrepresent true overall prevalence.[33] There are, of course, many reasons why a person with a severe respiratory pandemic illness may develop low mood or depression beyond the neurobiological effects of the infection. Nevertheless, it is possible that COVID-19 itself may directly lead to symptoms of depression, particularly as the risk of depressive symptoms may be increased with more severe COVID-19 illness.[34] The most plausible method of neurobiological depressogenesis in response to COVID-19 is via the (1) inflammatory response or (2) as a result of cerebrovascular damage secondary to systemic endotheliopathy, poststroke depression, or hypoxic brain injury.

Inflammatory cytokines have been postulated to cause depressive symptoms for decades,[35] and one evolutionary model of depression suggests that social withdrawal and "forced rest," both symptoms that overlap with those seen in depression, are a useful adaptive response to an infection or injury.[36] There has been evidence to support the hypothesis: chronic inflammatory conditions such as rheumatoid arthritis are associated with high levels of depression,[37] and administration of proinflammatory cytokines (eg, IFN-α–based immunotherapy in chronic hepatitis C) can induce depressive symptoms in humans and animals.[38] Some data have suggested that the degree of inflammation in COVID-19 is correlated with the extent of depressive symptoms,[39] although this has not always been replicated.[40] It remains to be established whether cytokines play a causal role in depressive illness in COVID-19 and other inflammatory conditions or whether they simply represent epiphenomena without major significance (or, more likely, that the bidirectional relationship is complicated and not yet fully understood).

As has been noted, patients with COVID-19 are predisposed to cerebrovascular pathology, including acute stroke.[8] It is well known that the incidence of depression is high following stroke.[41] In addition, multiple neuroimaging studies in patients with COVID-19 (typically severe cases) have consistently shown structural brain lesions, particularly in white matter tracts.[42] It is possible that this structural damage predisposes individuals to a depression in which vascular or structural changes are a contributing factor: a “vascular depression.” The vascular depression hypothesis posits that cerebrovascular damage, or vascular insufficiency, leads to disruption in cerebral functioning, especially of frontostriatal circuits, which predispose to low mood.[43]

In addition, it was noted in previous coronavirus epidemics that cases of acute affective disorders, including mania, arose in the context of systemically administered corticosteroid (eg, dexamethasone, prednisolone) therapy.[3] Following large randomized controlled trials that supported their use, corticosteroids are now routinely prescribed to hospitalized patients with COVID-19.[44] Corticosteroids are known to cause a spectrum of neuropsychiatric side effects, including acute mania and depression, which occur in an estimated 6% of prescriptions.[45] The mechanisms by which steroids induce affective symptoms remain unclear, although disruptions to the hypothalamic-pituitary-adrenal axis are commonly seen in depression,[46] and it is hypothesized that glucocorticoids may cause altered neurotransmitter and neuroreceptor gene transcription.[47] Nevertheless, despite these plausible assertions, there have only been sporadic reports of mania in hospitalized patients with COVID-19,[48] which have not been replicated in other samples.[4,49]

Psychosis

Psychosis has long been associated with viral illness, and as far back as the seventeenth century, certain respiratory infections including influenza were linked with acute psychotic disorders.[50,51] At the height of the 1918 to 1919 Spanish Influenza pandemic, hundreds of cases of postpsychotic influenza were reported.[50] In COVID-19, the incidence of psychotic disorders is estimated at around 1%, increasing to 3% for those with (ICU) admission and 7% in those with delirium.[52] The factors implicated in the genesis of psychotic symptoms in COVID-19 is likely to be multifactorial and center around physiologic and psychological stress.[6]

An additional factor for consideration is the confounding of true psychotic symptoms by the presence of delirium. Psychotic features are often present in delirium, and diagnosis of a true psychotic disorder may be difficult or even impossible in the acute illness phase. However, cases published earlier in the pandemic reported psychotic disorders in patients who have screened negative for delirium and without grossly abnormal inflammatory profiles.[48] Another important confounder may be the use of corticosteroids in treating COVID-19, which are well documented to precipitate delirium and hallucinations.[45] In summary, despite substantial evidence for biological plausibility implicating SARS-CoV-2 in the generation of psychotic illnesses, a temporal, definitive association is far from proved, especially because potential confounders such as delirium and treatment side effects are unaccounted for.

Nevertheless, immunopsychiatric research has implicated inflammatory processes in the development of psychosis,[53] and epidemiologic studies have shown robust associations between viral infections and subsequent development of psychosis, either in childhood or via maternal infection in utero.[54,55] A small subset of psychoses are autoimmune in origin, and the development of autoantibodies to receptors has been associated with acute viral infection. Nevertheless, this represents a small subset of psychotic patients and most of the patients tested will be negative for autoantibodies.[56] Cell or antibody-mediated postinfectious psychosis is therefore a potential, albeit likely rare, mechanism for the pathogenesis of COVID-19 psychosis.

Encephalitis

Encephalitis is defined as inflammation of the brain parenchyma that occurs most often in response to pathogens, systemic inflammation, or autoimmune antibodies.[57] Encephalitis, as well as the related inflammatory syndrome of acute disseminated encephalomyelitis,[58] has been reported to occur in patients with COVID-19.[59] In order for cerebral inflammation to occur, either pathogens or inflammatory mediators (or both) must enter the central nervous system, for example, via disruptions in the BBB. Although in theory this disruption could also allow for the migration of SARS-CoV-2 into the cerebral parenchyma infection (as seen in, for example, herpes simplex encephalitis), this has not yet been borne out by most data.[9]

Instead, there are data suggesting the presence of anti-SARS-CoV-2 antibodies[30] as well as autoantibodies, such as antineuronal,[60] antiglial,[60] and anti-NDMAR antibodies[60] in the cerebrospinal fluid of patients with neurologic symptoms associated with COVID-19. High-affinity SARS-CoV-2-neutralizing antibodies have been shown to cross-react with self-antigens found in the central nervous system.[61] These findings support the possibility of autoimmune-mediated encephalitis in a tiny minority of patients with severe COVID-19, although it should be emphasized that the presence of autoantibodies alone does not necessarily imply direct pathogenicity. Nevertheless, clinical series have shown improvement in patients with COVID-19–related encephalitis treated with immunotherapy, which does suggest a role for a host immune response in some patients.[62]

Cerebrovascular pathology

Patients with COVID-19 have been found to be susceptible to cerebrovascular pathology, including acute stroke.[8] Stroke occurs in approximately 1% to 3% of hospitalized patients with COVID-19 and 6% of those admitted to ICU.[63] Stroke can result in significant neuropsychiatric complications, with around one-third of stroke survivors experiencing anxiety, depression, or apathy.[64] COVID-19–associated strokes have been suggested to be more likely to present with large vessel occlusion, multiterritory involvement, and involvement of otherwise uncommonly affected vasculature than is typically, with clinically observed neurologic deficit typically being severe.[63]

Although neuroimaging findings in COVID-19 have often been heterogenous and nonspecific,[65] gray matter lesions occur most frequently in the temporal and precentral gyrus and bilateral thalamus, whereas white matter lesions occur most frequently in the corticospinal tract and corpus callosum.[42] Changes in thalamocortical connectivity have the potential to impair regulation of arousal and consciousness[66] and therefore may be responsible for observed symptoms such as agitation, disorientation, confusion, and loss of consciousness.[67] Corpus callosum injury impairs interhemispheric communication, potentially causing disconnection syndrome with neurocognitive deficits.[42]

Endotheliopathy (ie, a disruption of endothelial cells responsible for maintaining vascular integrity) in COVID-19 has been identified as a substantial contributor to development of thrombotic complications such as stroke.[68] Because SARS-CoV-2 particles infiltrate endothelial cells of the cerebral vasculature, there is activation of macrophages, neutrophils, complement pathways, and thrombin production; together, these encourage deposition of microthrombi.[69] Cerebral postmortem studies demonstrate acute hypoxic-ischemic injury from micro- and macroinfarcts, as well as hemorrhage and mild-to-moderate inflammation,[70] although correlation between histopathological findings and SARS-CoV-2 RNA in brain has been lacking.[71]

Patients with severe COVID-19 are at risk of hypoxic-ischemic brain injury both from the direct viral effects on pulmonary tissue, the inflammatory sepsis response (including hypotension),[72] as well as iatrogenic factors such as intubation.[73] Cerebral microhemorrhages have also been reported in cases of patients with severe COVID-19 requiring intensive care.[74] It has been suggested that these may arise secondary to hypoxia-induced cerebral vasodilatation and release of cytokines, reactive oxygen species, and vascular endothelial growth factor, as a similar pattern has been observed in individuals with non–COVID-19–related respiratory failure and critical illness.[75] Although the long-term effects of cerebral microhemorrhages in patients with COVID-19 are uncertain, in other diseases independent association has been observed between microhemorrhages and cognitive impairment and disability.[76]

What are the Mechanisms Behind the Longer Term Neuropsychiatric Complications of COVID-19?

Long COVID

Many patients who are infected with COVID-19 will experience persistent neuropsychiatric symptoms such as sleep disturbance, fatigue, cognitive difficulties, anxiety, and posttraumatic stress symptoms, depression, and myalgia.[77] Although, as yet, there is no universally agreed-on definition for this syndrome, which is thought to affect around 10% of COVID-19 survivors, it is currently most often referred to as long COVID.[14] The exact symptomology of long COVID is not yet clear with patients often reporting varied, relapsing-remitting symptoms[78] and the presence of symptoms varying depending on the methodology used to capture them as well as the populations studied.[77,79] Given the heterogeneity and unknowns that characterize current understanding of long COVID, mechanistic hypothesis remains speculative at present. Current understanding suggests at least 3 possible mechanistic hypotheses: (1) functional impairment akin to "post-ICU syndrome" (see later discussion), (2) lingering inflammation and immune dysfunction initially precipitated by the acute infection, and (3) physiologic changes induced by SARS-CoV-2, including persistence of the virus after the acute illness.[80] Regardless of the primary mechanistic pathway, symptoms in a subset of patients may be prolonged in part due to nonvolitional attentional diversion and somatic hyperawareness that arises secondary to the symptoms.

Intuitively, we might expect to see long COVID overrepresented in patients who have been hospitalized by severe acute COVID-19. Indeed, in some studies, length of hospitalization with COVID-19 has been identified as a predictor of greater impairment in functional status[81]; this indicates that prolonged symptoms that persist could in part demonstrate a broader post-ICU syndrome, a constellation of symptoms found in many patients following a critical illness, which is driven by factors such as prolonged deconditioning and the stress of responding to a life-threatening illness.[82] The story, however, is a little more complex, and many suffer with debilitating long COVID symptoms that emerge after a relatively "mild" acute COVID-19 illness[2,77]; indeed, one study found a correlation between a weaker anti-SARS-CoV-2 response and long COVID,[83] which indicates that long COVID is likely a heterogenous illness that includes a large proportion of patients who suffer with a phenotypical distinct entity to post-ICU syndrome.[77]

One theory suggests that the neuroendocrine and inflammatory effects of infection can mediate symptoms of withdrawal and fatigue, consistent with an evolutionary perspective which emphasizes the survival benefit gained from withdrawal to convalesce from a pathogenic illness (as discussed earlier). Furthermore, the physical and psychological exhaustion from the infection may lead to deconditioning, as was seen in severe acute respiratory syndrome (SARS, a coronavirus).[3]

Initial attempts have been made to establish biomarkers that may help us understand the underlying pathophysiology of long COVID. In patients discharged from hospital, lymphopenia and elevated D-dimer and C-reactive protein levels were found in a minority.[84] This persistence of derangement in biomarkers, particularly those associated with inflammation, indicate that long COVID symptoms could be related to a lingering "tail" and an abnormal inflammatory response to an infection.[85,86]

Some investigators have suggested that long COVID symptoms may linger due to the prolonged presence of SARS-CoV-2 after the acute illness, partly as some data have indicated that SARS-CoV-2 RNA continues to be found in bodily fluids after the acute illness (particularly in stool samples) and that B-cell somatic hypermutations continue months after exposure, suggesting an ongoing and evolving immune response to a persistent virus.[87] Nevertheless, there is no consensus on this hypothesis, particularly because it has not previously been considered relevant in previous coronavirus infections, and the presence of viral RNA does not necessarily translate into clinical relevance.[88]

Overall, firm evidence for the underlying neurobiology of long COVID is unclear, and the literature lacks large-scale prospective studies. The evidence so far is mixed, indicating possible avenues for further exploration, for example, whether increased inflammation during the infective phase of COVID-19 may predispose to more severe symptoms and that those with "long COVID" may have high to normal levels of inflammatory markers that exacerbate their symptoms. These increased inflammatory markers may or may not interact with the nervous system to drive abnormalities and autonomic dysfunction that drive symptoms.[89] All of these physiologic mechanisms must be seen in the biopsychosocial context where the experience of COVID-19 infection and its psychological effects may influence lingering symptoms.

Neurocognitive syndromes

Longer term neurocognitive impairment resulting from COVID-19 is likely to occur in some patients. Indeed, data from the SARS epidemic indicated that some hospitalized patients had impairments of memory, attention, concentration, or mental processing speed at 1-year follow-up[3]; this has been replicated in several studies in COVID-19, albeit many with shorter follow-up periods.[19,90] Whether or not these cognitive abnormalities are specific to COVID-19 can be contested, as cognitive deficits following many severe illnesses requiring intensive care (intensive therapy unit) admission are well recognized.[91] Nevertheless, as with many other long COVID symptoms, data suggest that the degree of longer-term cognitive impairment is not always related to the severity of the acute COVID-19 illness.[92]

Longer term neurocognitive syndromes following acute COVID-19 are likely to be seen in 3 distinct but overlapping patient groups: (1) those with postdelirium cognitive impairment, driven by central nervous system inflammation,[39] (2) those without preceding delirium, suggesting other mechanisms of cognitive deficit such as hypoxic brain insults,[93] and (3) those with a milder course of illness with alternate mechanisms of cognitive impairment.

It is well established that delirium is a risk factor for the subsequent development of neurocognitive impairment and dementia and can precipitate a stepwise, irretrievable decline in cognition in people who already have a dementia diagnosis or with mild cognitive impairment.[94] This suggests that we may see a sharp increase in the incidence of dementia as a result of COVID-19 over the coming years.

Neurocognitive deficits postdischarge from COVID-19 illness have been associated with low blood oxygenation as well as the presence of acute respiratory distress syndrome, which may indicate hypoxic brain insults in pathogenesis of persisting cognitive deficits.[90] It is known that medial temporal brain regions (including the hippocampus, which has a key role in short-term memory) are particularly sensitive to hypoxaemia,[95] and subtle neuroimaging changes across the brain, including in the hippocampus, have been found in patients who were hospitalized with severe COVID-19.[96] Other neuroimaging studies in COVID-19 have shown areas of brain hypometabolism in many brain regions, including limbic and paralimbic areas, brainstem, and cerebellum on positron emission tomography scans. The presence of these markers of brain hypometabolism have been associated with persistent cognitive abnormalities postacute COVID-19 illness.[97]

Finally, cognitive and attentional deficits, known by some as "brain fog," is a common feature of long COVID.[98] The mechanisms whereby these subjective cognitive changes arise have yet to be fully understood and will likely be complex and multifactorial. Nevertheless, it is likely that a proportion of patients, particularly those in younger age demographics than typically affected by dementias, will have symptoms indicating functional cognitive disorder, which, as with any functional disorder, may arise from an acute physical illness such as COVID-19. Functional cognitive disorders cause distress and disability; however, they do not represent a degenerative brain disorder.[99] Similar functional cognitive symptoms have been seen in other conditions such as functional neurologic disorder, chronic fatigue syndrome/myalgic encephalomyelitis (CFS/ME), and fibromyalgia.[100]

In utero effects

COVID-19 may adversely affect neonatal outcomes, with reported higher rates of fetal distress, low birth weight, intrauterine growth restriction, and increased rates of preterm births.[101] Some have suggested that this may translate into increased risk of neurodevelopmental and neuropsychiatric disorders, although at present these hypotheses are speculative.[102] Maternal infection with other viruses (eg, herpes simplex, rubella, poliovirus, Zika, and influenza) have been associated with increased risk of neurodevelopmental disorders,[103] including, for example, autism spectrum disorder (ASD).[104] Some of the strongest evidence linking maternal viral infections with schizophrenia to date is from the 1964 rubella pandemic, in which there was a 10- to 15-fold increased risk of schizophrenia spectrum disorders in offspring born to mothers who contracted the virus.[105]

Mechanisms behind these putative effects are broadly 2-fold: either via immune constituents or maternal hormones interacting with fetal neurogenesis. Elevated levels of immunoglobulin G (IgG) and IgM, which occur in viral infections, may cross into placental circulation, leading to disruption in neuronal development.[106] As has been noted, SARS-CoV-2 may elicit a Th17 (IL-17) immune response, and studies in mouse models show administration of IL-17 produces an autismlike phenotype and behavior in offspring.[107] Similarly, the physiologic, metabolic, and endocrine correlates of maternal physiologic stress, which may occur in the context of a viral illness, have been noted to be associated with increased risk of neurodevelopmental outcomes in offspring, including ASD[103] and schizophrenia.[108] Whether or not these factors will be relevant to the offspring of mothers who are COVID-19 positive is not yet known.[109]

SUMMARY

It has been well established that many patients with COVID-19 illness will develop neuropsychiatric complications. The neurobiology behind these acute complications is continuing to emerge, and emphasis is now placed on inflammatory and parainfectious systemic effects of COVID-19 illness as opposed to direct viral neurotropism. Beyond the COVID-19 pandemic, research into this area may help to elucidate mechanisms by which other viral illnesses may contribute to illnesses such as psychosis, cognitive impairment, and CFS/ME.

Many patients will experience long-lasting neuropsychiatric difficulties following COVID-19. These patients fall roughly into 2 distinct but overlapping groups: those who had a severe COVID-19 illness with acute neuropsychiatric complications and those with "milder" COVID-19 illnesses, who nevertheless have lasting neuropsychiatric effects. Finally, it has been speculated (although far from proved) that offspring born to mothers who had COVID-19 may be more at risk of neurodevelopmental conditions, principally autism spectrum disorder and schizophrenia spectrum disorders.

In clinical practice, patients can be reassured that it is most likely that the SARS-CoV-2 virus will not directly infect their central nervous system; however, physicians are encouraged to be alert to the common neuropsychiatric manifestations. Delirium is particularly common, and in some patients will be the sole presenting syndrome of SARS-CoV-2 infections. Finally, patients should be strongly advised to follow public health advice on COVID-19 transmission and to receive an SARS-CoV-2 vaccination whenever possible, as this is the most effective way of reducing risk of neuropsychiatric complications associated with COVID-19.

CLINICS CARE POINTS

- Patients in clinic can be reassured that it is very unlikely that the SARS-CoV-2 virus will directly infect their central nervous system.
- Nevertheless, do not forget the brain when dealing with acute COVID-19. Delirium is particularly common and in some patients will be the sole presenting syndrome of SARS-CoV-2 infections.
- Patients should be strongly advised to follow public health advice on COVID-19 transmission and to receive an SARS-CoV-2 vaccination whenever possible, as this is the most effective way of reducing risk of neuropsychiatric complications associated with COVID-19.

REFERENCES

1. Worldometer. COVID-19 CORONAVIRUS PANDEMIC. Available at: https://www.worldometers.info/coronavirus/. Accessed July 22, 2021.

2. Butler M, Pollak TA, Rooney AG, et al. Neuropsychiatric complications of covid-19. BMJ 2020;m3871. https://doi.org/10.1136/bmj.m3871.
3. Rogers JP, Chesney E, Oliver D, et al. Psychiatric and neuropsychiatric presentations associated with severe coronavirus infections: a systematic review and meta-analysis with comparison to the COVID-19 pandemic. Lancet Psychiatry 2020;7(7):611–27. https://doi.org/10.1016/S2215-0366(20)30203-0.
4. Rogers JP, Watson C, Badenoch J, et al. The neurology and neuropsychiatry of COVID-19: a systematic review and meta-analysis of the early literature reveals frequent CNS manifestations and key emerging narratives. Published online February 26, 2021. doi:10.1101/2021.02.24.21252335
5. Mondal R, Ganguly U, Deb S, et al. Meningoencephalitis associated with COVID-19: a systematic review. J Neurovirol 2021;27(1):12–25. https://doi.org/10.1007/s13365-020-00923-3.
6. Watson CJ, Thomas RH, Solomon T, et al. COVID-19 and psychosis risk: Real or delusional concern? Neurosci Lett 2021;741:135491. https://doi.org/10.1016/j.neulet.2020.135491.
7. Kennedy M, Helfand BKI, Gou RY, et al. Delirium in Older Patients With COVID-19 Presenting to the Emergency Department. JAMA Netw Open 2020;3(11):e2029540. https://doi.org/10.1001/jamanetworkopen.2020.29540.
8. Siow I, Lee KS, Zhang JJY, et al. Stroke as a Neurological Complication of COVID-19: A Systematic Review and Meta-Analysis of Incidence, Outcomes and Predictors. J Stroke Cerebrovasc Dis 2021;30(3):105549.
9. Solomon T. Neurological infection with SARS-CoV-2 — the story so far. Nat Rev Neurol 2021;17(2):65–6.
10. Bourgonje AR, Abdulle AE, Timens W, et al. Angiotensin-converting enzyme 2 (ACE2) and the pathophysiology of coronavirus disease 2019. J Pathol 2020;251(3):228–48.
11. Xydakis MS, Dehgani-Mobaraki P, Holbrook EH, et al. Smell and taste dysfunction in patients with COVID-19. Lancet Infect Dis 2020;20(9):1015–6.
12. Tiwari SK, Wang S, Smith D, et al. Revealing Tissue-Specific SARS-CoV-2 Infection and Host Responses using Human Stem Cell-Derived Lung and Cerebral Organoids. Stem Cell Rep 2021;16(3):437–45.
13. Douaud G, Lee S, Alfaro-Almagro F, et al. Brain Imaging before and after COVID-19 in UK Biobank. Neurology 2021. https://doi.org/10.1101/2021.06.11.21258690.
14. Sykes DL, Holdsworth L, Jawad N, et al. Post-COVID-19 Symptom Burden: What is Long-COVID and How Should We Manage It? Lung 2021. https://doi.org/10.1007/s00408-021-00423-z.
15. Slooter AJC, Otte WM, Devlin JW, et al. Updated nomenclature of delirium and acute encephalopathy: statement of ten Societies. Intensive Care Med 2020;46(5):1020–2.
16. Inouye SK, Westendorp RGJ, Saczynski JS. Delirium in elderly people. Lancet Lond Engl 2014;383(9920):911–22.
17. van Gool WA, van de Beek D, Eikelenboom P. Systemic infection and delirium: when cytokines and acetylcholine collide. Lancet Lond Engl 2010;375(9716):773–5.
18. Pun BT, Badenes R, Heras La Calle G, et al. Prevalence and risk factors for delirium in critically ill patients with COVID-19 (COVID-D): a multicentre cohort study. Lancet Respir Med 2021;9(3):239–50.
19. Helms J, Kremer S, Merdji H, et al. Neurologic Features in Severe SARS-CoV-2 Infection. N Engl J Med 2020;382(23):2268–70.

20. Mattace-Raso F, Polinder-Bos H, Oosterwijk B, et al. Delirium: A Frequent Manifestation in COVID-19 Older Patients. Clin Interv Aging 2020;15:2245–7.
21. Varatharaj A, Thomas N, Ellul MA, et al. Neurological and neuropsychiatric complications of COVID-19 in 153 patients: a UK-wide surveillance study. Lancet Psychiatry 2020. Avaialble at: https://www.journals.elsevier.com/the-lancet-psychiatry.
22. Mehta P, McAuley DF, Brown M, et al. COVID-19: consider cytokine storm syndromes and immunosuppression. Lancet 2020;395(10229):1033–4.
23. Cheng X-W, Lu J, Wu C-L, et al. Three fatal cases of pandemic 2009 influenza A virus infection in Shenzhen are associated with cytokine storm. Respir Physiol Neurobiol 2011;175(1):185–7.
24. Channappanavar R, Perlman S. Pathogenic human coronavirus infections: causes and consequences of cytokine storm and immunopathology. Semin Immunopathol 2017;39(5):529–39.
25. Sinha P, Matthay MA, Calfee CS. Is a "Cytokine Storm" Relevant to COVID-19? JAMA Intern Med 2020;180(9):1152.
26. Ghazavi A, Ganji A, Keshavarzian N, et al. Cytokine profile and disease severity in patients with COVID-19. Cytokine 2021;137:155323.
27. Del Valle DM, Kim-Schulze S, Huang H-H, et al. An inflammatory cytokine signature predicts COVID-19 severity and survival. Nat Med 2020;26(10):1636–43.
28. Yang C, Yang Y, DeMars KM, et al. Genetic Deletion or Pharmacological Inhibition of Cyclooxygenase-2 Reduces Blood-Brain Barrier Damage in Experimental Ischemic Stroke. Front Neurol 2020;11:887.
29. Buzhdygan TP, DeOre BJ, Baldwin-Leclair A, et al. The SARS-CoV-2 spike protein alters barrier function in 2D static and 3D microfluidic in vitro models of the human blood-brain barrier. Biorxiv Prepr Serv Biol 2020. https://doi.org/10.1101/2020.06.15.150912. 101680187.
30. Alexopoulos H, Magira E, Bitzogli K, et al. Anti–SARS-CoV-2 antibodies in the CSF, blood-brain barrier dysfunction, and neurological outcome: Studies in 8 stuporous and comatose patients. Neurol - Neuroimmunol Neuroinflammation 2020;7(6):e893.
31. Matschke J, Lütgehetmann M, Hagel C, et al. Neuropathology of patients with COVID-19 in Germany: a post-mortem case series. Lancet Neurol 2020; 19(11):919–29.
32. Cunningham C. Systemic inflammation and delirium: important co-factors in the progression of dementia. Biochem Soc Trans 2011;39(4):945–53.
33. Deng J, Zhou F, Hou W, et al. The prevalence of depression, anxiety, and sleep disturbances in COVID-19 patients: a meta-analysis. Ann N Y Acad Sci 2021; 1486(1):90–111.
34. Perlis RH, Ognyanova K, Santillana M, et al. Association of Acute Symptoms of COVID-19 and Symptoms of Depression in Adults. JAMA Netw Open 2021;4(3): e213223.
35. Lee C-H, Giuliani F. The Role of Inflammation in Depression and Fatigue. Front Immunol 2019;10:1696. https://doi.org/10.3389/fimmu.2019.01696.
36. Miller AH, Raison CL. The role of inflammation in depression: from evolutionary imperative to modern treatment target. Nat Rev Immunol 2016;16(1):22–34.
37. Nerurkar L, Siebert S, McInnes IB, et al. Rheumatoid arthritis and depression: an inflammatory perspective. Lancet Psychiatry 2019;6(2):164–73.
38. Machado MO, Oriolo G, Bortolato B, et al. Biological mechanisms of depression following treatment with interferon for chronic hepatitis C: A critical systematic review. J Affect Disord 2017;209:235–45.

39. Gennaro MM, Mariagrazia P, De Lorenzo R, et al. Persistent psychopathology and neurocognitive impairment in COVID-19 survivors: effect of inflammatory biomarkers at three-month follow-up. Brain Behav Immun 2021. https://doi.org/10.1016/j.bbi.2021.02.021.
40. Serrano García A, Montánchez Mateo J, Franch Pato CM, et al. Interleukin 6 and depression in patients affected by Covid-19. Med Clínica Engl Ed 2021. https://doi.org/10.1016/j.medcle.2020.11.013.
41. Lenzi GL, Altieri M, Maestrini I. Post-stroke depression. Rev Neurol (Paris) 2008; 164(10):837–40.
42. Parsons N, Outsikas A, Parish A, et al. Modelling the Anatomic Distribution of Neurologic Events in Patients with COVID-19: A Systematic Review of MRI Findings. AJNR Am J Neuroradiol 2021. https://doi.org/10.3174/ajnr.A7113.
43. Herrmann LL, Le Masurier M, Ebmeier KP. White matter hyperintensities in late life depression: a systematic review. J Neurol Neurosurg Psychiatry 2007;79(6): 619–24.
44. The WHO Rapid Evidence Appraisal for COVID-19, Therapies (REACT) Working Group, Sterne JAC, Murthy S, et al. Association Between Administration of Systemic Corticosteroids and Mortality Among Critically Ill Patients With COVID-19: A Meta-analysis. JAMA 2020;324(13):1330.
45. Dubovsky AN, Arvikar S, Stern TA, et al. The Neuropsychiatric Complications of Glucocorticoid Use: Steroid Psychosis Revisited. Psychosomatics 2012;53(2): 103–15.
46. Pariante CM, Lightman SL. The HPA axis in major depression: classical theories and new developments. Trends Neurosci 2008;31(9):464–8.
47. Datson NA, Morsink MC, Meijer OC, et al. Central corticosteroid actions: Search for gene targets. Eur J Pharmacol 2008;583(2–3):272–89.
48. Iqbal Y, Al Abdulla MA, Albrahim S, et al. Psychiatric presentation of patients with acute SARS-CoV-2 infection: a retrospective review of 50 consecutive patients seen by a consultation-liaison psychiatry team. BJPsych Open 2020; 6(5):e109.
49. Butler M, Delvi A, Mujic F, et al. Reduced Activity in an Inpatient Liaison Psychiatry Service During the First Wave of the COVID-19 Pandemic: Comparison With 2019 Data and Characterization of the SARS-CoV-2 Positive Cohort. Front Psychiatry 2021;12:619550.
50. Kępińska AP, Iyegbe CO, Vernon AC, et al. Schizophrenia and Influenza at the Centenary of the 1918-1919 Spanish Influenza Pandemic: Mechanisms of Psychosis Risk. Front Psychiatry 2020;11:72.
51. Yolken RH, Torrey EF. Are some cases of psychosis caused by microbial agents? A review of the evidence. Mol Psychiatry 2008;13(5):470–9.
52. Taquet M, Geddes JR, Husain M, et al. 6-month neurological and psychiatric outcomes in 236 379 survivors of COVID-19: a retrospective cohort study using electronic health records. Lancet Psychiatry 2021;8(5):416–27.
53. Najjar S, Steiner J, Najjar A, et al. A clinical approach to new-onset psychosis associated with immune dysregulation: the concept of autoimmune psychosis. J Neuroinflammation 2018;15(1):40.
54. Khandaker GM, Zimbron J, Dalman C, et al. Childhood infection and adult schizophrenia: A meta-analysis of population-based studies. Schizophr Res 2012;139(1–3):161–8.
55. Khandaker GM, Zimbron J, Lewis G, et al. Prenatal maternal infection, neurodevelopment and adult schizophrenia: a systematic review of population-based studies. Psychol Med 2013;43(2):239–57.

56. Pollak TA, Lennox BR, Müller S, et al. Autoimmune psychosis: an international consensus on an approach to the diagnosis and management of psychosis of suspected autoimmune origin. Lancet Psychiatry 2020;7(1):93–108.
57. Ellul MA, Benjamin L, Singh B, et al. Neurological associations of COVID-19. Lancet Neurol 2020;19(9):767–83.
58. McCuddy M, Kelkar P, Zhao Y, et al. Acute Demyelinating Encephalomyelitis (ADEM) in COVID-19 Infection: A Case Series. Neurology 2020. https://doi.org/10.1101/2020.07.15.20126730.
59. Pilotto A, Masciocchi S, Volonghi I, et al. Clinical Presentation and Outcomes of Severe Acute Respiratory Syndrome Coronavirus 2–Related Encephalitis: The ENCOVID Multicenter Study. J Infect Dis 2021;223(1):28–37.
60. Franke C, Ferse C, Kreye J, et al. High frequency of cerebrospinal fluid autoantibodies in COVID-19 patients with neurological symptoms. Brain Behav Immun 2021;93:415–9.
61. Kreye J, Reincke SM, Prüss H. Do cross-reactive antibodies cause neuropathology in COVID-19? Nat Rev Immunol 2020;20(11):645–6.
62. Cao A, Rohaut B, Le Guennec L, et al. Severe COVID-19-related encephalitis can respond to immunotherapy. Brain 2020;2. https://doi.org/10.1093/brain/awaa337. awaa337.
63. Vogrig A, Gigli GL, Bnà C, et al. Stroke in patients with COVID-19: Clinical and neuroimaging characteristics. Neurosci Lett 2021;743:135564.
64. Ferro JM, Caeiro L, Figueira ML. Neuropsychiatric sequelae of stroke. Nat Rev Neurol 2016;12(5):269–80.
65. Jensen-Kondering U, Neumann A, Margraf NG, et al. Cerebral Imaging in Patients with COVID-19 and Neurological Symptoms: First Experience from two University Hospitals in Northern Germany. ROFO Fortschr Geb Rontgenstr Nuklearmed 2020. https://doi.org/10.1055/a-1265-7209.
66. Edlow BL, Takahashi E, Wu O, et al. Neuroanatomic connectivity of the human ascending arousal system critical to consciousness and its disorders. J Neuropathol Exp Neurol 2012;71(6):531–46.
67. Kremer S, Lersy F, Anheim M, et al. Neurologic and neuroimaging findings in patients with COVID-19: A retrospective multicenter study. Neurology 2020;95(13):e1868–82.
68. Goshua G, Pine AB, Meizlish ML, et al. Endotheliopathy in COVID-19-associated coagulopathy: evidence from a single-centre, cross-sectional study. Lancet Haematol 2020;7(8):e575–82.
69. Meinhardt J, Radke J, Dittmayer C, et al. Olfactory transmucosal SARS-CoV-2 invasion as a port of central nervous system entry in individuals with COVID-19. Nat Neurosci 2021;24(2):168–75.
70. Mukerji SS, Solomon IH. What can we learn from brain autopsies in COVID-19? Neurosci Lett 2021;742:135528.
71. Lee M-H, Perl DP, Nair G, et al. Microvascular Injury in the Brains of Patients with Covid-19. N Engl J Med 2021;384(5):481–3.
72. Smith M, Meyfroidt G. Critical illness: the brain is always in the line of fire. Intensive Care Med 2017;43(6):870–3.
73. Baker HA, Safavynia SA, Evered LA. The ‘third wave’: impending cognitive and functional decline in COVID-19 survivors. Br J Anaesth 2021;126(1):44–7.
74. Conklin J, Frosch MP, Mukerji SS, et al. Susceptibility-weighted imaging reveals cerebral microvascular injury in severe COVID-19. J Neurol Sci 2021;421:117308.

75. Fanou EM, Coutinho JM, Shannon P, et al. Critical Illness-Associated Cerebral Microbleeds. Stroke 2017;48(4):1085–7.
76. Werring DJ, Frazer DW, Coward LJ, et al. Cognitive dysfunction in patients with cerebral microbleeds on T2*-weighted gradient-echo MRI. Brain J Neurol 2004; 127(Pt 10):2265–75.
77. Badenoch JB, Rengasamy ER, Watson CJ, et al. Persistent Neuropsychiatric Symptoms after COVID-19: A Systematic Review and Meta-Analysis. Psychiatry Clin Psychol 2021. https://doi.org/10.1101/2021.04.30.21256413.
78. Ladds E, Rushforth A, Wieringa S, et al. Persistent symptoms after Covid-19: qualitative study of 114 “long Covid” patients and draft quality principles for services. BMC Health Serv Res 2020;20(1):1144.
79. Davis HE, Assaf GS, McCorkell L, et al. Characterizing long COVID in an international cohort: 7 months of symptoms and their impact. Eclinicalmedicine 2021;101019. https://doi.org/10.1016/j.eclinm.2021.101019.
80. Nalbandian A, Sehgal K, Gupta A, et al. Post-acute COVID-19 syndrome. Nat Med 2021;27(4):601–15.
81. Taboada M, Cariñena A, Moreno E, et al. Post-COVID-19 functional status six-months after hospitalization. J Infect 2021;82(4):e31–3.
82. Myers EA, Smith DA, Allen SR, et al. Post-ICU syndrome: Rescuing the undiagnosed. J Am Acad Physician Assist 2016;29(4):34–7.
83. García-Abellán J, Padilla S, Fernández-González M, et al. Antibody Response to SARS-CoV-2 is Associated with Long-term Clinical Outcome in Patients with COVID-19: a Longitudinal Study. J Clin Immunol 2021. https://doi.org/10.1007/s10875-021-01083-7.
84. Mandal S, Barnett J, Brill SE, et al. ‘Long-COVID’: a cross-sectional study of persisting symptoms, biomarker and imaging abnormalities following hospitalisation for COVID-19. Thorax 2021;76(4):396–8.
85. Doykov I, Hällqvist J, Gilmour KC, et al. ‘The long tail of Covid-19’ - The detection of a prolonged inflammatory response after a SARS-CoV-2 infection in asymptomatic and mildly affected patients. F1000Research. 2021;9:1349.
86. Phetsouphanh C, Darley D, Howe A, et al. Immunological dysfunction persists for 8 Months following initial mild-moderate SARS-CoV-2 infection. Infectious Diseases (except HIV/AIDS); 2021. https://doi.org/10.1101/2021.06.01.21257759.
87. Zheng S, Fan J, Yu F, et al. Viral load dynamics and disease severity in patients infected with SARS-CoV-2 in Zhejiang province, China, January-March 2020: retrospective cohort study. BMJ 2020;m1443. https://doi.org/10.1136/bmj.m1443.
88. Altmann DM, Boyton RJ. Decoding the unknowns in long covid. BMJ 2021;4:n132. https://doi.org/10.1136/bmj.n132.
89. Dani M, Dirksen A, Taraborrelli P, et al. Autonomic dysfunction in ‘long COVID’: rationale, physiology and management strategies. Clin Med 2021;21(1):e63–7.
90. Ferrucci R, Dini M, Groppo E, et al. Long-Lasting Cognitive Abnormalities after COVID-19. Brain Sci 2021;11(2):235.
91. Colbenson GA, Johnson A, Wilson ME. Post-intensive care syndrome: impact, prevention, and management. Breathe 2019;15(2):98–101.
92. Del Brutto OH, Wu S, Mera RM, et al. Cognitive decline among individuals with history of mild symptomatic SARS-CoV-2 infection: A longitudinal prospective study nested to a population cohort. Eur J Neurol 2021. https://doi.org/10.1111/ene.14775.

93. Alemanno F, Houdayer E, Parma A, et al. COVID-19 cognitive deficits after respiratory assistance in the subacute phase: a COVID-rehabilitation unit experience. PLoS One 2021;16(2):e0246590.
94. O'Keeffe S, Lavan J. The Prognostic Significance of Delirium in Older Hospital Patients. J Am Geriatr Soc 1997;45(2):174–8.
95. Hossmann KA. The hypoxic brain. Insights from ischemia research. Adv Exp Med Biol 1999;474:155–69.
96. Qin Y, Wu J, Chen T, et al. Long-term micro-structure and cerebral blood flow changes in patients recovered from COVID-19 without neurological manifestations. J Clin Invest 2021;25. https://doi.org/10.1172/JCI147329.
97. Guedj E, Campion JY, Dudouet P, et al. 18F-FDG brain PET hypometabolism in patients with long COVID. Eur J Nucl Med Mol Imaging 2021;26. https://doi.org/10.1007/s00259-021-05215-4.
98. Boldrini M, Canoll PD, Klein RS. How COVID-19 Affects the Brain. JAMA Psychiatry 2021. https://doi.org/10.1001/jamapsychiatry.2021.0500.
99. McWhirter L, Ritchie C, Stone J, et al. Functional cognitive disorders: a systematic review. Lancet Psychiatry 2020. https://doi.org/10.1016/S2215-0366(19)30405-5.
100. Teodoro T, Edwards MJ, Isaacs JD. A unifying theory for cognitive abnormalities in functional neurological disorders, fibromyalgia and chronic fatigue syndrome: systematic review. J Neurol Neurosurg Psychiatry 2018;89(12):1308–19.
101. Smith V, Seo D, Warty R, et al. Maternal and neonatal outcomes associated with COVID-19 infection: A systematic review. PLoS One 2020;15(6):e0234187.
102. Cavalcante MB, de Melo Bezerra Cavalcante CT, Sarno M, et al. Maternal immune responses and obstetrical outcomes of pregnant women with COVID-19 and possible health risks of offspring. J Reprod Immunol 2021;143:103250. https://doi.org/10.1016/j.jri.2020.103250.
103. Zimmer A, Youngblood A, Adnane A, et al. Prenatal exposure to viral infection and neuropsychiatric disorders in offspring: A review of the literature and recommendations for the COVID-19 pandemic. Brain Behav Immun 2021;91:756–70.
104. Atladóttir HÓ, Thorsen P, Østergaard L, et al. Maternal Infection Requiring Hospitalization During Pregnancy and Autism Spectrum Disorders. J Autism Dev Disord 2010;40(12):1423–30.
105. Brown AS. Nonaffective Psychosis After Prenatal Exposure to Rubella. Am J Psychiatry 2000;157(3):438–43.
106. Buka SL. Maternal Infections and Subsequent Psychosis Among Offspring. Arch Gen Psychiatry 2001;58(11):1032–7.
107. Choi GB, Yim YS, Wong H, et al. The maternal interleukin-17a pathway in mice promotes autism-like phenotypes in offspring. Science 2016;351(6276):933–9.
108. Khashan AS, Abel KM, McNamee R, et al. Higher Risk of Offspring Schizophrenia Following Antenatal Maternal Exposure to Severe Adverse Life Events. Arch Gen Psychiatry 2008;65(2):146.
109. Barisic A. Conceived in the covid-19 crisis: impact of maternal stress and anxiety on fetal neurobehavioral development. J Psychosom Obstet Gynaecol 2020;(bu1, 8308648):1. https://doi.org/10.1080/0167482X.2020.1755838.

Inpatient Psychiatry During COVID-19: A Systems Perspective

Joshua Berezin, MD, MS[a], Flavio Casoy, MD[b,1], Matthew D. Erlich, MD[a], Yamilette Hernandez, BS[b,1], Thomas E. Smith, MD[b,*]

KEYWORDS

• COVID-19 • Inpatient psychiatry • Health care system • Telehealth
• Infection control

KEY POINTS

- A nonuniform pandemic affecting a nonuniform health care system makes it challenging for mental health providers to adapt to the rapidly shifting demands of the COVID-19 pandemic.
- Public and not-for-profit community health care settings and academic medical centers coordinated across systems to expand medical capacity and preserve space for acute psychiatric treatment.
- Regulations were extensively relaxed to allow hospitals and other providers to rapidly adapt to the COVID-19 pandemic.
- Use of telehealth increased in acute inpatient programs during the COVID-19 pandemic.

INTRODUCTION

Mirroring the public mental health system as a whole, the United States lacks a uniform approach to inpatient psychiatric care. Instead, inpatient care reflects a miscellany of tradition, laws, regulations, resource availability, and common practices. Inpatient practices vary not just between states but across municipalities and hospital systems, where different inpatient units can have widely disparate cultures, values, and outcomes.

Even if COVID-19 had affected the United States uniformly, these differences would have bred disparate responses. But the initial stage of the COVID-19 pandemic was anything but uniform.[1] Its effects came in waves that varied in time, place, and intensity. An ever-evolving pandemic with discordant results colliding with a nonuniform,

[a] New York State Office of Mental Health, 330 Fifth Avenue – 9th Floor, New York, NY 10001, USA; [b] New York State Office of Mental Health
[1] Present address: 1051 Riverside Drive, Unit 100, New York, NY 10032.
* Corresponding author. 1051 Riverside Drive, Unit 100, New York, NY 10032.
E-mail address: thomas.smith@nyspi.columbia.edu

Psychiatr Clin N Am 45 (2022) 45–55
https://doi.org/10.1016/j.psc.2021.11.002
psych.theclinics.com

heterogenous mental health system makes it challenging to describe a unified view of how the inpatient psychiatric system responded to COVID-19.

Numerous reports have described how individual hospitals responded to the pandemic, but few describe how these changes played out across a system of care. In this report the authors use New York State (NYS), and New York City (NYC) in particular, as a case study in how an inpatient psychiatry system of care reacted and adjusted to COVID-19. NYS has a robust inpatient psychiatric system, and NYC was one of the epicenters of the first COVID-19 outbreak in the Spring of 2020. The NYS response included a range of coordinated planning and regulatory efforts to preserve and create medical and intensive care unit (ICU) capacity; maintain access to acute psychiatric services; and redefine inpatient psychiatric care.

BACKGROUND: ACUTE PSYCHIATRIC SERVICES IN THE NEW YORK CITY METROPOLITAN AREA

In 2018, NYS had an estimated 7467 adult inpatient psychiatric beds (47.8/100,000 adults) and 1606 child and adolescent beds (38.2/100,000 children).[2] At that time NYC had an estimated 3763 adult beds (55.2/100,000 adults) and 468 child and adolescent beds (26.0/100,000 children). Most of these beds were in 36 NYC public or nonprofit community hospitals and are referred to here as "acute" beds or units to distinguish them from the State-run psychiatric hospitals described later. These community hospital units have an average length of stay of 1 to 2 weeks. Patients are typically admitted either from medical emergency rooms with varying degrees of dedicated psychiatric space or from 1 of 16 Comprehensive Psychiatric Emergency Programs. These are specifically designated settings with requirements for staffing, specialized resources, and the legal authority to admit people for 72-hour observation.

Seven NYS Office of Mental Health (OMH) State-operated adult, civil Psychiatric Centers (PCs) serve more than 12 million residents of the greater NYC metropolitan area, 1 in each of the 5 boroughs of NYC and 2 in surrounding suburban counties. These PCs rarely take admissions directly from the community; instead, they are centers of intermediate care and primarily serve people with persistent severe symptoms that cannot be adequately addressed in the acute care system and thus require further specialized treatment. In contrast to the relatively brief length of stay at the acute care hospitals, the average length of stay in these PCs varies from 6 to 12 months.

INITIAL RESPONSE TO THE COVID-19 SPRING 2020 SURGE IN NEW YORK: PRESERVING MEDICAL CAPACITY

COVID-19 was first identified in Wuhan, Hubei Province, China at the end of 2019. By March 11, 2020, the World Health Organization declared COVID-19 a pandemic, as it spread across continental boundaries and began to affect every state in the United States.[3] New York State Governor Andrew Cuomo declared a state of emergency in response to COVID-19 on March 7, 2020. By March 22nd, the New York City area accounted for half of the cases in the United States and roughly 5% of cases globally.[4]

The initial days and weeks of the outbreak were chaotic and fluid, with rapidly mounting death tolls. It was unclear how long and severe the initial wave of infection would be, and there was real fear that hospitals would become overwhelmed by acutely ill patients with COVID-19 and run out of space, supplies, and staff.[5] In this context, the mounting priority for individual hospitals, and the system as a whole, was to create medical and ICU capacity. Governor Cuomo ordered elective surgeries to be canceled across the state on March 7, 2020[6] and furthermore required hospitals to maintain 30% ICU available capacity at all times.[7]

Hospitals responded by shifting space and staffing, which included repurposing of inpatient psychiatry services and staff. During the first wave of the pandemic, NYC acute care hospitals closed an estimated 20% of their inpatient psychiatric beds to accommodate the need for increased medical capacity.[8] Some of these units were converted from psychiatric to medical capacity, whereas others were used for ancillary purposes (supplies, operation centers, staff respite, and so forth) or held vacant in anticipation of further surges of patients presenting for intensive medical care.

Although there was no unified or centrally managed process for unit closures and reallocation of staff, there was significant coordination and cooperation across the system. Some large hospital systems apportioned closures based on medical demand, so that hospitals in COVID-19 hotspots could allocate more resources toward medical capacity, whereas other hospitals within their system maintained more of their psychiatric capacity and could take on the closed hospital's demand for psychiatric care. In one case, this coordination occurred across hospital systems when one hospital was forced to close all of its emergency and inpatient psychiatric capacity. Recognizing that a nearby hospital was likely to see increased demand for psychiatric services, the hospitals agreed to share staff during this unique and unprecedented situation.

The NYS OMH fostered cross-system collaboration in multiple ways. Although NYS OMH collected data on inpatient capacity and utilization before COVID-19, the reporting mechanisms were not designed to account for the rapidly changing situation during the outbreak. NYS OMH was in frequent contact with hospitals from across the city and NYC metropolitan area to quantify the extent of inpatient closures and changes. During the pandemic, NYS OMH hosted weekly calls with directors of inpatient psychiatric programs to discuss service needs and infection control procedures.

To relieve the pressure on the system, NYS OMH rapidly responded in the 7 adult, civil State-operated PCs that serve the New York City metropolitan area. One of these PCs had recently completed construction on a new inpatient building when the COVID-19 pandemic struck. This building was repurposed as a medical facility for patients with COVID-19, managed by a community hospital system, for the duration of the pandemic in NYS. None of the other PCs were equipped to provide medical or ICU capacity. They did, however, support the "decanting" of patients from the acute care system. Rather than adding bed capacity, per se, the PCs accomplished this by working with the outpatient system to increase the pace of appropriate discharges and by creating swing space in offline wards. Before COVID-19, acute care hospitals would apply directly to one of the state-operated PCs to transfer patients with refractory symptoms. During the spring 2020 COVID-19 surge, this process was centralized, simplified, and expedited. The centralization allowed the NYS OMH Central Office to review applications and match referrals to the next available bed across the PC system.

These adjustments allowed for timely collaboration with acute care hospitals, particularly the NYC public hospital system, which has psychiatric inpatient programs at 11 of its hospitals. The NYC public hospital system converted approximately 30% of its adult inpatient capacity, 40% of its child and adolescent capacity, and 100% of its detox units to COVID-19–related medical services.[8] During the initial course of the outbreak, NYS OMH and the NYC public hospital system collaborated to transfer an estimated 90 adult psychiatric inpatients from acute to state-operated hospitals. Across all NYC metropolitan area ("Downstate") acute hospitals, before COVID-19, approximately 35 to 45 adult individuals without a forensic legal status were accepted into inpatient units at civil, state-operated PCs each month. In March of 2020, this same population increased to 85 and further increased in April to 133. During the entire first wave of COVID-19 (March through end of May 2020), the state-operated PCs accepted 263 transfers from acute care hospitals and forensic settings, approximately double the number from the similar period in 2019.

MAINTAINING ACCESS TO ACUTE PSYCHIATRIC SERVICES

Although unit closures and transferring patients to PCs helped to create medical and ICU capacity across the system, most psychiatric inpatient beds remained available for admissions during COVID-19. Those remaining units made numerous adjustments to operating procedures to maintain staff and patient safety. Hospital psychiatric staff were likely especially concerned after hearing reports in the popular media of large outbreaks in psychiatric settings internationally.[9,10] NYS hospitals adopted various strategies to prevent similar outbreaks. Early in the pandemic, testing for the COVID-19 virus was limited.[11] One NYC hospital reported that during the initial COVID-19 outbreak, 9.9% of patients were COVID-19 positive at the time of admission, and 76.1% of those positive cases were either asymptomatic or unable to report symptoms due to psychiatric issues.[12] Some hospital systems created specific dedicated units for people who had confirmed or suspected COVID-19. These units allowed other hospitals in their system to isolate COVID-19 positive patients. For example, after outbreaks on both of their inpatient units, one hospital converted the unit with the larger outbreak into a COVID-19 positive unit and the other unit into a COVID-19 negative unit.[13] They used strict personal protective equipment (PPE) guidelines for staff and used videoconferencing for therapeutic interactions whenever possible (and for all family-patient interactions). Another community hospital psychiatric program developed a detailed algorithm for screening, testing, isolation, and infection control and also created a holding area for people awaiting test results and then admitted to either COVID-19 positive or negative units.[14] A community hospital in the Bronx similarly created a "Person Under Investigation" area along with a COVID-19 positive unit.[15] Similar to other hospitals, as testing became increasingly available, they described the progression from symptom-based testing to universal testing before admission.

Other hospitals created quarantine procedures within their units so that COVID-19 positive and negative patients did not mix. For example, one hospital's voluntary unit was able to provide individual rooms to all patients, whereas another unit in their system designated 2 communal rooms for COVID-19 positive patients. With these precautions in place, transmission of the COVID-19 virus in the hospital psychiatric programs was low (just 3% of total identified cases).[16]

All psychiatric programs grappled with maintaining infection control procedures with an acutely psychiatrically ill population. Communal meals, group activities, and visitation were all curtailed or modified, as programs tried to enforce masking and social distancing. One NYC community hospital implemented telepsychiatry on its COVID-19 positive inpatient unit.[17] Dispensing of medications, vital signs, laboratory draws, and routine checks remained in-person but tablets were provided to patients for meetings with the treatment team, virtual visits with family and friends in the community, and behavioral health–oriented apps. Another community hospital similarly created detailed infection control and programming protocols for its 35-bed COVID-19 positive unit and also distributed tablets to their patients.[18] The hospital psychiatric program admitted a total of 48 patients in April and May of 2020, 8 of whom were subsequently transferred for acute medical care; all staff working on the unit remained COVID-19 negative.

REDEFINING INPATIENT PSYCHIATRIC CARE

To further reduce pressure on community hospital acute psychiatric programs that were struggling to rapidly implement infection control protocols and, in many places, managing shortages of staff and PPE, NYS OMH relaxed regulatory standards for inpatient programs in late March 2020. These changes remained in effect throughout the spring of 2020.

To facilitate infection control protocols, programs were permitted to cancel therapeutic, rehabilitative, and recreational groups and allow patients to remain in their rooms throughout the day. Programs were also advised to consider plans in which nursing staff and one psychiatrist remained on-site to handle emergencies while the rest of the treatment team provided telehealth services. Because a federal and state public health emergency declaration was declared, documentation requirements were significantly relaxed, for example, the requirement was waived for written, multidisciplinary treatment plans. Instead of writing daily comprehensive progress notes, treatment teams were only required to write admission notes, discharge notes detailing course of treatment, and brief notes detailing clinically relevant events. Each patient was required to have at least one medical record notation per day, not one per treating professional.

Discharge planning requirements were adjusted to fit the reality of an outpatient system that was also rapidly adapting to the pandemic. Inpatient providers continued to attempt scheduling a discharge appointment within 7 days of discharge, but if an outpatient provider was not available or was unable to accommodate the patient, NYS OMH staff provided assistance locating available outpatient providers. In the event the outpatient treatment could not be located, inpatient teams were encouraged to provide a larger supply of medications and remain available to the patient for refills and other clinical emergencies pending engagement to ambulatory care. For higher risk patients, the inpatient team was asked to proactively remain in contact with the patient after discharge pending continuation of outpatient care. NYS OMH leveraged several Assertive Community Treatment teams to provide critical time intervention services to individuals who presented to psychiatric emergency departments to reduce the need for inpatient readmissions.

Regulations on the use of telehealth for psychiatric treatment were relaxed across multiple treatment settings, including inpatient care. These regulatory changes remained in effect through the duration of the declared State and Federal emergency periods. Telehealth evaluations were permitted for involuntary inpatient holds or assisted outpatient treatment; outside of the emergency period, these evaluations are required to be in-person. Rules requiring an in-person evaluation by a physician for seclusion or restraint orders were also relaxed to allow an in-person evaluation by a nurse practitioner or physician assistant with telephonic consultation with a physician. However, telehealth-only evaluations for seclusion or restraint orders were not permitted.

IMPACT OF COVID-19 SPRING 2020 SURGE ON NEW YORK STATE ACUTE PSYCHIATRIC SERVICE SYSTEM

Despite early capacity concerns, the NYS inpatient psychiatric system continued to serve individuals needing acute inpatient care during the initial COVID-19 wave. In addition to the measures described earlier, several factors helped the system remain functional. First, COVID-19 infections peaked the week of April 5, 2020, and COVID-19 hospitalizations began steadily decreasing by April 13, 2020.[19,20] The peaking of the pandemic precluded further psychiatric inpatient unit closures. Second, fewer people presented for acute psychiatric services during the height of the pandemic. Preliminary NYS Medicaid data suggest that in April of 2020, approximately 14,000 Medicaid enrollees received an inpatient or emergency department mental health service compared with 21,000 enrollees in April 2019. There were anecdotal reports that

Emergency Medical Service crews were reluctant to transport non-COVID-19–related emergencies to hospitals during this time. Furthermore, people with psychiatric issues (as the general population) likely wanted to avoid hospitals to limit their exposure to COVID-19. However, it is worth reiterating that COVID-19 was not evenly distributed across time, space, or racial and socioeconomic lines.[21] So although as a whole, the system remained intact, the situation at individual hospitals was difficult at times.[22]

As the spring COVID-19 surge abated in NYC, some inpatient capacity came back online, whereas other units remained closed for various reasons. Some hospitals had converted their psychiatric units into full-scale medical units and needed to rerenovate to make the unit safe for psychiatric patients again. Other units were held offline in the event of another surge or remained closed due to staffing issues. When the second surge hit in October of 2020, the system responded in a similar but attenuated fashion. Some units closed again to reallocate staff to other parts of the hospital. Because of operations from the initial surge that remained in place through the winter of 2020, OMH's state-operated PCs did not need to expand capacity, and more widespread testing allowed for easier infection control protocols than in the spring.

COVID-19S EFFECT ON INPATIENT CARE BEYOND NEW YORK CITY

As the pandemic progressed, the popular press reported in March 2020 on outbreaks at psychiatric facilities first in Washington State.[23] By April, NBC News was reporting "more than 1450 COVID-19 cases at state mental health facilities in 23 states and Washington, D.C."[24] Another media report highlighted hospital and governmental bureaucracy, lack of testing and PPE, a focus on reimbursement rather than treatment, and a lack of guidelines as drivers of outbreaks on psychiatric inpatient units.[25]

There was, however, an informal network of providers that shared strategies over social media on how to prevent and control outbreaks on inpatient psychiatric units.[26] These strategies focused on testing, admission protocols, social distancing, limitations on groups, visitation restrictions, and infection control. Initial ideas about best practices also came out of the international community.[27–29] By midsummer more guidelines were being published in academic journals. Li, for example, suggested strategies related to screening, PPE, visitor policies, staffing, use of telepsychiatry, and adjustments to programming.[30]

As of 2021, published reports describing the impact of the COVID-19 pandemic on hospital psychiatric inpatient care largely focused on how individual hospitals and inpatient units responded. Less attention has been paid to the type of collaborations and interactions that occurred across networks and systems of behavioral health care. One exception is Angelino and colleagues' description of the development of a COVID-19–dedicated unit that served as a hub for the entire state of Maryland.[31]

On the individual hospital level, the strategies used were largely consistent with those adopted by NYC hospitals. COVID-19–dedicated units were established in Massachusetts,[32] Washington State,[33] Pennsylvania,[34] and Connecticut.[35] Other units managed outbreaks by closing to new admissions and initiating mitigation efforts.[36] As in NYC, telepsychiatry became a crucial tool for maintaining operations on some inpatient units. Kalin and colleagues, for example, describe a blended model where rounding and team meetings were completed via telepsychiatry, physicians were available for specific situations such as physical examinations, and nurses led behavioral emergency responses with physicians available via video.[37] Similarly, Heyman-Kantor and colleagues described how nurses remained in-person with physicians generally performing remote evaluations but having at least one physician available for in-person evaluation when necessary.[38] Krass and colleagues described a mix of telepsychiatry for therapy and evaluation with in-person programming on a COVID-19 positive adolescent unit.[34] Reflecting on the use of telepsychiatry on inpatient units, Morris and Hirschtritt suggest that telepsychiatry could help in future outbreaks with staffing, safety (in terms of both infection control and violence reduction), maintaining connections in the community, and developing the capacity for immediate consultation during crises.[39]

Statistics reported from across the United States also generally mirrored those reported in NYC. Various hospitals reported decreased census in line with most reports from NYS.[35,40] Some hospitals that treated COVID-19 positive patients on psychiatric inpatient units reported that they did not have to transfer patients to medical units due to COVID-19 symptoms.[34,35] Similar to NYC, rates of positive tests were relatively low, with Li and colleagues, for example, reporting 5.9% positive test rate among all tests and a 10.2% positive rate among people suspected of having COVID-19.[35] One outbreak at a state psychiatric hospital in the South provided a cautionary tale; despite following CDC guidelines, 78% (51/70) of test results in a building with an outbreak were positive; the investigators urged mask wearing and universal testing of staff to prevent similar outbreaks in other hospitals.[41]

OTHER ISSUES SURROUNDING INPATIENT PSYCHIATRY DURING COVID-19

COVID-19 brought to the fore ethical issues in all aspects of medicine, and psychiatric inpatient care was no exception. Barnett noted that the risk that a patient involuntarily committed to a psychiatric unit could infect others, or become infected themselves, added an additional level of complexity to an already fraught ethical framework around involuntary commitment.[42] Similarly, Bojdani and colleagues encouraged hospital providers to disclose this potential additional risk to patients before admission as part of a risks and benefits discussion.[32] Other investigators highlighted the ethical issues involved with capacity to refuse COVID-19 testing or appropriate monitoring[43] and how to enforce infection control policies as having patients wear masks and stay in their rooms.[44,45]

COVID-19 highlighted the need to think of inpatient psychiatry in the context of the full array of community services. Various investigators pointed out that disposition became very challenging during COVID-19 due to limitations in outpatient and residential services brought about by the pandemic.[30,32] In particular, Millard and colleagues discuss challenges with discharge related both to delays in testing and the investigators' impression that congregate settings were being more stringent than CDC guidelines suggested.[46]

SUMMARY

The COVID-19 pandemic provided valuable lessons on how inpatient psychiatric systems of care can respond to public health emergencies. Although it may seem trivial, having a convening entity that maintains contacts with each hospital within a region is a key step that can be accomplished during nonemergent times. Centralization allows for system-wide planning instead of each hospital reacting on an individual basis; this is not specific to COVID-19; for example, if a hospital decides to change its inpatient capacity, that decision has ripple effects across the community. However, the surrounding hospitals may be part of different hospital systems, making it difficult to formulate a plan that is coherent for the entire community. During COVID-19 there was more cooperation than usual, but even then, decisions were largely undertaken within rather than among hospital systems. Developing a better system to track hospital capacity and demand is not only critical in a public health emergency but would improve the overall resiliency and adaptability of the mental health system. Improved coordination would also facilitate dissemination of information and clinical best practices that could save lives during an emergency. The response to COVID-19 also demonstrated that oversight agencies can act rapidly to provide regulatory relief that preserves providers' fiscal viability and allows them to adapt to ever-changing and complex demands of a pandemic or other similar emergency.

Acute psychiatric services in NYS and nationally are typically not closely linked to outpatient and residential services. From a systems perspective, when inpatient beds close, the logical next step is to ensure that resources in the community are sufficient to provide for the needs that were previously met with inpatient hospitalization; this suggests a shifting of resources from inpatient to outpatient settings. The pandemic provided a condensed lesson in some of the difficulties of achieving that type of coordination in the current psychiatric care system. During the height of the pandemic, there were efforts to ease access to high-intensity outpatient services and housing settings. But those efforts required coordination across multiple government and nonprofit agencies, slowing down any progress. Moreover, NYS had the advantage of having a very large state-operated, mental health system with considerable capacity that could absorb patients from community hospitals. A more integrated system could allow for more nimble and creative approaches.

Finally, the details of what actually happens on inpatient units also changed during the pandemic. Some of these changes, as limitations in group therapy, seem countertherapeutic and should not persist in a postpandemic world. Others, as the wider implementation of telepsychiatry, have potential benefits and drawbacks that need to be further evaluated.

COVID-19 had profound impacts on every level of inpatient psychiatry: patients, providers, units, hospitals, systems of care, and society as a whole. It behooves us to take heed of the lessons learned from the pandemic and to answer the myriad clinical, ethical, and systems questions that it raised. Doing so will help during the next emergency but should also allow us to design a more rational, effective, and compassionate system of care.

CONFLICT OF INTEREST

None reported.

REFERENCES

1. Yong E. America's patchwork pandemic is fraying even further. The Atlantic; 2020. Available at: https://www.theatlantic.com/health/archive/2020/05/patchwork-pandemic-states-reopening-inequalities/611866/. Accessed July 2, 2021.
2. County OMH. Capacity and utilization data book calendar years 2017-2018 2019. Available at: https://omh.ny.gov/omhweb/special-projects/dsrip/docs/county_utilization_data_book.pdf. Accessed July 2, 2021.
3. Cucinotta D, Vanelli M. WHO declares COVID-19 a pandemic. Acta Biomed 2020;91(1):157–60.
4. McKinley J. New York City region is now an epicenter of the coronavirus pandemic. The New York Times. Available at: https://www.nytimes.com/2020/03/22/nyregion/Coronavirus-new-York-epicenter.html. Accessed July 2, 2021.
5. Brian M, Goldstein J, Rothfeld M, et al. 'Deluge' of cases begins hitting hospitals. The New York Times. Available at: https://www.nytimes.com/2020/03/20/nyregion/ny-coronavirus-hospitals.html. Accessed July 2, 2021.

6. Executive Order 202.10: Continuing temporary suspension and modification of laws relating to the disaster emergency. In: State NY, editor. 2020.
7. Amid Ongoing COVID-19 Pandemic. Governor cuomo outlines additional guidelines for when regions can re-open. 2020. Available at: https://www.governor.ny.gov/news/amid-ongoing-covid-19-pandemic-governor-cuomo-outlines-additional-guidelines-when-regions-can. Accessed July 2, 2021.
8. Smith T, Sullivan A, Druss B. Redesigning public mental health systems post-COVID-19. Psychiatr Serv 2021;72(5):602–5.
9. Kim M. 'It was a medical disaster': How a South Korean psychiatric ward became a 'medical disaster' when coronavirus hit. Washington Post. Available at: https://www.washingtonpost.com/world/asia_pacific/how-a-south-korean-psychiatric-ward-became-a-medical-disaster-when-coronavirus-hit/2020/02/29/fe8f6e40-5897-11ea-8efd-0f904bdd8057_story.html. Accessed 06/23/2021.
10. Xiang YT, Zhao YJ, Liu ZH, et al. The COVID-19 outbreak and psychiatric hospitals in China: managing challenges through mental health service reform. Int J Biol Sci 2020;16(10):1741–4.
11. Andrews MNY. Leads the nation in COVID-19 tests, but testing Still Doesn't Meet demand. Kaiser Health News. Available at: https://khn.org/news/n-y-leads-the-nation-in-covid-19-tests-but-the-effort-still-lags-behind-demand/. Accessed July 2, 2021.
12. Brody BD, Shi Z, Shaffer C, et al. COVID-19 infection rates in patients referred for psychiatric admission during a regional surge: The case for universal testing. Psychiatry Res 2021;298:113833.
13. Spitzer Sverd S, Gardner LE, Cabassa JA, et al. A Bronx tale: Exposure, containment and care on inpatient psychiatry units during COVID-19. Gen Hosp Psychiatry 2021;69:121–3.
14. Brody BD, Parish SJ, Kanellopoulos D, et al. A COVID-19 testing and triage algorithm for psychiatric units: One hospital's response to the New York region's pandemic. Psychiatry Res 2020;291:113244.
15. Sarcevic N, Popiel M. Maintaining a Bronx inpatient psychiatry service at full capacity during the COVID-19 pandemic. Perspect Psychiatr Care 2021. https://doi.org/10.1111/ppc.12751.
16. Zhang E, LeQuesne E, Fichtel K, et al. In-patient psychiatry management of COVID-19: rates of asymptomatic infection and on-unit transmission. BJPsych Open 2020;6(5):e99. https://doi.org/10.1192/bjo.2020.86.
17. Kanellopoulos D, Bueno Castellano C, McGlynn L, et al. Implementation of telehealth services for inpatient psychiatric Covid-19 positive patients: A blueprint for adapting the milieu. Gen Hosp Psychiatry 2021;68:113–4.
18. Mahgoub N, Agarkar S, Radosta M, et al. Inpatient psychiatry unit devoted to COVID-19 patients. Compr Psychiatry 2021;107:152237.
19. Thompson CN, Baumgartner J, Pichardo C, et al. COVID-19 Outbreak - New York City, February 29-June 1, 2020. MMWR Morb Mortal Wkly Rep 2020;69(46):1725–9.
20. Forward NY. Daily Hospitalization Summary by Region. Available at: https://forward.ny.gov/daily-hospitalization-summary-region. Accessed July 2, 2021.
21. Renelus BD, Khoury NC, Chandrasekaran K, et al. Racial Disparities in COVID-19 Hospitalization and In-hospital Mortality at the Height of the New York City Pandemic. J Racial Ethn Health Disparities 2020.
22. Dwyer J. One hospital was Besieged by the virus. Nearby was 'Plenty of space.'. The New York Times. May 14. Available at: https://www.nytimes.com/2020/05/14/nyregion/coronavirus-ny-hospitals.html. Accessed July 2, 2021.

23. Bellisle M. More than a dozen COVID-19 cases at psychiatric hospital. Associated Press. Available at: https://apnews.com/article/08d134a821beed752103666b22c34132. Accessed July 2, 2021.
24. Ramgopal K. Coronavirus in a psychiatric hospital: 'It's the worst of all worlds'. NBC News. Available at: https://www.nbcnews.com/health/mental-health/coronavirus-psychiatric-hospital-it-s-worst-all-worlds-n1184266. Accessed July 2, 2021.
25. Gessen M. Why psychiatric Wards are uniquely Vulnerable to the Coronavirus. The New Yorker; 2020. Available at: https://www.newyorker.com/news/news-desk/why-psychiatric-wards-are-uniquely-vulnerable-to-the-coronavirus. Accessed July 2, 2021.
26. Barnett B, Esper F, Foster CB. Keeping the wolf at bay: Infection prevention and control measures for inpatient psychiatric facilities in the time of COVID-19. Gen Hosp Psychiatry 2020;66:51–3.
27. D'Agostino A, Demartini B, Cavallotti S, et al. Mental health services in Italy during the COVID-19 outbreak. Lancet Psychiatry 2020;7(5):385–7.
28. Starace F, Ferrara M. COVID-19 disease emergency operational instructions for Mental Health Departments issued by the Italian Society of Epidemiological Psychiatry. Epidemiol Psychiatr Sci 2020;31:29–e116.
29. Fagiolini A, Cuomo A, Frank E. COVID-19 diary from a psychiatry department in Italy. J Clin Psychiatry 2020;81(3). https://doi.org/10.4088/JCP.20com13357.
30. Li L. Challenges and priorities in responding to COVID-19 in inpatient psychiatry. Psychiatr Serv 2020;71(6):624–6.
31. Angelino AF, Lyketsos CG, Ahmed MS, et al. Design and implementation of a regional inpatient psychiatry unit for patients who are positive for asymptomatic SARS-CoV-2. Psychosomatics 2020;61(6):662–71.
32. Bojdani E, Rajagopalan A, Chen A, et al. COVID-19 pandemic: impact on psychiatric care in the United States. Psychiatry Res 2020;289:113069.
33. Constantino-Shor C, Rani G, Olin S, et al. Containment of a COVID-19 outbreak in an inpatient geriatric psychiatry unit. J Am Psychiatr Nurses Assoc 2021;27(1):77–82.
34. Krass P, Zimbrick-Rogers C, Iheagwara C, et al. COVID-19 outbreak among adolescents at an inpatient behavioral health hospital. J Adolesc Health 2020;67(4):612–4.
35. Li L, Roberts SC, Kulp W, et al. Epidemiology, infection prevention, testing data, and clinical outcomes of covid-19 on five inpatient psychiatric units in a large academic medical center. Psychiatry Res 2021;298:113776.
36. McGloin JM, Asokaraj N, Feeser B, et al. Coronavirus disease 2019 (COVID-19) outbreak on an inpatient psychiatry unit: mitigation and prevention. Infect Control Hosp Epidemiol 2021;1–2. https://doi.org/10.1017/ice.2021.233.
37. Kalin ML, Garlow SJ, Thertus K, et al. Rapid implementation of telehealth in hospital psychiatry in response to COVID-19. Am J Psychiatry 2020;177(7):636–7.
38. Heyman-Kantor R, Hardy N, Corcoran AR. Patient perspectives on telepsychiatry on the inpatient psychiatric unit during the COVID-19 pandemic. J Patient Exp 2020;7(5):677–9.
39. Morris NP, Hirschtritt ME. Telepsychiatry, hospitals, and the COVID-19 pandemic. Psychiatr Serv 2020;71(12):1309–12.
40. Ugueto AM, Zeni CP. Patterns of youth inpatient psychiatric admissions before and after the onset of the covid-19 pandemic. J Am Acad Child Adolesc Psychiatry 2021;60(7):796–8.

41. Thompson JW Jr, Mikolajewski AJ, Kissinger P, et al. An epidemiologic study of COVID-19 patients in a state psychiatric hospital: high penetrance with early CDC guidelines. Psychiatr Serv 2020;71(12):1285–7.
42. Barnett B. Meditations on involuntary civil commitment amid a pandemic. Psychiatr Serv 2020;71(9):979–80.
43. Fahed M, Barron GC, Steffens DC. Ethical and logistical considerations of caring for older adults on inpatient psychiatry during the COVID-19 pandemic. Am J Geriatr Psychiatry 2020;28(8):829–34.
44. Russ MJ, Sisti D, Wilner PJ. When patients refuse COVID-19 testing, quarantine, and social distancing in inpatient psychiatry: clinical and ethical challenges. J Med Ethics 2020;46(9):579–80.
45. London S. COVID-19, autonomy, and the inpatient psychiatric unit. Acad Psychiatry 2020;44(6):671–2.
46. Millard H, Wilson C, Fortunati F, et al. COVID-19 psychiatric patients: impact of variability in testing on length of hospital stay and disposition back to congregate care settings. Psychiatry Res 2020;292:113324.

Transformation of Outpatient Psychiatry

Manu S. Sharma, MD[a,*], Mara De Maio, PhD[b], Kevin Young, PhD[c,d], John Santopietro, MD[a,e,f,g]

KEYWORDS

- Outpatient psychiatry • Telehealth • COVID-19 • Barriers

KEY POINTS

- Most patients are able to engage productively via telepsychiatry, although specific strategies, implemented by providers/systems, can increase likelihood of successful treatment.
- Telepsychiatry has the potential to increase access to services, particularly when accommodations for those populations with unique needs are used.
- The pandemic has forced health care systems to take important steps to improve access and safety, and many of these changes should become standard practice.
- The pandemic has helped highlight the potential of innovative approaches to practice; we must move forward with openness while relying on science to guide practice.

BACKGROUND

The first cases of the severe acute respiratory syndrome coronavirus 2 (SARS-CoV-2) were reported in December 2019 in Wuhan, Hubei Province, China.[1] Within a matter of 3 months, the novel coronavirus disease 2019 (COVID-19) was declared a pandemic by the World Health Organization (WHO).[2] Over the following year, in the United States (US) alone, around 33 million individuals contracted SARS-CoV-2, and there were greater than 550,000 recorded deaths.[3] Every aspect of human life was affected. To curb the spread of the virus, numerous public health measures were adopted, to varying degrees and durations across all the states. These included but were not limited to mask mandates, work from home orders, closures of schools and nonessential businesses, and travel restrictions.[4] Health care systems and Public Health Departments worldwide had to adapt to the changing health care needs of the population. In the

[a] Yale School of Medicine, 1450 Chapel Street, New Haven, CT-06511, USA; [b] Child and Adolescent Services, Institute of Living, 200 Retreat Avenue, Terry Building 2nd floor, Hartford, CT 06106, USA; [c] Psychology Training, Institute of Living, 200 Retreat Avenue, Terry Building 2nd floor, Hartford, CT 06106, USA; [d] Psychiatry, University of Connecticut School of Medicine; [e] University of Connecticut School of Medicine, Farmington, CT 06032, USA; [f] Hartford HealthCare; [g] Behavioral Health Network, Hartford, CT, USA
* Corresponding author.
E-mail address: manu.s.sharma@yale.edu

Psychiatr Clin N Am 45 (2022) 57–69
https://doi.org/10.1016/j.psc.2021.11.003 psych.theclinics.com

early days of the pandemic, many US hospitals struggled with a shortage of personal protective equipment (PPE) and other critical resources.[5] Hospital systems worked hard to expand critical care and emergency services, infrastructure, and staffing; canceled or delayed elective procedures; and revamped infection control protocols and policies to protect their staff and patients.[6]

As the hospitals grappled with the consequences of the COVID-19 pandemic, another silent epidemic was brewing. With school closures and stay-at-home orders, more people became socially isolated. An estimated 9.6 million individuals experienced job loss and loss of their ability to support themselves and their families.[7] Millions of individuals lost access to their friends or loved ones, and a large proportion of the population experienced some form of socioeconomic distress, particularly individuals of color.[8] Historically, periods of socioeconomic stress have been associated with an increase in the incidence and prevalence of mental health disorders. Past studies have shown a significant increase in reports of symptoms of anxiety, depression, posttraumatic stress disorder, and increased suicide rates during and after epidemics (up to 3 years) caused by respiratory viruses (eg, influenza A/H1N1, Middle East respiratory syndrome). Women, elderly, migrant workers, and students were found to be most vulnerable to the mental health consequences of such epidemics.[9] Early studies have shown similar trends during the ongoing COVID-19 pandemic. For example, a nationally representative survey of more than 1400 adults in the US showed a nearly 3 times increase in the self-reported symptoms of depression as compared with prepandemic times.[10] Similarly, there has been an increase in reports of psychiatric symptoms for health care workers and individuals suffering from COVID-19 along with worsening of psychiatric symptoms in individuals with preexisting psychiatric disorders.[11,12] The epidemiologic patterns of such changes in the incidence and prevalence of mental health disorders as a result of COVID-19 pandemic are detailed in other articles in this issue. In the following article, the authors focus on the impact of the ongoing COVID-19 pandemic on the practice of outpatient (OP) psychiatry.

THE EARLY CHALLENGE

COVID-19 pandemic posed several unique challenges to the practice of OP psychiatry. In the initial phase of the pandemic, the absence of known effective treatment and vaccines meant that public health measures were our best hope for containing the morbidity and mortality associated with the infection. Most OP practices had to adhere to mask mandates and social distancing guidelines. For example, when the patient presented for their visit, they would be expected to wear masks, the psychiatrist had to wear appropriate PPE, and the office had to be reconfigured, when possible, to maintain 6 feet distance. At the Behavioral Health Network (BHN), Hartford Healthcare (the largest integrated network providing behavioral health services in the New England region), the following protocols were adopted to help provide safe and efficient OP psychiatric care to our patients:

- All patients were prescreened for symptoms of COVID-19 before ambulatory treatment session.
- All patients remained masked at all times while in the clinic.
- Changes were made to ensure social distancing. Offices and group therapy rooms were reconfigured to ensure social distancing. The number of patients attending group therapy sessions in the same room was reduced. To accommodate remaining patients, make-shift trailers were used to provide group therapy.
- Patients were encouraged to follow hand hygiene guidelines. Flyers with Centers for Disease Control and Prevention (CDC) guidance about hand washing/hygiene

were placed throughout the clinic. Hand sanitizing stations were set up at the entrance of the clinic, offices, group therapy rooms, and waiting rooms.
- All staff wore appropriate PPE at all times.
- Surfaces in group therapy rooms and offices were sanitized after every session.
- Staff sanitized commonly touched surfaces (railings, doorknobs, chairs) in the common clinic areas once every 2 hours.

The COVID-19 safety protocols were a difficult adjustment for the staff and patients. Of all medical specialties, psychiatry is extremely reliant on the development of the appropriate therapeutic alliance and a large body of literature emphasizes the role of therapeutic alliance in determining treatment outcomes.[13] Wearing PPE added an extra layer of difficulty in developing a personal connection and alliance. From the perspective of the psychiatrist, it became more difficult to observe facial expressions, pick up nonverbal cues, make an appropriate estimation of affective states, and perform accurate mental status examination.[14–16] Wearing masks during clinical encounters also often resulted in reduced efficacy of communication and patient's perception of empathy.[17]

As the pandemic progressed, many OP psychiatric practices were left with no option but to start using telepsychiatry services to provide OP psychiatric care. There were several barriers that had limited the wide-scale adoption of Telepsychiatry practices before the COVID-19 pandemic. In accordance with the Center for Medicare and Medicaid Services (CMS) rules, Medicare beneficiaries had to reside in designated rural/remote areas to be considered eligible to receive telehealth services. These individuals were expected to travel to rural clinics/community mental health centers to receive telehealth services. The professionals providing the medical services had to be located in their clinic or hospital. In other words, they could not provide services from their residence. More importantly, in order to establish care with a provider, the rules mandated an initial in-person visit, and only follow-up visits were allowed using telehealth. CMS introduced sweeping reforms of these rules in March 2020.[18] The change in rules allowed for the expansion of telehealth services across America. Providers were permitted to provide telehealth services from home, and rules requiring an initial in-person visit to establish care were waived. Under the new rules, Medicare started reimbursing E-Visits (asynchronous patient-initiated communication using online patient portals), audio-only visits, and telehealth visits at the same rate as in-person visits. The patients could receive telehealth services in the comfort of their home, anywhere in America, as the requirement for a rural residence was also relaxed.[19] At the same time, the US Department of Health and Human Services issued a notice that relaxed the enforcement of the Health Insurance Portability and Accountability Act of 1996, which allowed providers to use numerous online platforms such as Microsoft Teams, Zoom for Healthcare, and Cisco WebEx to provide telehealth services under the good faith provisions during the pandemic.[20] Another important regulatory change happened when the Ryan Haight Online Pharmacy Consumer Protection Act of 2008 was relaxed. In accordance with this public health emergency exception, the rule that required in-person visits for prescription of controlled substances was waived.[21] These changes allowed for the rapid expansion of telehealth services. Within the first 3 months of the announcement, CMS reported that more than 9 million individuals had received telehealth services.[19]

TELEPSYCHIATRY BECOMES THE NORM

Telepsychiatry lent itself very well to the public health mandates during the pandemic. It allowed for the patients and psychiatrists to receive and provide services, respectively, from their homes, reducing the risk of unnecessary exposure. As the year progressed, telepsychiatry became the default for providing OP psychiatric services. In the BHN, the number of telepsychiatry visits increased from a mere 356 in 2019 to 419,549 in the year 2020. Similar massive increases in telehealth visits were recorded in health systems across the country,[22] with one CDC report noting a 154% increase in the latter half of March 2020 when compared with the same time in 2019.[23] Interestingly, according to early CMS data, the rates of utilization of telehealth services did not vary by demographic variables such as gender, age, place of residence (urban vs rural), race, or ethnicity.[19]

The utilization of telepsychiatry services was already increasing in the US before the pandemic. According to publicly available data, in 2017, around 29.2% of facilities offering mental health services also offered telepsychiatry options; this had increased from about 15.2% in 2010. Also, the facilities that offered telehealth services were more likely to be funded by federal/local government sources, be a part of clinics offering other primary care services, and were less likely to be State or Medicaid funded.[24] There was a growing body of literature that showed that telepsychiatry was well-liked by patients, offered a reliable way to accurately assess psychiatric symptoms, had similar outcomes, and was more cost-efficient when compared with face-to-face clinical interactions.[25,26] Studies cited difficulty in developing rapport, picking up on nonverbal cues/body language, concerns about privacy, concerns about the ability to manage clinical emergencies, and technological barriers (internet speeds, appropriate telepsychiatry platforms) as the main concerns raised by patients and clinicians when participating in telepsychiatry visits.[27]

Through the experience gained in the initial days of the rapid transition to telepsychiatry, most health systems identified best practices to help provide the highest level of care during these challenging times. At the BHN, education modules were created to train staff to use telepsychiatry platforms. Each site identified champions who volunteered to train staff in using the telepsychiatry platform and who were available to troubleshoot when needed. Appropriate education material was created for patients and distributed through letters, emails, patient portals, and phone calls. Preappointment reminder calls, traditionally about 24 to 48 hours before the scheduled appointment, had been a common practice in many OP clinics. The amended workflow included offering the patient a telehealth visit during this call. The staff helped patients download the appropriate telehealth application/platform onto their smartphone/computer. They often did practice runs with the patients to help them troubleshoot and reduce their anxiety about the upcoming appointments. Furthermore, additional calls and attempts to reach out were made to patients and families to help improve engagement in psychiatric appointments at a time where everyone had competing demands, such as homeschooling, childcare, and work.

Concerns about risk mitigation and crisis management led to the development of protocols that improved clinician's ability to locate patients in crisis and direct emergency services as needed. In addition, at the BHN, we found that telepsychiatry allowed us to leverage new resources during crisis. During one telepsychiatry session, a patient indicated that she had tied a noose in the hours preceding the appointment and had put it around her neck—but subsequently had hidden it in her room. In addition to other risk mitigation strategies, the astute clinician was able to bring family directly into the session, and with the patient, disclose the location of the noose so that family could remove it and then the family could join in safety planning, including further lethal means restriction.

The disparities in Internet access/smartphone usage are important to note. To overcome technological barriers, special on-site rooms were set up for patients who did not have access to smartphones, computers, or the Internet, which allowed them to participate in telepsychiatry visits. These rooms, in most clinics, were modified clinical offices with a computer. Before the scheduled visit, the on-site staff who came into work on a rotation schedule would sanitize the surfaces in the room and set up the computer for the visit. Once the patient arrived, he/she/they were screened for COVID symptoms and then guided into the special room. The room would be sanitized again after the visit. This reduced the possibility of exposure for staff and patient and helped the patient receive needed psychiatric care when they did not have access to computers, smartphones, or the Internet. The patients were also given the option of participating in a telephone-only visit when they were unable to participate in a synchronous video-conferencing visit.

The American Psychiatric Association developed and distributed a Telepsychiatry Toolkit, which provided specific guidelines for the practice of telepsychiatry. For example, it outlined best practices for psychiatrists where they were advised to start the visit by confirming the patient's name and exact location of the patient (in case the psychiatrist needed to dispatch emergency services to the location). During telephone-only visits, the psychiatrists were encouraged to have access to another phone line to allow them to call emergency services if needed while continuing to keep the patient engaged on the first line.[28] The Canadian College of Family Physicians and the UK The National Institute for Health and Care Excellence also developed similar guidelines to help physicians adapt to evolving regulatory and clinical needs.[29,30] These guidelines and toolkits have been regularly updated through the pandemic and offer a useful resource. The most updated versions can be easily accessed online by going to the respective Web sites (see references for Web site links).

Although telepsychiatry allowed the BHN to function and continue to serve patients, there were financial implications of the work, with solutions still evolving. In the early part of 2020, we had ~35,000 monthly appointments scheduled for behavioral health concerns. By summer 2020, and through the remainder of the year, we averaged ~41,500 monthly appointments, an increase of 18.6%. Although monthly no-shows more than doubled (3352–7186) in the second half of 2020 through early 2021, there was still a net increase in completed appointments after transitioning to telehealth dominated practice.

Clinics Care Points—Telepsychiatry

- Telepsychiatry has been proved to be an effective way to maintain and improve access to mental health services.
- Several best practice guidelines exist and continue to evolve and should be used in guiding future practice.
- Systems can support patients who lack access to technology by designating clinic space for patients to use as a hub to sit in while meeting virtually with clinicians.
- Telepsychiatry has proved to improve access, allows for effective care delivery, and concerns, such as risk mitigation processes, have been addressed—with new opportunities for enhancing care identified.

COVID-19 AND SPECIAL POPULATIONS

OP psychiatrists had the unique responsibility of treating some of the most vulnerable members of our society. Data from the CDC's National Syndromic Surveillance Program, which includes approximately 73% of emergency department visits nationally, found that mental health–related visits increased by 24% in children between ages 5 and 11 years and by 31% in children between ages 12 and 17 years across the same time points in 2019 and 2020.[31] Although this is consistent with lifespan mental health emergency department visit trends during that time,[32] not all hospital systems found the same pattern.[33] With mandated school closures, overnight, the children were deprived of the structure, supports, and social interactions they received at school. There was a significant increase in children experiencing symptoms of depression and anxiety. Children with preexisting psychiatric conditions displayed an increased likelihood of decompensation and needed a higher level of care.[34–36] Some data suggested that conducting telepsychiatry visits among children was more challenging than the adult population.

There was a reduction in the total number of child and adolescent visits when systems switched to the telehealth model, and this reduction was more pronounced for psychotherapy visits when compared with medication management visits.[37] To improve engagements and outcomes, psychiatrists and therapists developed new workflows and strategies. Locally, a clinician began sending postcards to patients a week after they get discharged from our intensive outpatient programs, and almost all of the children contacted her to express their gratitude for the gesture. In accordance with the guidance provided by the American Academy of Child and Adolescent Psychiatry, it was important to continue to include parents and occasionally teachers for information gathering and development of appropriate treatment plans. Telehealth technology made it easy to include both parents, even when they were at geographically different locations/cities. Teachers could also be added to the telehealth visits to gather needed information and to assess changes in behaviors during school hours. In keeping with the regulations regarding assent, it became important to conduct part of the assessment and treatment planning with the child alone. This planning could be facilitated by asking the parent/caregiver to leave the room and then confirming with the child that he/she/they are alone in the room.[38]

On the one hand, telepsychiatry platforms provided a window into the child's home environment. On the other hand, the psychiatrist had to put in extra effort to hold the child's attention and perform an appropriate mental status examination. In the course of a face-to-face visit, child psychiatrists would observe children playing with toys and had to pay special attention to eye contact and gestures and observe for possible motor abnormalities. This posed an extra challenge during telepsychiatry visits, and the psychiatrist had to seek extra co-operation from the parents/caregivers to allow for such assessment. The placement of the camera proved to be a crucial part of such visits. The psychiatrist had to ensure that the camera was positioned in such a way that they could carry a conversation with the parent but be able to observe the child play at the same time. The psychiatrist could ask the parents to reposition the camera, zoom when possible, to try and observe tics or other abnormal motor movements. When in doubt, the psychiatrist could always make arrangements for in-person follow-up visits when needed.[39,40]

On the other end of the spectrum, elderly patients were at increased risk of developing a serious illness, needing hospitalization, and had higher mortality rates.[41] Fortunately, there was extensive literature that provided the evidence base for the utilization of telehealth services for providing psychiatric care and neurocognitive testing in the geriatric population.[42] However, this population faced significant challenges that affected their ability to engage in telepsychiatry visits. They were less likely to have access to the needed smartphones/computers and were also more likely to have difficulty using technological software or platforms that were being used for telehealth visits.[43,44] Reduced visual acuity and hearing impairments also resulted in significant challenges in conducting these visits. It became important to involve family members of the elderly patients to help them engage in telepsychiatry visits. The front desk staff was instructed to expect to spend extra time to help the elderly patients set up the needed telehealth platform. Also, the elderly patients were encouraged to participate in practice runs to help them get familiar with the telehealth format and to troubleshoot before the actual visit. In case of hearing impairments, the psychiatrist augmented the communication by typing questions/instructions in a chat-box for the patients to read. Patients were encouraged to use headphones to help improve communication and reduce distractions. Readiness to engage in video conferencing visits was assessed at every visit, and appropriate alternatives were also provided (like telephone-only or in-person visits).

Individuals with substance use disorders were perhaps the most vulnerable to decompensation and relapse. Changes brought on by the pandemic resulted in social isolation and increased the burden of various psychosocial stressors, whereas access to life-saving treatment and harm reduction services was also reduced because of public health measures and an overburdened health care system. Risk of developing complications because of withdrawal and their risk of death by overdose increased substantially.[45] Many states responded by setting up hotlines for patients struggling with substance use disorders.[46] The relaxation of the Ryan Haight Online Pharmacy Consumer Protection Act of 2008 also helped further improve access.[21] In addition to using telepsychiatry, telephone calls, and text messaging, clinics also adapted by allowing for larger take-home Methadone doses, using smart lockboxes (that enabled them to dispense medications at preset times), prescribing Naloxone to every patient with an opiate use disorder, and favoring Suboxone over methadone in new patients presenting for treatment of Opiate use disorder.[47]

SES seems to have affected service utilization during the time of heightened telepsychiatry. Although an APA telehealth survey in June 2020 indicated reduced no-shows for telepsychiatry visits,[48] and other smaller studies found improved rates of attendance against both prepandemic and during pandemic in-office visits (ie, in one setting; 7.5% no-show telehealth vs 36.1% prepandemic and 29.8% during),[49] a review based on claims data indicated that patients with Medicare used services differently that those with commercial insurers during the shift toward telehealth.[50] In 2020, Medicaid beneficiaries used telehealth platforms for far fewer sessions than commercial or Medicare beneficiaries, despite high increases (from a low baseline) of use of telehealth in this group; this suggests that this group may have barriers to using telehealth that may require creative solutions, such as increasing access to, or training with, technology used for these visits.

In addition to the special considerations outlined earlier, it was important to take additional steps to ensure that OP psychiatrists were providing safe and efficient care. It became even more important to collaborate with local pharmacies/laboratories and encourage home delivery of medications, utilization of special packaging to avoid dose confusions, increased utilization of long-acting injectable antipsychotics, and performing appropriate laboratory tests to monitor drug levels, metabolic health, and absolute neutrophil counts for patients on clozapine.[51]

Clinics Care Points—Special Populations

- Treatment of children via telepsychiatry is enhanced via planning with parents (environment, distractors, and so forth), preserving one-to-one space for clinician and patient without the parent present, and flexibility (ie, working with family to help find best camera positions to allow meaningful mental status examination).
- Although age-related changes in perception and/or cognition can lead to a reduced experience for geriatric patients, the experience can be improved by

use of specific technology (ie, headphones) and involvement of family to help coordinate the visit.
- Treatment of individuals with opiate use disorders shifted toward suboxone>methadone, and rescue naloxone should be routinely prescribed for individuals in treatment.
- Increased collaboration between psychiatrists and pharmacies mitigates risk of dose confusion, compliance risks, and laboratory value monitoring.

INNOVATION AND DIGITAL PSYCHIATRY

The practice of psychiatry has not been immune to the disruptive forces of digital technologies that have been fueled by increasing access to smartphones/devices and the artificial intelligence revolution. There are more than 20,000 mental health apps available for download on any smart phone,[52] and venture capital companies have been investing billions of dollars in digital mental health companies.[53] The ongoing pandemic added fuel to the already raging fire, further accelerating the growth of digital psychiatry. Although telepsychiatry has consistently been shown to be a safe, efficient, and cost-effective way of providing psychiatric care,[25,26] it has failed to make a significant dent in access-related issues caused by the current and projected shortage of psychiatrists.[54] Innovative digital psychiatry solutions could, in the future, help bridge the gaps left behind by such shortages and augment the ability of psychiatrists to provide objective, high-quality care to a larger population.

Currently, digital psychiatry solutions range from simple phone apps that remind the patient to take medications on time or record mood to advanced chatbot–based applications that are capable of providing real-time therapy using advanced natural language processing algorithms. Most applications can be broadly divided into digital therapeutics, which include apps or devices that can be used to provide treatment to patients, and digital phenotyping solutions, which include apps or devices that can collect data, actively or passively, to help quantify psychiatric symptoms and provide clinical decision support. Self-help and mindfulness apps, such as Calm and Headspace, are perhaps some of the most well-known apps that saw an exponential increase in their downloads during the pandemic.[55] Although very preliminary evidence suggests that these apps have been helpful in the reduction of perceived stress in nonclinical populations,[56,57] there is next to no evidence to support the use of these applications in a clinical population.[58] There are a limited number of randomized clinical trials that explore the efficacy of smartphone-based cognitive behavioral therapy (CBT). Yet, there are several apps on the market that claim to provide evidence-based CBT for insomnia, depression, posttraumatic stress disorder, and anxiety. Unfortunately, initial evidence with regard to their efficacy has been underwhelming.[59,60] There are emerging companies that offer chatbot-based real-time online therapies. Using such apps, the patients are able to text their virtual therapist at any time. Some apps, such as WoeBot, use natural language processing to try and understand the text sent by the patient and respond immediately using preprogrammed answers that are based on CBT or supportive therapy principles. Other apps, such as Better-Help, use asynchronous replies from therapists to facilitate therapy. Initial evidence of the efficacy of such interventions is encouraging.[61]

Digital phenotyping refers to collecting data, actively or passively, using a digital device or a smartphone to help gain insight into various behaviors/psychiatric symptoms in an individual.[62] For example, researchers have used phone GPS data (to assess social interaction and movement), the volume of phone calls made and received, the content of text messages, and recorded voice samples in combination with self-reported symptoms scales to quantify psychiatric symptoms, predict the risk of hospitalizations, drug relapse, and provide clinical decision support.[63–65] It is not difficult to imagine augmenting the effectiveness of telepsychiatry and improving access to psychiatric services using innovative, economical, and scalable digital psychiatry solutions.

Clinics Care Points—Innovation

- Self-help apps are attractive and some highly used, although utility in reducing symptoms in patient populations is unclear.
- App delivered therapy via prerecorded modules, and artificial intelligence bot response is a developing area with mixed efficacy but clear potential.
- The role of technology in assessing patients and providing information about their behaviors (digital phenotyping) is rapidly expanding and will have a future role in assessment and treatment.
- These technologies provide additional data, not reliant on patient introspection or self-report, that can prove critical in appropriately titrating treatment.

SUMMARY

To say that the COVID-19 pandemic transformed the practice of OP psychiatry would be an understatement. We went from face-to-face interactions in clinics to online interactions using videoconferencing software, where both the patient and the psychiatrist were at their respective homes. We gained unprecedented access to the home environments of our patients and were able to meet their family members and occasionally their neighbors and pets. Small private practice clinics and large health care organizations alike displayed great grit and resilience in the way they adapted to the challenges of the pandemic. It is evident that we have seen just the tip of the iceberg when it comes to an understanding of the true psychological impact of the COVID-19 pandemic and what it would mean for the incidence and prevalence of psychiatric disorders in the future. The changes, or the lack there off, to the regulatory landscapes and reimbursement models, once the public health emergency ends, will determine the future of OP psychiatric practice. Concerns regarding poor reimbursement for telepsychiatry services, among other regulatory challenges, were cited as some of the main barriers to wide-scale adoption of such services across organizations,[27] despite many studies showing that such services improve access to care in a cost-effective way and hold the potential of alleviating some of the health disparities that plague our current system of health care.[66] Many state lawmakers are recognizing the positive impact of telehealth services and are already moving to make telehealth parity laws permanent to aid the ongoing expansion of telehealth services in the future.[67] It is hoped that the ongoing expansion of telepsychiatry services in combination with the revolution in digital psychiatry driven by increasing investments and technological advancements will result in increased access to high-quality, efficient, and equitable psychiatric care.

DISCLOSURE

The authors have nothing to disclose.

REFERENCES

1. Zhu N, Zhang D, Wang W, et al. A novel coronavirus from patients with pneumonia in China, 2019. N Engl J Med 2020;382(8):727–33. https://doi.org/10.1056/NEJMoa2001017.

2. Cucinotta D, Vanelli M. WHO declares COVID-19 a pandemic. Acta Biomed 2020;91(1):157–60. https://doi.org/10.23750/abm.v91i1.9397.
3. COVID-19 map. Johns Hopkins Coronavirus Resource Center. Available at: https://coronavirus.jhu.edu/map.html.
4. MultiState. COVID-19 policy tracker 2021. https://www.multistate.us/issues/covid-19-policy-tracker.
5. Sen-Crowe B, McKenney M, Elkbuli A. COVID-19 response and containment strategies in the US, South Korea, and Iceland: Lessons learned and future directions. Am J Emerg Med 2020;38(7):1537–9. https://doi.org/10.1016/j.ajem.2020.04.072.
6. Uppal A, Silvestri DM, Siegler M, et al. Critical care and emergency department response at the epicenter of the COVID-19 pandemic. Health Aff 2020;39(8):1443–9. https://doi.org/10.1377/hlthaff.2020.00901.
7. Bennet J. Fewer jobs have been lost in the EU than in the U.S. during the COVID-19 downturn. https://pewrsr.ch/3gdKH5u.
8. Center on budget and policy priorities: tracking the COVID-19 recession's effects on food, housing, and employment hardships.
9. Luo Y, Chua CR, Xiong Z, et al. A systematic review of the impact of viral respiratory epidemics on mental health: an implication on the coronavirus disease 2019 pandemic. Front Psychiatry 2020;11:565098. https://doi.org/10.3389/fpsyt.2020.565098.
10. Ettman CK, Abdalla SM, Cohen GH, et al. Prevalence of depression symptoms in us adults before and during the COVID-19 pandemic. JAMA Netw Open 2020;3(9):e2019686. https://doi.org/10.1001/jamanetworkopen.2020.19686.
11. Young KP, Kolcz DL, O'Sullivan DM, et al. Health care workers' mental health and quality of life during COVID-19: results from a mid-pandemic. Natl Surv *Psychiatr Serv* 2021;72(2):122–8. https://doi.org/10.1176/appi.ps.202000424.
12. Vindegaard N, Benros ME. COVID-19 pandemic and mental health consequences: Systematic review of the current evidence. Brain Behav Immun 2020;89:531–42. https://doi.org/10.1016/j.bbi.2020.05.048.
13. Stubbe DE. The therapeutic alliance: the fundamental element of psychotherapy. Focus (Madison) 2018;16(4):402–3. https://doi.org/10.1176/appi.focus.20180022.
14. Mehta UM, Venkatasubramanian G, Chandra PS. The "mind" behind the "mask": Assessing mental states and creating therapeutic alliance amidst COVID-19. Schizophr Res 2020;222:503–4. https://doi.org/10.1016/j.schres.2020.05.033.
15. Veluri N. Are masks impacting psychiatric inpatients' treatment? Psychiatry Res 2020;293:113459. https://doi.org/10.1016/j.psychres.2020.113459.
16. Pal A, Gupta P, Parmar A, et al. "Masking" of the mental state: Unintended consequences of personal protective equipment (PPE) on psychiatric clinical practice. Psychiatry Res 2020;290:113178. https://doi.org/10.1016/j.psychres.2020.113178.
17. Wong CKM, Yip BHK, Mercer S, et al. Effect of facemasks on empathy and relational continuity: a randomised controlled trial in primary care. BMC Fam Pract 2013;14:200. https://doi.org/10.1186/1471-2296-14-200.
18. COVID-19: president trump expands telehealth benefits for medicare beneficiaries during COVID-19 outbreak. Available at: https://www.cms.gov/outreach-and-educationoutreachffsprovpartprogprovider-partnership-email-archive/2020-03-17.
19. Verma S. Early impact of CMS expansion of medicare telehealth during COVID-19. Health Aff Blog 2020. https://doi.org/10.1377/hblog20200715.454789.

20. HHS. Notification of enforcement discretion for telehealth remote communications during the COVID-19 nationwide public health emergency. 2020. Available at: https://www.hhs.gov/hipaa/for-professionals/special-topics/emergency-preparedness/notification-enforcement-discretion-telehealth/index.html.
21. Chen JA, Chung W-J, Young SK, et al. COVID-19 and telepsychiatry: early outpatient experiences and implications for the future. Gen Hosp Psychiatry 2020;66: 89–95. https://doi.org/10.1016/j.genhosppsych.2020.07.002.
22. Esper GJ, Sweeney RL, Winchell E, et al. Rapid systemwide implementation of outpatient telehealth in response to the COVID-19 pandemic. J Healthc Manag 2020;65(6):443–52. https://doi.org/10.1097/JHM-D-20-00131.
23. Koonin LM, Hoots B, Tsang CA, et al. Trends in the use of telehealth during the emergence of the COVID-19 Pandemic — United States, January–March 2020. MMWR Morb Mortal Wkly Rep 2020;69(43):1595–9. https://doi.org/10.15585/mmwr.mm6943a3.
24. Spivak S, Spivak A, Cullen B, et al. Telepsychiatry use in U.S. mental health facilities, 2010–2017. Psychiatr Serv 2020;71(2):121–7. https://doi.org/10.1176/appi.ps.201900261.
25. Hubley S, Lynch SB, Schneck C, et al. Review of key telepsychiatry outcomes. World J Psychiatry 2016;6(2):269. https://doi.org/10.5498/wjp.v6.i2.269.
26. Hilty DM, Ferrer DC, Parish MB, et al. The effectiveness of telemental health: a 2013 review. Telemed J E Health 2013;19(6):444–54. https://doi.org/10.1089/tmj.2013.0075.
27. Cowan KE, McKean AJ, Gentry MT, et al. Barriers to use of telepsychiatry: clinicians as gatekeepers. Mayo Clin Proc 2019;94(12):2510–23. https://doi.org/10.1016/j.mayocp.2019.04.018.
28. APA's Telepsychiatry Toolkit. Available at: https://www.psychiatry.org/psychiatrists/practice/telepsychiatry/toolkit.
29. Covid-19: remote consultations. NICE. Available at: https://www.nice.org.uk/guidance/ng163/resources/%0Dbmj-visual-summary-for-remote-consultations-pdf-8713904797.
30. Telemedicine Essentials. The College of family physicians of Canada. Available at: https://www.cfp.ca/sites/default/files/pubfiles/PDF Documents/Blog/telehealth_tool_eng.pdf.
31. Leeb RT, Bitsko RH, Radhakrishnan L, et al. Mental health–related emergency department visits among children aged <18 years during the COVID-19 pandemic — United States, January 1–October 17, 2020. MMWR Morb Mortal Wkly Rep 2020;69(45):1675–80. https://doi.org/10.15585/mmwr.mm6945a3.
32. Holland KM, Jones C, Vivolo-Kantor AM, et al. Trends in US emergency department visits for mental health, overdose, and violence outcomes before and during the COVID-19 pandemic. JAMA Psychiatry 2021;78(4):372. https://doi.org/10.1001/jamapsychiatry.2020.4402.
33. Leff RA, Setzer E, Cicero MX, et al. Changes in pediatric emergency department visits for mental health during the COVID-19 pandemic: a cross-sectional study. Clin Child Psychol Psychiatry 2021;26(1):33–8. https://doi.org/10.1177/1359104520972453.
34. Singh S, Roy D, Sinha K, et al. Impact of COVID-19 and lockdown on mental health of children and adolescents: a narrative review with recommendations. Psychiatry Res 2020;293:113429. https://doi.org/10.1016/j.psychres.2020.113429.
35. de Figueiredo CS, Sandre PC, Portugal LCL, et al. COVID-19 pandemic impact on children and adolescents' mental health: biological, environmental, and social factors. Prog Neuropsychopharmacol Biol Psychiatry 2021;106:110171. https://doi.org/10.1016/j.pnpbp.2020.110171.

36. Guessoum SB, Lachal J, Radjack R, et al. Adolescent psychiatric disorders during the COVID-19 pandemic and lockdown. Psychiatry Res 2020;291:113264. https://doi.org/10.1016/j.psychres.2020.113264.
37. Hoffnung G, Feigenbaum E, Schechter A, et al. Children and telehealth in mental healthcare: what we have learned from COVID-19 and 40,000+ sessions. Psychiatr Res Clin Pract 2021. https://doi.org/10.1176/appi.prcp.20200035.
38. Myers K, Cain S, Work Group on Quality Issues, American Academy of Child and Adolescent Psychiatry Staff. Practice parameter for telepsychiatry with children and adolescents. J Am Acad Child Adolesc Psychiatry 2008;47(12):1468–83. https://doi.org/10.1097/CHI.0b013e31818b4e13.
39. Gloff NE, LeNoue SR, Novins DK, et al. Telemental health for children and adolescents. Int Rev Psychiatry 2015;27(6):513–24. https://doi.org/10.3109/09540261.2015.1086322.
40. Goldstein F, Glueck D. Developing rapport and therapeutic alliance during telemental health sessions with children and adolescents. J Child Adolesc Psychopharmacol 2016;26(3):204–11. https://doi.org/10.1089/cap.2015.0022.
41. Yanez ND, Weiss NS, Romand J-A, et al. COVID-19 mortality risk for older men and women. BMC Public Health 2020;20(1):1742. https://doi.org/10.1186/s12889-020-09826-8.
42. Gentry MT, Lapid MI, Rummans TA. Geriatric telepsychiatry: systematic review and policy considerations. Am J Geriatr Psychiatry 2019;27(2):109–27. https://doi.org/10.1016/j.jagp.2018.10.009.
43. Delello JA, McWhorter RR. Reducing the digital divide. J Appl Gerontol 2017;36(1):3–28. https://doi.org/10.1177/0733464815589985.
44. Heinz M, Martin P, Margrett JA, et al. Perceptions of technology among older adults. J Gerontol Nurs 2013;39(1):42–51. https://doi.org/10.3928/00989134-20121204-04.
45. Alexander GC, Stoller KB, Haffajee RL, et al. An epidemic in the midst of a pandemic: opioid use disorder and COVID-19. Ann Intern Med 2020;173(1):57–8. https://doi.org/10.7326/M20-1141.
46. Samuels EA, Clark SA, Wunsch C, et al. Innovation during COVID-19: improving addiction treatment access. J Addict Med 2020;14(4):e8–9. https://doi.org/10.1097/ADM.0000000000000685.
47. Leppla IE, Gross MS. Optimizing medication treatment of opioid use disorder during COVID-19 (SARS-CoV-2). J Addict Med 2020;14(4):e1–3. https://doi.org/10.1097/ADM.0000000000000678.
48. Psychiatrists use of Telepsychiatry during COVID-19 Public Health Emergency. Policy recommendations. American Psychiatric Association; 2020.
49. Drerup B, Espenschied J, Wiedemer J, et al. Reduced no-show rates and sustained patient satisfaction of telehealth during the COVID-19 pandemic. Telemed J E Health 2021. https://doi.org/10.1089/tmj.2021.0002.
50. Davenport S, Melek S, Gray TJ. Behavioral healthcare utilization changes during the COVID-19 pandemic. An analysis of claims data through august 2020 for 12.5 million individuals. Milliman White Paper; 2021.
51. Hamada K, Fan X. The impact of COVID-19 on individuals living with serious mental illness. Schizophr Res 2020;222:3–5. https://doi.org/10.1016/j.schres.2020.05.054.
52. Pappas S. Providing care in innovative ways 2020. Available at: https://www.apa.org/monitor/2020/01/cover-trends-innovative-ways.
53. Shah RN, Berry OO. The rise of venture capital investing in mental health. JAMA Psychiatry 2021;78(4):351. https://doi.org/10.1001/jamapsychiatry.2020.2847.

54. Satiani A, Niedermier J, Satiani B, et al. Projected workforce of psychiatrists in the united states: a population analysis. Psychiatr Serv 2018;69(6):710–3. https://doi.org/10.1176/appi.ps.201700344.
55. Chapple C. Downloads of top English-language mental Wellness apps surged by 2 million in april amid COVID-19 pandemic.
56. Champion L, Economides M, Chandler C. The efficacy of a brief app-based mindfulness intervention on psychosocial outcomes in healthy adults: a pilot randomised controlled trial. PLoS One 2018;13(12):e0209482. https://doi.org/10.1371/journal.pone.0209482.
57. Huberty J, Green J, Glissmann C, et al. Efficacy of the mindfulness meditation mobile app “calm” to reduce stress among college students: randomized controlled trial. JMIR mHealth uHealth 2019;7(6):e14273. https://doi.org/10.2196/14273.
58. Lau N, O'Daffer A, Colt S, et al. Android and iPhone mobile apps for psychosocial wellness and stress management: systematic search in app stores and literature review. JMIR mHealth uHealth 2020;8(5):e17798. https://doi.org/10.2196/17798.
59. Rathbone AL, Clarry L, Prescott J. Assessing the efficacy of mobile health apps using the basic principles of cognitive behavioral therapy: systematic review. J Med Internet Res 2017;19(11):e399. https://doi.org/10.2196/jmir.8598.
60. Huguet A, Rao S, McGrath PJ, et al. A systematic review of cognitive behavioral therapy and behavioral activation apps for depression. PLoS One 2016;11(5): e0154248. https://doi.org/10.1371/journal.pone.0154248.
61. Vaidyam AN, Wisniewski H, Halamka JD, et al. Chatbots and conversational agents in mental health: a review of the psychiatric landscape. Can J Psychiatry 2019;64(7):456–64. https://doi.org/10.1177/0706743719828977.
62. Torous J, Kiang MV, Lorme J, et al. New tools for new research in psychiatry: a scalable and customizable platform to empower data driven smartphone research. JMIR Ment Health 2016;3(2):e16. https://doi.org/10.2196/mental.5165.
63. Andrea A, Agulia A, Serafini G, et al. Digital biomarkers and digital phenotyping in mental health care and prevention. Eur J Public Health 2020;30(Suppl_5). https://doi.org/10.1093/eurpub/ckaa165.1080.
64. Benoit J, Onyeaka H, Keshavan M, et al. Systematic review of digital phenotyping and machine learning in psychosis spectrum illnesses. Harv Rev Psychiatry 2020;28(5):296–304. https://doi.org/10.1097/HRP.0000000000000268.
65. Corcoran CM, Mittal VA, Bearden CE, et al. Language as a biomarker for psychosis: a natural language processing approach. Schizophr Res 2020;226:158–66. https://doi.org/10.1016/j.schres.2020.04.032.
66. Hirko KA, Kerver JM, Ford S, et al. Telehealth in response to the COVID-19 pandemic: implications for rural health disparities. J Am Med Inform Assoc 2020;27(11):1816–8. https://doi.org/10.1093/jamia/ocaa156.
67. Baumann BC, MacArthur KM, Michalski JM. The importance of temporary telehealth parity laws to improve public health during COVID-19 and future pandemics. Int J Radiat Oncol Biol Phys 2020;108(2):362–3. https://doi.org/10.1016/j.ijrobp.2020.05.039.

Psychiatry's Expanded Integration into Primary Care

Mark H. Duncan, MD*, Jennifer M. Erickson, DO[1], Denise Chang, MD[1], Ramanpreet Toor, MD[1], Anna D.H. Ratzliff, MD, PhD[1]

KEYWORDS

• COVID • Integrated care • Integrated behavioral care

KEY POINTS

- Integrated mental health care has been a leading strategy to improve access to psychiatric treatment.
- The pandemic disrupted current integrated care efforts at a systems level, team-based care level, scope of care level, and patient access to care level.
- Renewed efforts to build more flexible and resilient integrated programs can and should be done to not only prevent future disruptions in care but also meet the mental behavioral health needs of a broader population of patients.

INTRODUCTION

Integrated behavioral health care is broadly defined by the Agency for Healthcare Research and Quality as the care a patient experiences as a result of a team of primary care and behavioral health clinicians, working together with patients and families, using a systematic and cost-effective approach to provide patient-centered care for a defined population.[1] Arguably, this approach has become a leading strategy in the United States to meet the growing need for mental health treatment at the front lines of medicine resulting in increasing access to care, improving health outcomes, and reducing costs. The collaborative care model (CoCM) is the foremost example of integrated care that uses a team approach, where a primary care provider (PCP), a behavioral health care manager, and a consulting psychiatrist work together as a team to help provide mental health interventions to patients in a primary care setting. This model offers an opportunity for psychiatrists to leverage their skills to reach a larger population. Collaborative care has an extensive evidence base demonstrating improved patient outcomes compared with usual care for common mental health conditions seen in the primary

Department of Psychiatry and Behavioral Sciences, University of Washington, 4225 Roosevelt Way Northeast, Street 306, Seattle, WA 98105, USA
[1] Present address: 1959 NE Pacific Street, Box 356560, Seattle, WA 98195-6560.
* Corresponding author.
E-mail address: mhduncan@uw.edu

Psychiatr Clin N Am 45 (2022) 71–80
https://doi.org/10.1016/j.psc.2021.11.004
psych.theclinics.com

care setting.[2] Before the pandemic, the effectiveness of the CoCM in a clinical setting was impacted by implementation and sustainment challenges, nurturing of the relationship of the CoCM team members, the scope of the CoCM program, and how well patients and providers could access the program. Since the pandemic, each of those areas has been impacted in positive and negative ways. This article looks at prepandemic status of those areas of integrated care, followed by a close examination of the ways the pandemic disrupted those areas of integrated care. The final section describes what changes from the pandemic should be kept and what should not during this unique opportunity to re-envision integrated behavioral health.

THE PREPANDEMIC STATE OF INTEGRATED CARE

System Constraints

Lack of access to specialty mental health care was a driving force behind the development of integrated care in primary care settings, and in particular the CoCM. Despite CoCM's clear effectiveness, implementing a collaborative care program is complex and time consuming. Specifically, CoCM implementation requires buy in from organizational leaders and providers, and all team members need to have a clear understanding of the model and everyone's individual roles. It is also essential to have the appropriate infrastructure to support team-based care, including having the right systems and tools in place to complete the work (eg, a registry to track the patients, ways to effectively communicate among team members). Although implementing collaborative care is complicated, sustaining a collaborative care practice is equally challenging. Common issues include clinicians not having adequate time built into their schedules for team meetings and keeping the registry up to date, multiple competing priorities for the care manager or PCP, variable psychiatric consultant involvement, inconsistencies related to time devoted to caseload review, workflow logistics, staff turnover, and lack of patient engagement.[1,3] Thus, in the prepandemic state of integrated care there were significant hurdles in starting integrated care programs and sustaining these practices.

Although there are many existing barriers, there have been some recent prepandemic innovations and policy changes that have the potential to further help expand the use of CoCM and integrated care more broadly. This potential has been seen in two main areas. The first relates to the growing evidence for the effective use of telemedicine-based collaborative care services.[4,5] However, broad implementation of telehealth services for integrated care has been sluggish prepandemic likely because of multiple barriers including reimbursement, interstate licensing issues, technology limitations, and providers interest in its use.[6] Second, new CPT codes released by Centers for Medicare and Medicaid Services in 2017 were designed to financially support the types of services furnished through collaborative care. These new CoCM billing codes include reimbursement of direct patient care in addition to telephone visits and other non-face-to-face care, including electronic communication with the patient, care coordination on behalf of the patient, or time consulting with other team members, such as the psychiatrist and the PCP.[7] Unfortunately, numerous challenges in using those codes have hampered uptake and use, including the need to obtain patient consent before participation in CoCM, tracking time spent working with or on behalf of each patient, and monitoring the time spent billing thresholds.[8,9] Although implementation of either telehealth and/or the new CoCM billing codes come with their own challenges and complexities, organizations that were able to successfully implement one or both of these options before the onset of the pandemic would have likely seen less disruption in care for patients.

Team-Based Care

Team-based care has been a defining characteristic of the most effective integrated care models and is an essential feature in the CoCM. The prepandemic approach to integrated care was often a hybrid of models and used telehealth to a modest degree and mostly fell along the spectrum of basic collaboration to full integration as defined by the SAMSHA Standard Framework for Levels of Integrated Healthcare.[10]

- Basic collaboration or colocated model: In a colocated model the primary care and psychiatric teams work independently. Psychiatric providers see and treat patients directly. The communication among the providers happens as needed or when the patient is stabilized and handed back to the PCP. The care is usually provided in person and built around the in-person professional relationship between the mental health provider and the PCP. Curbside consultations in the hallway and workroom are a common aspect of this model and helps foster confidence in each other's skill set.[11]
- Full integration or the CoCM: In the CoCM, the psychiatric team includes a behavioral health provider or care manager in addition to the psychiatric consultant. One of the primary roles of a behavioral health provider is to coordinate care and help the communication between patient, psychiatric provider, and PCP. In this model psychiatric providers mostly provide care indirectly by reviewing patients with the behavioral health provider and rely on the information gathered by other team members. The psychiatric providers may work remotely in the model and may not have regular direct communication with the PCP.
- Combination: Many providers and systems have appreciated the familiarity of the professional community and shared responsibility these models have provided. This has often led to settling on a mix of both options.

Scope

Although integrated care has had a growing evidence base for the spectrum of mental health disorders, most implementation efforts have focused on depression and anxiety problems.[12] This is because depression and anxiety disorders are the most common mental health problems found in primary care.[13] From that point, a substantial evidence base for the integrated treatment of depression and anxiety disorders in primary care has emerged that has guided implementation efforts.[2] Unfortunately, this typically results in most patients with serious mental illness (SMI), such as bipolar disorder and schizophrenia, or substance use disorders (SUD), left to seek care in two different clinical settings: their primary care clinic, and their specialty clinic. This is unfortunate because patients with SMI and or SUDs could benefit from a more integrated care approach because of their high rates of chronic medical conditions, which are often undertreated.[14] In addition, clinics have often been inflexible in their willingness to expand beyond depression and anxiety because of the narrow scope of training of the integrated workforce.[15] Thus, the prepandemic state of integrated care has been defined by an often inflexible and narrow scope despite a much broader spectrum of mental health issues presenting in primary care.

Capacity/Access

Capacity and access have long been issues in psychiatry. One of the original goals of the CoCM was to reach patients where they typically receive care, which is in primary care. Several barriers exist when attempting to implement CoCM, which can hinder initial efforts at developing capacity. Although the CoCM is effective at treating a multitude of disorders and populations, the model does have several limits to access.

Access to the CoCM within a clinic is often dictated by the ability of the patient to meet with the care team. Before the pandemic, patients were required to physically come in person for most of their visits. Some iterations of the CoCM allowed for patients to be contacted via telephone for some sessions, but most models required greater than 50% in-person contact. There are some benefits to having patients physically present including providing structure to clinician-patient clinical interactions and the ability to fully assess patients for subtle examination findings. There are also significant challenges for patients. Presenting for any appointment requires patients to have access to transportation, flexibility in their work hours, and childcare or eldercare. These challenges often can become barriers to engagement in collaborative care. Furthermore, poor engagement with difficulty growing a caseload has been found to threaten sustainability of the entire program.[3]

HOW THE PANDEMIC DISRUPTED INTEGRATED CARE

System Constraints

As the pandemic started, health care organizations almost universally experienced a drop in visits and practices found themselves making rapid transitions to telehealth services to maintain access.[16,17] This transition was further supported by the declaration of a public health emergency and lifting of restrictions on payment for telehealth. With the transition to telehealth many changes to clinical workflow and operations were required, which significantly impacted the provision of integrated care. For example, many organizations likely saw a drop in screening rates for mental health conditions as a direct result of fewer patients presenting for in-person primary care visits. This had an impact on the integrated care workflow, because the mental health screening done at the primary care visit is often how patients are identified and then referred to the integrated care team. Similarly, measurement-based care is often dependent on the same screening workflows and likely would have been impacted leading to a reduction in tracking treatment outcomes on the individual and organizational levels. Eventually, some organizations were able to send screening questionnaires electronically and, in some situations, systems were further able to integrate these tools into the electronic medical record and have them sent out concurrently with telehealth visits. However, this type of integration takes time and resources, which many organizations have struggled with during the pandemic. In addition, this shift to telehealth may have adversely affected certain patients, particularly those patients that had difficulty accessing virtual care. This disparity further added to preexisting concerns around equity and access for disadvantaged populations.

Team-Based Care

With the COVID-19 pandemic, providers had to quickly adapt and learn how to provide patient care and communicate with primary care teams mostly via telemedicine. The institutions created training for providers to learn and use skills on the go, which otherwise would have taken months to adapt. This change had its benefits, but also added more complications to care and lead to the stress of a rapid change. In addition, previously colocated psychiatric providers moved to virtual care and were no longer physically present in the clinics. This made traditional integrated care collaboration harder among teammates with less curbside consultations. Now, outreach to PCPs needed to be more intentional to build those relationships. In addition, communication using technology (eg, emails, text messages) increased and likely added more work for providers. Social distancing during stressful times among providers also led to social isolation and decreased peer support and affected building relationships with new providers in the clinic. This is all in the context of the worsening of provider's mental health during the pandemic with higher rates of depression and anxiety most notably in the front-line workers.[18] There has also been an increase in burnout rates among providers leading to the loss of team members potentially derailing integrated care efforts. In some places providers needed to be reassigned to different departments with limited resources and increased need. In most cases, team-based care would be considered somewhat immune to some of these problems, but the disruption of established work routines, the added stress of a crisis, and the potential loss of team members revealed the multiple ways the pandemic disrupted team-based care.

Scope

As pandemic restrictions began to be implemented and telehealth ramped up, outpatient and inpatient care for SMI and SUD were reduced.[19] Community mental health centers were found to lack the necessary equipment to deliver telehealth and had reduced delivery of mental health services because of staff illness or lack of childcare.[20] Substance use treatment centers faced similar problems resulting in having to restrict new admissions.[21] At the same time, telehealth stripped away the physical separation that partly defined specialty care and thus highlighted the similarities between integrated care and specialty care to a greater degree. Whether a psychiatrist worked out of the specialty mental health clinic or the primary care clinic, both visits happened over telehealth and the clinician would use the same clinical skills. Support staff services were reduced at both sites often resulting in similar levels of care being offered as defined by clinical contacts, therapy performed, and medication management offered. This reduced access and reduction in service offerings was likely a significant contributor to pushing existing integrated care models to expand their scope of care because there were limited options to refer people to specialty clinics that were not able to offer a higher level of care. Clinician inertia caused by previous limitations in training were overlooked out of necessity and offered an important opportunity to recognize the inherent generalizability of their clinical skillset.

Capacity/Access

The concept of using telemedicine as part of, or as augmentation to integrated care is not new and has been successfully deployed for the last few decades.[5,22–24] However, it took the COVID-19 pandemic to force systems to embrace telemedicine in all areas of the medical system including mental health.[16] In a recent analysis of telehealth claims during the pandemic the transition to telehealth was dramatic, with mental and behavioral telehealth claims far outpacing all other insurance claims by a factor of five, peaking at more than 5 million in April 2020.[25] Telehealth seems to offer improved access for patients with logistical barriers, competing such demands as work schedules, and mobility problems.[26] It also offered the opportunity to use technology to provide appointments for patients who would have canceled their appointment or even fill an appointment slot that became empty at the last minute. Along with the rest of medicine all aspects of integrated care were converted to remote care. In particular, the pandemic facilitated the growth of indirect integrated care efforts, such as eConsults, Project ECHO, and psychiatric consultation hotlines providing an unprecedented level of access to psychiatric care.[22,27,28] The full impact on telemedicine interventions during COVID is still being studied. However, overall, these efforts seem similar to what was seen before COVID but on a significantly larger scale: decreased wait times to see specialists, decreased no-show rates, and decreased travel times.[22,29]

THE POSTPANDEMIC STATE OF INTEGRATED CARE

System Flexibility

Before the pandemic, integrated care, and CoCM in particular, had emerged as arguably the most evidence-based approach to address common mental health issues in primary care settings. That said, the complexities of implementation and reimbursement issues, including restrictions around telehealth reimbursement, likely slowed the adoption of this model to a significant extent, and kept it from expanding to include regular telehealth integration. Although the pandemic made the biggest impact by temporarily eliminating telehealth reimbursement restrictions, it also highlighted the vulnerabilities of a complex program, such as integrated care, to adapt to change, and the need for a broader population lens to address patients who may not even be on the integrated care radar. It is clear integrated care and CoCM are the right direction to proceed, but there are a few essential changes that should be retained from the pandemic that further enhance the impact of CoCM at a systems level. In particular, the reimbursement for telehealth needs to continue and the regulatory restrictions remain lifted to help facilitate the ongoing use and development and innovation of telehealth.[29] Furthermore, the lessons learned around reimbursement and implementation should not be lost when it comes to the need to simplify CoCM billing codes, where expanded use of these billing codes could further help support and sustain CoCM programs. Workflows should become more adaptable, being flexible enough to incorporate in-person and virtual visits. This helps meet the varying needs of an organization's patient population. Finally, an integrated care team should view their population of patients as the same population as the clinic at large and have access to the population management tools to accompany this vision. In particular, this approach can leverage the positive impact that CoCM can have on reducing disparities in providing effective mental health care to at-risk populations.[30]

Team-Based Care

Team-based care has become the default approach to integrated care and has occurred through onsite and telehealth options. In addition to treating patients, integrated team-based care has helped improve the knowledge and confidence of the PCPs in treating mental health disorders partly because of those incidental conversations during colocated care.[31] Unfortunately, with the transition to telehealth the collaboration between team members has been altered and led some teams to take more intentional steps to maintain the team dynamic. Using technology to do informal educational sessions, offering office hours for clinic providers to drop-in, and prompt replies to questions over the electronic health record have become regular tasks for the consulting psychiatrist and might be worthwhile maintaining. Several qualitative studies found collaboration is improved by a supportive clinic culture, minimizing power dynamics among staff, and constant informal shared communication.[32] At the same time telepsychiatry often limits communication to written form, which may pose challenges for collaboration that requires planning to overcome.[33] Building in time to allow members of the team to use technology to provide ongoing contact, education, and communication is important to maintain a resilient and effective collaborative care team.

Scope

It is clear the pandemic placed pressures on all integrated care teams to expand their scope of treatment to help meet the increased need across the spectrum of mental illness. However, it is not clear how these teams responded, despite the evidence that collaborative care can address the spectrum of mental illness. That said, the disruption introduced a moment in time where practices had to be more flexible just to keep seeing the patients they normally see and potentially see some of the patients who had nowhere else to go. This moment in time should be examined and that imposed flexibility fostered as the pandemic begins to recede. Integrated care teams should look at what types of patients they saw during this time, how those patients did, and how long they followed them for. They should ask if there were any differences in the type of care they delivered and how the existing skill set of the team was adequate or not. In many cases teams may be surprised to realize that they were able to provide the care needed across the spectrum of mental health problems and that many of the therapeutic skills and case management skills were applicable.

Capacity/Access

How patients and providers access each other has been changed by the pandemic. Telepsychiatry adoption across the US hospital system was low and has significant variations state to state.[34] Despite this, many systems have successfully pivoted to incorporate some form of telemedicine. An academic center that converted to telepsychiatry self-surveyed during and after the process. They found that their providers adapted quickly to virtual platforms, noted potential advantages to the modalities, and even suggested that virtual care would be a permanent component of their practice in the future.[35] It is unlikely that telepsychiatry will return to prepandemic utilization levels. With this in mind, it is important to revisit the integrated care model and key strategies that helped maintain access to integrated care. One strength of collaborate care is in multiple team member assessments that go into making a provisional diagnosis and ongoing communications/collaboration. Now, with telehealth, the psychiatrist can offer an accessible diagnostic evaluation, and patients have more options to make it to their appointments. Although this increase in access offers opportunities, it also presents challenges. One of the markers of sustainability of a collaborative care program was psychiatrist engagement.[3] New vigilance is needed to be in place for psychiatrists to remain connected to the team and patients while offering teleappointments. In the end, the stronger the integrated team, the better capacity one has. Finally, emerging integrated care efforts through the expanded use of technology, such as ECHO programs, provider consult hotlines, or eConsults, is building capacity within the existing workforce and should continue. These models offer the potential for further innovation in capacity/access.

SUMMARY

Many of the changes we have discussed have supported more flexible approaches to delivering integrated care. For example, the rapid transition to telehealth required new workflows to offer more options to collect the information needed to deliver a strong measurement-based treat-to-target approach. Another example is the ability to deliver a hybrid of telehealth and direct service, which could allow for improved engagement in visits. Engagement is an important target in integrated mental health because close follow-up after initial visit has been shown to be associated with better depression outcomes in the CoCM.[36] The continued use of a variety of communication channels, such as televideo and even telephone, is helpful for facilitating important collaborative care functions, such as the psychiatric case review process. Continued flexibility in how teams can deliver this important structure in the CoCM is associated with improved depression outcomes.[37] Each of these examples highlights that the opportunity of the postpandemic state is to continue to creatively create workflows that deliver core components of quality care with the resources available to the clinic.

The pandemic has highlighted the need for more efficient and scalable ways to deliver mental health care and this represents an opportunity to continue to highlight the need for new and more adaptable models of integrated health. Continuing to silo mental health care makes it challenging to adapt to the needs of the population and is less flexible in cases like a public health emergency. Implementing an integrated care model allows for adaptable, scalable, and sustainable practice that adequately addresses the growing mental health needs of the public.[38] The pandemic has only underscored the need for improved mental health access, and with an ongoing shortage of mental health providers, integrated care brings specialty expertise directly into the primary care setting where most patients are being seen for mental health care. Combining the fact that there is now widespread adoption of telehealth services and evidence that the CoCM is effectively delivered remotely, this provides an additional option for systems to deliver integrated care. This is a particularly important time for practices to invest in careful monitoring of their newly implemented collaborative care programs and invest in thoughtful sustainment of these efforts because it can take up to 2 years for organizations to achieve meaningful population-level improvement in depression outcomes.[39] Practices may need to consider how to build larger caseloads, aim to have a full-time behavioral health care manager, and engage in continuous quality improvement to achieve strong depression outcomes because these factors have been associated with more sustainable programs.[3] Lastly, with the ability to use CoCM billing codes to capture the time of the behavioral health care manager over a calendar month, CoCM teams could have more flexibility to engage with patients that is more financially sustainable and resilient to future disruptions. As health care systems begin to return to more normal routines, there is the opportunity to consider which of the many rapid changes that needed to be made to function during the pandemic should be kept.

CLINICS CARE POINTS

- Potential pitfalls of a CoCM program clinicians not having adequate time built for team meetings and maintaining the registry competing priorities for the care manager or PCP variable psychiatric consultant involvement not using the Collaborative Care CPT codes scope of Collaborative Care program is inflexibly narrow difficulty in building a caseload due to rigidity in patients accessing the program
- Emerging Strategies to build a resilient and flexible CoCM program Use the CoCM CPT codes to allow for more flexible service delivery instead of relying on fee-for-service codes.
- Leverage telehealth options for patient visits and psychiatric consultation Nurture the integrated team through educational updates, informal office hours/curbsides, and program updates
- Support skill development and clinical confidence of team members to support a broader spectrum of mental health problems.

DISCLOSURE

Dr A.D.H. Ratzliff receives Royalties from Wiley for Integrated Care book. No disclosures for the rest of the authors.

REFERENCES

1. Peek C. National integration academy council, *Lexicon for behavioral Health and primary care integration: concepts and definitions developed by expert consensus*. Rockville, MD: Agency for Healthcare Research and Quality; 2013.
2. Archer J, Bower P, Gilbody S, et al. Collaborative care for depression and anxiety problems. Cochrane Database Syst Rev 2012;10:CD006525.
3. Moise N, Shah RN, Essock S, et al. Sustainability of collaborative care management for depression in primary care settings with academic affiliations across New York State. Implement Sci 2018;13(1):128.
4. Fortney JC, Pyne JM, Edlund MJ, et al. A randomized trial of telemedicine-based collaborative care for depression. J Gen Intern Med 2007;22(8):1086–93.
5. Fortney JC, Pyne JM, Turner EE, et al. Telepsychiatry integration of mental health services into rural primary care settings. Int Rev Psychiatry 2015;27(6):525–39.
6. May C, Gask L, Atkinson T, et al. Resisting and promoting new technologies in clinical practice: the case of telepsychiatry. Soc Sci Med 2001;52(12):1889–901.
7. Press MJ, Howe R, Schoenbaum M, et al. Medicare payment for behavioral health integration. N Engl J Med 2017;376(5):405–7.
8. Cross DA, Qin X, Huckfeldt P, et al. Use of Medicare's behavioral health integration service codes in the first two years: an observational study. J Gen Intern Med 2020;35(12):3745–6.
9. Carlo AD, Drake L, Ratzliff ADH, et al. Sustaining the Collaborative Care Model (CoCM): billing newly available CoCM CPT codes in an academic primary care system. Psychiatr Serv 2020;71(9):972–4.
10. Heath B, Wise Romero P, Reynolds KA. In: SAMHSA-HRSA, editor. Standard framework for levels of integrated healthcare. Washington DC: Center for Integrated Health Solutions; 2013.
11. Erickson JM, Ratzliff A. Integrated care. In: Lavakumar M, Rosenthal LJ, Rabinowitz T, editors. Fundamentals of consultation liaison psychiatry: principles and practice. Hauppauge, New York: Nova Science Pub Inc; 2019. p. 51.
12. Beil H, Feinberg RK, Patel SV, et al. Behavioral health integration with primary care: implementation experience and impacts from the state innovation model round 1 states. Milbank Q 2019;97(2):543–82.
13. Ustün TB, Goldberg D, Cooper J, et al. New classification for mental disorders with management guidelines for use in primary care: ICD-10 PHC chapter five. Br J Gen Pract 1995;45(393):211–5.
14. Park J, Svendsen D, Singer P, et al., Morbidity and Mortality, People with Serious Mental Illness 2006, National Association of State Mental Health Program Directors(NASMHPD), Medical Directors Council; Alexandria, VA.
15. Mundon CR, Anderson ML, Najavits LM. Attitudes toward substance abuse clients: an empirical study of clinical psychology trainees. J Psychoactive Drugs 2015;47(4):293–300.
16. Mehrotra A, Chernew M, Linetsky D, et al., The impact of COVID-19 on outpatient visits in 2020: visits remained stable, despite a late surge in cases, The Commonwealth Fund; New York, New York.
17. Shapiro PA, Brahmbhatt K, Caravella R, et al. Report of the Academy of consultation-liaison psychiatry task force on lessons learned from the COVID-19 pandemic: executive summary. J Acad Consult Liaison Psychiatry 2021; 62(4):377–86.
18. Unutzer J, Kimmel RJ, Snowden M. Psychiatry in the age of COVID-19. World Psychiatry 2020;19(2):130–1.

19. Bojdani E, Rajagopalan A, Chen A, et al. COVID-19 pandemic: impact on psychiatric care in the United States. Psychiatry Res 2020;289:113069.
20. CBHA summary of CBHA member survey on the effects of COVID-19. Sacramento, California.
21. Kedia SK, Schmidt M, Dillon PJ, et al. Substance use treatment in Appalachian Tennessee amid COVID-19: challenges and preparing for the future. J Subst Abuse Treat 2021;124:108270.
22. Hilt RJ. Telemedicine for child collaborative or integrated care. Child Adolesc Psychiatr Clin N Am 2017;26(4):637–45.
23. Hilty DM, Rabinowitz T, McCarron RM, et al. An update on telepsychiatry and how it can leverage collaborative, stepped, and integrated services to primary care. Psychosomatics 2017;59(3):227–50.
24. Waugh M, Calderone J, Brown Levey S, et al. Using telepsychiatry to enrich existing integrated primary care. Telemed J E Health 2019;25(8):762–8.
25. Group TC. Telehealth impact: claims data analysis. McLean, Virginia: COVID-19 Healthcare Coalition; 2021.
26. Sugarman DE, Horvitz LE, Greenfield SF, et al, Horvitz LE, Greenfield SF,. Clinicians' perceptions of rapid scale-up of telehealth services in outpatient mental health treatment. Telemed J E Health 2021;27(12):1399–408.
27. Komaromy M, Bartlett J, Manis K, et al. Enhanced primary care treatment of behavioral disorders with ECHO case-based learning. Psychiatr Serv 2017;68(9):873–5.
28. Di Carlo F, Sociali A, Picutti E, et al. Telepsychiatry and other cutting-edge technologies in COVID-19 pandemic: bridging the distance in mental health assistance. Int J Clin Pract 2021;75(1):e13716.
29. Wahezi S, Kohan L, Cornett E, et al. Telemedicine and current clinical practice trends in a COVID-19 pandemic. Best Pract Res Clin Anaesthesiol 2020;35(3):307–19.
30. Angstman KB, Phelan S, Myszkowski MR, et al. Minority primary care patients with depression: outcome disparities improve with collaborative care management. Med Care 2015;53(1):32–7.
31. Turkozer HB, Ongur D. A projection for psychiatry in the post-COVID-19 era: potential trends, challenges, and directions. Mol Psychiatry 2020;25(10):2214–9.
32. Morgan S, Pullon S, McKinlay E. Observation of interprofessional collaborative practice in primary care teams: an integrative literature review. Int J Nurs Stud 2015;52(7):1217–30.
33. Bjorkquist C, Forss M, Samuelsen F. Collaborative challenges in the use of telecare. Scand J Caring Sci 2019;33(1):93–101.
34. Li Z, Harrison SE, Li X, et al. Telepsychiatry adoption across hospitals in the United States: a cross-sectional study. BMC Psychiatry 2021;21(1):182.
35. Parikh SV, Taubman DS, Grambeau M, et al. Going virtual during a pandemic: an academic psychiatry department's experience with telepsychiatry. Psychopharmacol Bull 2021;51(1):59–68.
36. Bao Y, Druss BG, Jung HY, et al. Unpacking collaborative care for depression: examining two essential tasks for implementation. Psychiatr Serv 2016;67(4):418–24.
37. Sowa NA, Jeng P, Bauer AM, et al. Psychiatric case review and treatment intensification in collaborative care management for depression in primary care. Psychiatr Serv 2018;69(5):549–54.
38. Carlo AD, Barnett BS, Unützer J. Harnessing Collaborative Care to Meet Mental Health Demands in the Era of COVID-19. JAMA Psychiatry 2021;78(4):355–6.
39. Carlo AD, Jeng PJ, Bao Y, et al. The learning curve after implementation of collaborative care in a state mental health integration program. Psychiatr Serv 2019;70(2):139–42.

The Impact of Coronavirus Disease 2019 on US Emergency Departments

Manuel G. Alvarez Romero, BA[a], Chandra Penthala, BA[a], Scott L. Zeller, MD[b,c,*], Michael P. Wilson, MD, PhD[a,d]

KEYWORDS

- Behavioral emergencies • COVID-19 • Emergency department • Hospitalization
- Mental health • Pandemic

KEY POINTS

- Behavioral emergencies in the United States are increasing with some studies even reporting a doubling in the number of people experiencing symptoms related to mental health conditions, although visits to US EDs decreased during the COVID-19 pandemic.
- Emergency departments have experienced substantial volume changes throughout the coronavirus disease 2019 (COVID-19) pandemic.
- Health care professionals, especially those working in emergency department, have been mentally and financially challenged by the effects of the COVID-19 pandemic.

INTRODUCTION

The emergence of a fast-spreading, novel infectious respiratory virus in late 2019 caused alarm among public health officials, health care providers, and the general public. The World Health Organization declared the coronavirus disease 2019 (COVID-19) outbreak a pandemic on March 11, 2020, and by that date, several countries around the world were already confronting the rapid spread of the novel coronavirus (COVID-19) within their borders. In the United States, one of the initial and immediate impacts of this declaration, and of the emergency declaration by the US government[1] 2 days later on March 13, was an overall decrease in the number of patients presenting for emergency care.[2,3] This overall decrease in patient volume early in the pandemic was in stark contrast to a common trend that emergency departments (EDs) have experienced in recent years before the pandemic: substantial overcrowding.[4]

[a] Department of Emergency Medicine, University of Arkansas for Medical Sciences, 4301 W. Markham Street, Slot #584, Little Rock, AR 72205, USA; [b] Department of Psychiatry, University of California-Riverside, Riverside, CA, USA; [c] Acute Psychiatry, Vituity, Emeryville, CA, USA; [d] Department of Psychiatry, University of Arkansas for Medical Sciences, 4301 W. Markham Street, Slot #584, Little Rock, AR 72205, USA
* Corresponding author. 21-C Orinda Way #221, Orinda, CA 94563.
E-mail address: scott.zeller@vituity.com

Psychiatr Clin N Am 45 (2022) 81–94
https://doi.org/10.1016/j.psc.2021.11.005

The impact of COVID-19 on EDs is unprecedented in modern times. The first part of this article provides an overview of the major changes experienced by EDs both before COVID-19 and during the peak of the COVID-19 pandemic, including some of the major challenges in caring for patients with behavioral emergencies. The second part of this article discusses strategies for rational ED management of these patients during the pandemic and postpandemic periods. As the impact of COVID-19 on medical practice may continue for some time and thus influence the care of psychiatric patients in EDs for the foreseeable future, it is important to consider the impact of these changes on care for patients with behavioral emergencies.

EMERGENCY DEPARTMENT TRENDS BEFORE CORONAVIRUS DISEASE 2019

Before COVID-19, EDs provided more than half of all medical care in the United States,[5] and despite the fact that emergency medicine only became an official specialty in 1979, these have long been recognized as the primary clinical setting in which patients received emergency care.[6] The onset of the COVID-19 pandemic represented the first decrease in visits to US EDs, which before that time had experienced increases in patient volumes for decades. Between 2010 and 2014, for instance, the rate of increase in overall ED utilization was greater than the growth rate of the US population.[7] In particular, EDs experienced large increases in patient volumes in patients with behavioral emergencies.[8,9] Between 2006 and 2014, for instance, ED visits for behavioral emergencies overall increased by 44%, whereas visits by patients for some behavioral emergencies, such as suicidal ideation and self-harm, more than quadrupled.[10] Before COVID-19, resources to treat this patient population did not keep up with the demand. According to a 2016 American College of Emergency Physicians (ACEP) survey, for example, only 17% of emergency physicians had on-call psychiatrists to consult, whereas 11% of respondents reported having no specialist at all to consult for any patient with mental health conditions or substance abuse issues.[10]

EMERGENCY DEPARTMENT CHANGES IN PATIENT VOLUMES DURING CORONAVIRUS DISEASE 2019

In the early stages of its spread, limited information on this novel disease was available to both public health officials and health care providers.[11] In geographic areas with high rates of COVID-19 infection, some health systems implemented outdoor facilities for treating patients with symptoms of COVID-19 infection.[12] Federal agencies, like the Centers for Disease Control and Prevention (CDC), state public health departments, and private organizations, issued numerous recommendations and mandates intended to limit the spread of the virus in the community.[13,14] Although these changes were presumably made to limit the spread of COVID-19, many changes may have unfortunately had some unintentional consequences as well, such as leading people to delay emergency care and preventing others from receiving ongoing treatment.[15]

Despite efforts by public health officials and others to assure the public that they could safely seek emergency care, many individuals began delaying treatment of many important health concerns such as ischemic heart disease.[16] In sharp contrast to decades of growth, some initial reports indicated that EDs in the United States experienced as much as a 50% decrease in utilization during the early pandemic period.[15] In one study at a community hospital in California, for instance, qualitative interviews with patients about changes in behavior and attitude toward hospital use revealed that patients experienced an overwhelming sense of fear.[15] This fear, as stated by the patients, prevented them from seeking emergency care. Specifically, these patients expressed fears of contracting COVID-19 in hospitals, unfamiliarity with the efforts implemented by the hospital to limit the spread of COVID-19, and uncertainty about the urgency of their particular medical concern.[15] Collectively, these fears potentially contributed to the significant reduction in ED volumes early the pandemic as discussed earlier.

CORONAVIRUS DISEASE 2019 IMPACTS ON MENTAL HEALTH PRESENTATIONS TO US EMERGENCY DEPARTMENTS

In addition to reductions in the number of individuals seeking emergency care, the COVID-19 pandemic and some of the public health measures implemented to reduce the spread of the virus may have simultaneously exacerbated the severity of ongoing substance use (see section "Coronavirus disease 2019 impacts on substance use disorders"), symptoms of preexisting mental health conditions, and increased the rates of newly arising behavioral health diagnoses (see later). Most mitigation measures, for instance, involved loss of social connections[17] by limiting or restricting public gatherings, closing numerous businesses and schools, limiting outdoor activity, and prohibiting individuals from gathering in large groups, which may have worsened symptoms in patients with preexisting mental health conditions. One study analyzed self-reported responses from an online mental health questionnaire and concluded that respondents with a diagnosed psychiatric disorder had significantly worse anxiety and depression symptoms.[18] In addition, 17.9% of respondents with a diagnosed psychiatric disorder reported an increase in suicidal ideation severity compared with only 3.8% of respondents without a diagnosed psychiatric disorder who reported an increase.[18]

At the same time, individuals experienced increasing stressors, such as fear of COVID-19 infection, loss of income, and social isolation.[19] The combination of additional stressors, worsened symptoms in patients with preexisting disease, and increased rates of new diagnoses were catastrophic for the mental health of many individuals.[20] According to surveys administered by the CDC in June 2020, for instance, 40.9% of respondents reported having experienced symptoms related to several behavioral health conditions, including depressive disorder and substance use disorder.[21]

At the same time, EDs experienced reductions in presentations for behavioral health issues,[22,23] although the percent decrease in psychiatric-related visits to general EDs may have been less than the overall decrease in patient visits for other conditions in some locations within the United States.[24,25] In one survey of billing data from 141 EDs in 16 states, for instance, the greatest decrease was seen in the nonemergent encounters, with the smallest decrease for substance abuse visits.[24] Given the increase in rates of anxiety/depression and the increase in drug overdose deaths, however, the smaller decreases in presentations for behavioral health emergencies is not comforting and likely represents a large underutilization of the ED for this group of patients.

The decrease in utilization of mental health services has been reported across different types of facilities providing emergency care. One study comparing patient volume and dispositions in Veteran's Affairs (VA) psychiatric EDs from March to August 2020 to the same period from 3 prior years, for instance, measured an overall decrease in visits with the greatest decrease in April 2020 during the pandemic. This decrease in VA psychiatric ED visits coincided with a peak in COVID-19 cases, suggesting that veterans may have postponed mental health and substance use treatment during that time. If so, this may potentially foreshadow the increased demand for mental health and substance use services in the future, although likely in patients with worsened or more severe disease.[26]

In contrast to adults, the number of mental health-related ED visits among pediatric patients had a more variable course, with fluctuations during the COVID-19 pandemic. According to the CDC's National Syndromic Surveillance Program, mental health-related ED visits among children were higher during the January 1 to March 15, 2020, period than during the similar period in the preceding year.[27] Similarly, one pediatric ED recorded significantly higher rates of suicidal ideation and attempts from February to March 2020 and during the month of July 2020 when compared with the same months in the preceding year.[28] However, pediatric ED visits decreased by 43% from mid-March to early April during the peak of the pandemic but then gradually increased through October 2020.[27]

THE INCREASE IN DOMESTIC VIOLENCE DURING CORONAVIRUS DISEASE 2019

In addition to contributing to an increased rate of new behavioral health diagnoses and the association with worsened symptoms in patients with preexisting behavioral health diagnoses, the increased time at home may have contributed to an increase in domestic violence incidents.[29] Domestic violence has been increasing throughout many countries since the onset of the pandemic.[30] Some COVID-19 mitigation measures, including shelter-in-place mandates, coupled with stress induced by social isolation and financial insecurity have perpetuated domestic violence incidents. Countries across Europe, Asia, South America, and agencies in the United States have reported increased incidents of domestic violence, and some perpetrators have used the fears surrounding the COVID-19 virus to torment their victims.[30]

CORONAVIRUS DISEASE 2019 IMPACTS ON SUBSTANCE USE DISORDERS

The United States experienced an unprecedented increase in overdose deaths during the pandemic, with approximately a 60% increase in drug deaths in May 2020 compared with the previous year.[31] Opioids are predominantly involved in overdose deaths in the United States, accounting for 70.6% of all overdose deaths in 2019.[32] One study examining opioid overdose deaths in Cook County, Illinois, before, during, and after an 11-week COVID-19 stay-at-home order, for instance, found that opioid-related deaths increased during the stay-at-home order period.[33] Another study using medical examiner data in San Francisco documented decreases in deaths for opioids and cocaine but a significant increase for deaths attributable to fentanyl.[34] These findings further support the theory that individuals may be delaying treatment of substance use disorders, particularly opioid use disorder, which is similar to the delay in seeking medical care for other conditions. There is also evidence that individuals may be increasingly misusing drugs to cope with COVID-19 stressors. Specifically, surveys conducted on US adults during the COVID-19 pandemic recorded increased behavioral health concerns with initiation of or increase in substance use.[35] According to Millennium Health, there was a sharp increase in the positivity rate for several substances, including nonprescribed fentanyl and methamphetamine, after the declaration of the COVID-19 national emergency on March 13, 2020, by the US government.[36]

INCREASED SUSCEPTIBILITY OF PATIENTS WITH PREEXISTING MENTAL HEALTH CONDITIONS TO CORONAVIRUS DISEASE 2019

Paradoxically, although the number of patients with behavioral health emergencies presenting to EDs decreased during the COVID-19 pandemic,[37] there is some evidence that patients with preexisting mental health conditions are at higher risk of contracting COVID-19 and have poorer outcomes if they do become infected. In one study, a preexisting psychiatric diagnosis was independently associated with an increased risk of contracting COVID-19.[38] Patients with schizophrenia, for instance, experience a greater risk of contracting and transmitting COVID-19 during the pandemic, perhaps in part because of the lower awareness of risk and fewer barriers to adequate infection control.[39] In addition, many patients with mental health conditions, including those with schizophrenia, have a greater number of medical comorbidities such as substance use disorders. According to a meta-analysis of worldwide studies, more than 60% of people with schizophrenia are frequent smokers,[40] placing them at higher risk of disease progression and poor outcomes from COVID-19. In one study, schizophrenia ranked only second to age in significance of association with mortality among patients with confirmed COVID-19.[41]

In another study, researchers analyzed the association of being recently diagnosed with a mental health disorder such as attention-deficit/hyperactivity disorder, bipolar disorder, depression, and schizophrenia with the risk of contracting COVID-19 and the related mortality. Patients recently diagnosed with a mental disorder had a significantly increased risk of contracting COVID-19 with the strongest association being with depression and schizophrenia. The COVID-19-related mortality rate for patients recently diagnosed with a mental disorder was nearly double (8.5% versus 4.7%) that of patients with COVID-19 without a mental disorder.[42] The bidirectional association between COVID-19 and psychiatric disorders makes mental health an especially vulnerable and integral aspect of COVID-19 health outcomes.[38]

The reduction in ED presentations for medical conditions may have also had deleterious effects on patients with preexisting behavioral health diagnoses. As the COVID-19 pandemic has caused an economic recession and disrupted outpatient mental health services, preexisting mental health conditions could worsen, leading to patients with greater agitation during an ED encounter. Furthermore, other COVID-19 data suggest that individuals with milder symptoms have refrained from visiting EDs, whereas those who have visited EDs actually presented more severe forms of agitation and delirium.[43]

IMPACTS OF CORONAVIRUS DISEASE 2019 ON PERSISTENT NEUROPSYCHIATRIC SYMPTOMS

Although transmitted via the respiratory system, it has long been recognized that COVID-19 does not remain confined to the upper respiratory tract. In an early study of 214 patients from Wuhan, China, 36.4% had central nervous system (CNS) symptoms or disorders.[44] Subsequent articles[45–47] have reported the existence of symptoms after resolution of COVID-19 infection, often termed "long-haul COVID." Although the most common symptoms reported are related to the respiratory nature of the virus such as dyspnea, patients in one study experienced psychiatric symptoms, such as anxiety and depression, after a COVID-19 diagnosis.[38] In one retrospective cohort study, the most common psychiatric disorder diagnoses within 3 months after COVID-19 infection were anxiety, insomnia, and dementia.

The cause of psychiatric symptoms in long-haul COVID is unclear, and puzzlingly, it does not seem related to the initial severity of the disease. Previous reports in other novel coronavirus diseases such as Middle East respiratory syndrome have linked psychiatric symptoms like depression to the severity of distress experienced by the patient during illness,[48] but psychiatric symptoms in COVID-19 may instead be related to the severity of the initial inflammatory response.[49] Regardless, when considering the state of current evidence on the psychological effects of COVID-19, further research is urgently needed to improve treatment and therapeutic options.[50]

RESULTING FINANCIAL CHALLENGES TO HOSPITALS

Although the COVID-19 pandemic was associated with worsening symptoms in patients with preexisting behavioral health conditions, increased rates of new diagnoses of mental health and substance use conditions, and poorer outcomes for patients with behavioral health conditions infected with COVID-19, many hospitals, especially those in rural areas,[51] have paradoxically experienced financial difficulties, because reductions in overall patient volumes also had unfortunate consequences for hospital finances. A survey conducted by the ACEP examined the financial impact of COVID-19 on emergency medicine group practices and individual emergency medicine physicians, finding that approximately 21% of surveyed hospitals had to layoff physicians.[52] In addition, those surveyed had a substantial level of uncertainty about the future,[52] leading to the startling conclusion that the emergency medicine workforce may have actually contracted in the midst of a devastating pandemic.

In addition to EDs, hospitals as a whole also suffered financially. The American Hospital Association (AHA), for instance, estimated a $202.6 billion loss between the months of March and June 2020, and another $120.5 billion loss from July to December 2020.[53] This financial loss may have disproportionately affected rural hospitals with a poorer payer mix.[51] This financial impact could have long-term implications on hospital survival. A June 2020 survey by the AHA showed that 67% of hospitals indicated that they did not think they would achieve baseline patient volumes by the end of 2020.[53] Alarmingly, an additional 30% of hospitals reported that the time frame for returning to baseline patient volumes was unknown, or they never expect to return to baseline volumes.[53]

INCREASED STRESS AMONG EMERGENCY DEPARTMENT PHYSICIANS AND STAFF

In addition to economic uncertainty caused by layoffs of medical staff, frontline workers experienced increased symptoms of burnout[54]; this may have resulted from many factors, including the perception that these workers were being tasked with saving lives without appropriate resources. In many locations, a global surge in demand for personal protective equipment (PPE) limited the supply available to health care workers[55] and many staff were asked to continue reusing an N95 respirator until visibly soiled. The uncertainty of a novel virus combined with the possibility of infection significantly increased distress among staff. In one study, 74% of surveyed health care workers reported high amounts of distress,[56] and in another study, almost 50% of respondents reported moderate to severe symptoms of burnout.[54] ED physicians and other providers reported numerous fears, including the possibility of inadvertently infecting themselves or other family members[57]; moral distress from ethical dilemmas, such as decisions on how best to allocate ventilators to intubated patients[58]; and health care disparities due to racial and structural inequalities, which may have imposed further emotional distress related to social justice and human rights.

One positive change for health care workers may have been the widespread measures, implemented by US hospitals, which were intended to slow the spread of the COVID-19 virus. Using CDC recommendations,[13] many hospitals implemented both widespread structural and process changes, including increased use of telehealth,[59] utilization of health screening stations at hospital entrances,[13] mandatory face masks,[14] and limitations on both the number of visitors per patient, which may have increased difficulty in obtaining collateral information,[60] and visitation times.[61] Some research, however, has suggested that these measures have been greeted in a generally positive manner among the public and health care workers.[62] Perhaps more importantly, they may have been effective in detecting and reducing transmission of

COVID-19 in the health care environment. One study, for instance, found that 84.2% of COVID-19 cases were detected at the ED triage by using the official screening criteria followed by broader internal screening criteria.[63] The combined sensitivity of triage plus internal screening was significantly higher than the official screening criteria (84.3% versus 48.6%), suggesting the utility of layered screening. In the same study, surveillance of patients and ED staff who were potentially exposed to a patient with confirmed COVID-19 detected no cases of nosocomial transmission, which the investigators attributed to enhanced safety protocols and appropriate use of PPE by ED staff.[63]

EMERGENCY DEPARTMENT MANAGEMENT STRATEGIES FOR THE PATIENT WITH MENTAL HEALTH CONDITION DURING CORONAVIRUS DISEASE 2019

Despite the seemingly insurmountable challenges posed by the COVID-19 pandemic reviewed earlier, there are several strategies, which although relatively underresearched during the pandemic and postpandemic periods, are thought to be effective for management of behavioral emergencies.[64] Prepandemic, several researchers advocated for methods to improve the care of these patients in the ED, particularly the development of educational training programs for EDs, the initiation of compassionate patient-centered psychotherapeutic interventions early in the ED course, and the development of outpatient mental health treatment capabilities that are able to accept ED referral.[64] The implementation of these strategies is likely still effective in the pandemic and postpandemic periods. In one study, about 16% of COVID-19-positive patients aged 65 years or older presenting to the ED with delirium experienced symptoms of agitation.[65]

Even before COVID-19, emergency care staff often experienced verbal abuse or violent assault. Expert recommendations for pharmacologic management of agitation have not substantially changed since the 2012 BETA project, in part because of the difficulty in performing prospective randomized trials of agitated patients.[66] In patients with agitation both from psychiatric and nonpsychiatric causes (such as hypoxemia resulting from severe COVID-19 disease), verbal deescalation remains first-line therapy. If needed, antipsychotics or other calming medication should be administered orally,[67] with second-generation antipsychotics being preferred.[68,69] Although underresearched, COVID-19 is likely to accelerate the need for these ED interventions, not replace them.

As a result of the pandemic, there has been a renewed focus on the importance of proper identification and treatment of behavioral health issues in the ED through appropriate screening, intervention, and referral. Given the many precipitating factors related to COVID-19, EDs may simply not find it feasible to continue boarding psychiatric patients without treatment for long periods. Unfortunately, admission to psychiatric inpatient facilities also presents challenges. Many inpatient units are constructed with communal areas. Although this may promote therapeutic interactions,[70] it may also paradoxically increase the risk for spread of any respiratory disease. In some cases, it may be difficult for patients to properly adhere to mitigation measures, such as requirements for masking.

In an effort to further limit the spread of COVID-19 within the health care setting, some hospitals across the United States have implemented the use of rapid COVID-19 testing before a patient can be admitted to psychiatry services.[71] A positive test result can change the course of treatment of the patient, because patients are typically admitted to a dedicated COVID-19 unit or other unit with the capability for enhanced infectious diseases protocols. The need to isolate COVID-19-positive patients receiving psychiatric care may also lead to increased stressors for these patients.[72]

EMERGENCY DEPARTMENT MENTAL HEALTH INNOVATIONS DURING THE PANDEMIC

One positive development for the care of emergency psychiatric patients during the pandemic was the acceleration of interest and demand for innovative approaches to treat this population in EDs. As health systems reviewed their ED capacity with an eye toward possible COVID surges, the persistent phenomena of "boarding"—otherwise medically stable emergency psychiatric patients remaining in the ED for long hours, awaiting transfer to an elusive inpatient psychiatric hospital bed—seemed an ideal target for improvement.

As many patients nationwide boarding in EDs had historically been referred directly to psychiatric facilities by the ED staff, without any evaluation by mental health professionals, the improved strategy of addition of on-demand emergency telepsychiatry consultations had become more commonplace over the past decade.[73] On-demand emergency telepsychiatry offered the chance for a timely expert psychiatrist consultation at an ED patient's bedside over videoconferencing, allowing for greater possibility of recommendations for discharges or alternative dispositions besides inpatient hospitalization, which then could lead to reduced lengths of stay and enhanced bed turnover.[74] On-demand emergency telepsychiatry may be more cost-effective than hiring an onsite specialist and allows a single psychiatrist to see patients at multiple hospitals in one shift without transportation delays or wasted intervals between consultations.[75] However, although on-demand emergency telepsychiatry had been proved as relatively safe, effective, and well-accepted by patients for several years, regulations nationwide had still often been a barrier.[76] New policies allowing wider use of telemedicine during the pandemic opened the door for far more EDs to commence with on-demand emergency telepsychiatry programs, improving access to psychiatric care while also reducing percentages of psychiatric hospitalizations and boarding times.[77,78]

In another recent innovation, owing to the recognition that standard EDs may be a suboptimal environment for psychiatric emergency care, several hospitals looking to prepare for surges during the pandemic created external mental-health-only observation units, to which medically clear ED psychiatric patients could be swiftly moved for targeted care with trained personnel, thus opening up beds in the ED for nonpsychiatric emergency patients.[79,80] These programs, also known as EmPATH units (Emergency Psychiatry Assessment, Treatment and Healing units) feature a more spacious, calming, and homelike atmosphere,[81] with prompt access to psychiatric providers, and have been demonstrated to alleviate most emergency psychiatric patient conditions to subacute status in less than 24 hours; this has resulted in a reported 70% or more of individuals, who in previous protocols would have been boarding in EDs awaiting inpatient admission, instead being discharged to community levels of care, preserving the limited inpatient beds for those patients with truly no alternative to psychiatric hospitalization.[82]

The authors are aware of several EmPATH units that were able to assist their affiliated EDs even further during the pandemic, and that was via moving medically stable and asymptomatic, yet COVID test-positive acute psychiatric patients out of the ED into specific isolation rooms in the EmPATH unit reserved for this purpose. In relocating these patients from the hectic ED into a more serene setting, the psychiatric professionals on the EmPATH unit could commence psychiatric interventions and better assess these patients for an appropriate and swift disposition, either discharging to home for quarantining, or transfer to an inpatient psychiatric ward reserved for patients with COVID. In doing this ED capacity was increased, whereas the EmPATH unit was used for the primary purpose of the patient visit—psychiatric assessment and treatment—all while maintaining safety protocols.

EXPECTATIONS FOR THE NEAR FUTURE

As the nation comes out of the pandemic and lockdowns, there are indications that the next wave of impact for hospitals may be one of dramatically increasing numbers of behavioral health emergency patients presenting to EDs, many of whom delayed seeking assistance previously due to infection concerns.[83,84] Thus the true overall mental health consequences of COVID-19 for EDs may be yet to be fully determined.

SUMMARY

The ability to address mental health and substance abuse issues in the ED became more difficult during the COVID-19 pandemic. Challenges to appropriate care of these patients, reviewed in this article, include the underutilization of EDs during the peak of the pandemic, COVID-19-related financial challenges, and increased stress among ED staff. Unfortunately, these changes occurred at a time when many EDs across the country were already facing numerous challenges, ranging from overcrowding to the need for additional resources.

Much of the prepandemic research on the proper approach to behavioral health patients likely remains valid but may have to be flexibly implemented alongside strategies intended to limit the spread of COVID-19. During the pandemic, many EDs used alternative facility space, implemented entrance screening stations, and limited patient visitations. Although some impacts of the COVID-19 pandemic on EDs may resolve in the postpandemic period, many challenges will remain. Thus, health care providers will still need to look to innovative strategies and implement appropriate solutions for the ongoing issues in emergency psychiatry.

DISCLOSURE

Dr M.P. Wilson is an Associate Editor of the Journal of Emergency Medicine. Drs M.P. Wilson and S.L. Zeller are editors of the 2017 book *The Diagnosis and Management of Agitation*. The authors have no other relevant financial interests to disclose.

REFERENCES

1. Bragg L. President Trump Declares State of Emergency for COVID-19. National Conference of State Legislatures. 2020. Available at: https://www.ncsl.org/ncsl-in-dc/publications-and-resources/president-trump-declares-state-of-emergency-for-covid-19.aspx. Accessed June 25, 2021.
2. Hartnett, Kathleen P, Kite-Powell A, et al. Impact of the COVID-19 Pandemic on Emergency Department Visits. Morb Mortal Wkly Rep 2020;69(23):699–704. Available at: cdc.gov/mmwr/volumes/69/wr/pdfs/mm6923e1-H.pdf.
3. Boserup B, McKenney M, Elkbuli A. The impact of the COVID-19 pandemic on emergency department visits and patient safety in the United States. Am J Emerg Med 2020;38(9):1732–6.
4. Morley C, Unwin M, Peterson GM, et al. Emergency department crowding: A systematic review of causes, consequences and solutions. PLoS One 2018; 13(8):1–42.

5. Marcozzi D, Carr B, Liferidge A, et al. Trends in the Contribution of Emergency Departments to the Provision of Hospital-Associated Health Care in the USA. Int J Heal Serv 2018;48(2):267–88.
6. Suter RE. Emergency medicine in the United States: a systemic review. World J Emerg Med 2012;3(1):5–10.
7. Hooker EA, Mallow PJ, Oglesby MM. Characteristics and Trends of Emergency Department Visits in the United States (2010–2014). J Emerg Med 2019;56(3): 344–51.
8. Larkin GL, Claassen CA, Emond JA, et al. Trends in U.S. emergency department visits for mental health conditions, 1992 to 2001. Psychiatr Serv 2005;56(6): 671–7.
9. Pandya A, Larkin GL, Randles R, et al. Epidemiological trends in psychosis-related Emergency Department visits in the United States, 1992-2001. Schizophr Res 2009;110:28–32.
10. Zeller S. Pandemic Creates Far-Reaching Challenges for Behavioral Healthcare. 2021. Available at: https://www.vituity.com/blog/pandemic-creates-far-reaching-challenges-for-behavioral-healthcare/. Accessed February 17, 2021.
11. Yee J, Unger L, Zadravecz F, et al. Novel coronavirus 2019 (COVID-19): Emergence and implications for emergency care. J Am Coll Emerg Physicians Open 2020;1(2):63–9.
12. Konda SR, Dankert JF, Merkow D, et al. COVID-19 Response in the Global Epicenter: Converting a New York City Level 1 Orthopedic Trauma Service into a Hybrid Orthopedic and Medicine COVID-19 Management Team. J Orthop Trauma 2020;34(8):411–7.
13. Centers for Disease Control and Prevention. Interim infection prevention and control recommendations for healthcare personnel during the coronavirus disease 2019 (COVID-19) pandemic 2020. Available at: https://www.cdc.gov/coronavirus/2019-ncov/hcp/infection-control-recommendations.html. Accessed April 13, 2021.
14. Advani SD, Smith BA, Lewis SS, et al. Universal masking in hospitals in the COVID-19 era: Is it time to consider shielding? Infect Control Hosp Epidemiol 2020;41(9):1066–7.
15. Wong L, Hawkins J, Langness S, et al. Where Are All the Patients? Addressing Covid-19 Fear to Encourage Sick Patients to Seek Emergency Care. NEJM Catal 2020;. https://catalyst.nejm.org/doi/abs/10.1056/CAT.20.0193.
16. Porter A, Brown C, Tilford M, et al. Association of the COVID-19 pandemic and dying at home due to ischemic heart disease. Prev Med 2021;153:106818.
17. Saeri AK, Cruwys T, Barlow FK, et al. Social connectedness improves public mental health: Investigating bidirectional relationships in the New Zealand attitudes and values survey. Aust N Z J Psychiatry 2018;52(4):365–74.
18. Robillard R, Daros AR, Phillips JL, et al. Emerging New Psychiatric Symptoms and the Worsening of Pre-existing Mental Disorders during the COVID-19 Pandemic: A Canadian Multisite Study: Nouveaux symptômes psychiatriques émergents et détérioration des troubles mentaux préexistants pendanturant la p. Can J Psychiatry 2021;1–12.
19. Simon N, Saxe G, Marmar C. Mental Health Disorders Related to COVID-19–Related Deaths. JAMA 2020;324(15):1493–4.
20. Holingue C, Kalb LG, Riehm KE, et al. Mental distress in the United States at the beginning of the covid-19 pandemic. Am J Public Health 2020;110(11):1628–34.

21. Czeisler MÉ, Lane RI, Petrosky E, et al. Mental Health, Substance Use, and Suicidal Ideation During the COVID-19 Pandemic — United States, June 24–30, 2020. Morb Mortal Wkly Rep 2020;69(32):1049–57.
22. Westgard BC, Morgan MW, Vazquez-Benitez G, et al. An Analysis of Changes in Emergency Department Visits After a State Declaration During the Time of COVID-19. Ann Emerg Med 2020;76(5):595–601.
23. Baugh JJ, White BA, McEvoy D, et al. The cases not seen: Patterns of emergency department visits and procedures in the era of COVID-19. Am J Emerg Med 2020. https://doi.org/10.1016/j.ajem.2020.10.081.
24. Lucero AD, Lee A, Hyun J, et al. Underutilization of the emergency department during the covid-19 pandemic. West J Emerg Med 2020;21(6):15–23.
25. Goldenberg MN, Parwani V. Psychiatric emergency department volume during Covid-19 pandemic. Am J Emerg Med 2021;41:233–4.
26. Mitchell L, Fuehrlein B. Patient Volume and Dispositions in a VA Psychiatric Emergency Room During COVID-19. Community Ment Health J 2021. https://doi.org/10.1007/s10597-021-00778-w.
27. Leeb RT, Bitsko RH, Radhakrishnan L, et al. Mental Health–Related Emergency Department Visits Among Children Aged <18 Years During the COVID-19 Pandemic — United States, January 1–October 17, 2020. Morb Mortal Wkly Rep 2020;69(45):1675–80.
28. Hill RM, Rufino K, Kurian S, et al. Suicide Ideation and Attempts in a Pediatric Emergency Department Before and During COVID-19. Pediatrics 2021;147(3). e2020029280.
29. Kofman YB, Garfin DR. Home Is Not Always a Haven: The Domestic Violence Crisis Amid the COVID-19 Pandemic. Psychol Trauma Theory, Res Pract Policy 2020;12(S1):S199–201.
30. Campbell AM. An increasing risk of family violence during the Covid-19 pandemic: Strengthening community collaborations to save lives. Forensic Sci Int Rep 2020;2. https://doi.org/10.1016/j.fsir.2020.100089.
31. Friedman J, Akre S. COVID-19 and the Drug Overdose Crisis: Uncovering the Deadliest Months in the United States, January–July 2020. Am J Public Health 2021. https://doi.org/10.2105/ajph.2021.306256.
32. Centers for Disease Control and Prevention. Drug Overdose Deaths. Available at: https://www.cdc.gov/drugoverdose/deaths/index.html. Accessed June 28, 2021.
33. Mason M, Welch S, Arunkumar P, et al. Opioid Overdose Deaths Before, During, and After an 11-Week COVID-19 Stay-at-Home Order — Cook County, Illinois, January 1, 2018–October 6, 2020. MMWR Morb Mortal Wkly Rep 2021;70(10):362–3.
34. Appa A, Rodda LN, Cawley C, et al. Drug Overdose Deaths before and after Shelter-in-Place Orders during the COVID-19 Pandemic in San Francisco. JAMA Netw Open 2021;4(5):e2110452.
35. McKnight-Eily LR, Okoro CA, Strine TW, et al. Racial and Ethnic Disparities in the Prevalence of Stress and Worry, Mental Health Conditions, and Increased Substance Use Among Adults During the COVID-19 Pandemic — United States, April and May 2020. MMWR Morb Mortal Wkly Rep 2021;70(5):162–6.
36. Wainwright JJ, Mikre M, Whitley P, et al. Analysis of Drug Test Results Before and After the US Declaration of a National Emergency Concerning the COVID-19 Outbreak. JAMA 2020;324(16):1674–7.
37. Di Lorenzo R, Frattini N, Dragone D, et al. Psychiatric emergencies during the covid-19 pandemic: A 6-month observational study. Neuropsychiatr Dis Treat 2021;17:1763–78.

38. Taquet M, Luciano S, Geddes JR, et al. Bidirectional associations between COVID-19 and psychiatric disorder: retrospective cohort studies of 62 354 COVID-19 cases in the USA. Lancet Psychiatry 2021;8:130–40.
39. Kozloff N, Mulsant BH, Stergiopoulos V, et al. The COVID-19 global pandemic: Implications for people with schizophrenia and related disorders. Schizophr Bull 2020;46(4):752–7.
40. de Leon J, Diaz FJ. A meta-analysis of worldwide studies demonstrates an association between schizophrenia and tobacco smoking behaviors. Schizophr Res 2005;76:135–57.
41. Nemani K, Li C, Olfson M, et al. Association of Psychiatric Disorders with Mortality among Patients with COVID-19. JAMA Psychiatry 2021;78(4):380–6.
42. Wang QQ, Xu R, Volkow ND. Increased risk of COVID-19 infection and mortality in people with mental disorders: analysis from electronic health records in the United States. World Psychiatry 2021;20:124–30.
43. Wong AH, Roppolo LP, Chang BP, et al. Management of agitation during the COVID-19 pandemic. West J Emerg Med 2020;21(4):795–800.
44. Mao L, Wang M, Chen S, et al. Neurologic Manifestations of Hospitalized Patients with Coronavirus Disease 2019 in Wuhan, China: a retrospective case series study. JAMA Neurol 2020;77:683–90.
45. Rubin R. As Their Numbers Grow, COVID-19 “Long Haulers” Stump Experts. JAMA - J Am Med Assoc 2020;324(14):1381–3.
46. Callard F, Perego E. How and why patients made Long Covid. Soc Sci Med 2021; 268:113426.
47. Baig AM. Chronic COVID syndrome: Need for an appropriate medical terminology for long-COVID and COVID long-haulers. J Med Virol 2021;93(5):2555–6.
48. Kim HC, Yoo SY, Lee BH, et al. Psychiatric findings in suspected and confirmed Middle East Respiratory Syndrome patients quarantined in hospital: A retrospective chart analysis. Psychiatry Investig 2018;15(4):355–60.
49. Yong SJ. Long COVID or post-COVID-19 syndrome: putative pathophysiology, risk factors, and treatments. Infect Dis 2021;1–18.
50. Holmes EA, O'Connor RC, Perry VH, et al. Multidisciplinary research priorities for the COVID-19 pandemic: a call for action for mental health science. The Lancet Psychiatry 2020;7(6):547–60.
51. Fried JE, Liebers DT, Roberts ET. Sustaining Rural Hospitals after COVID-19: The Case for Global Budgets. JAMA 2020;324(2):137–8.
52. ACEP Now. ACEP Surveys Members About COVID-19. ACEP Now. 2020. Available at: https://www.acepnow.com/article/acep-surveys-members-about-covid-19/. Accessed April 9, 2021.
53. American Hospital Association. Hospitals and Health Systems Face Unprecedented Financial Pressures Due to COVID-19. 2020. Available at: https://www.aha.org/system/files/media/file/2020/06/aha-covid19-financial-impact-report.pdf. Accessed June 25, 2021.
54. Chor WPD, Ng WM, Cheng L, et al. Burnout amongst emergency healthcare workers during the COVID-19 pandemic: A multi-center study. Am J Emerg Med 2020. https://doi.org/10.1016/j.ajem.2020.10.040.
55. Cook TM. Personal protective equipment during the coronavirus disease (COVID) 2019 pandemic – a narrative review. Anaesthesia 2020;75(7):920–7.
56. Shechter A, Diaz F, Moise N, et al. Psychological distress, coping behaviors, and preferences for support among New York healthcare workers during the COVID-19 pandemic. Gen Hosp Psychiatry 2020;66:1–8. https://doi.org/10.1016/j.genhosppsych.2020.06.007.

57. Shreffler J, Petrey J, Huecker M. The impact of COVID-19 on healthcare worker wellness: A scoping review. West J Emerg Med 2020;21(5):1059–66.
58. White DB, Lo B. A Framework for Rationing Ventilators and Critical Care Beds During the COVID-19 Pandemic. JAMA 2020;323(18):1773–4.
59. Centers for Disease Control and Prevention. Using Telehealth to Expand Access to Essential Health Services during the COVID-19 Pandemic. 2020. Available at: https://www.cdc.gov/coronavirus/2019-ncov/hcp/telehealth.html.
60. Petrik ML, Billera M, Kaplan Y, et al. Balancing Patient Care and Confidentiality: Considerations in Obtaining Collateral Information. J Psychiatr Pract 2015; 21(3):220–4.
61. Centers for Disease Control and Prevention. Management of Visitors to Healthcare Facilities in the Context of COVID-19: Non-US Healthcare Settings. 2020. Available at: https://www.cdc.gov/coronavirus/2019-ncov/hcp/non-us-settings/hcf-visitors.html.
62. Saadatjoo S, Miri M, Hassanipour S, et al. Knowledge, attitudes, and practices of the general population about Coronavirus disease 2019 (COVID-19): a systematic review and meta-analysis with policy recommendations. Public Health 2021;194:185–95.
63. Wee LE, Fua TP, Chua YY, et al. Containing COVID-19 in the Emergency Department: The Role of Improved Case Detection and Segregation of Suspect Cases. Acad Emerg Med 2020;27(5):379–87.
64. Larkin GL, Beautrais AL, Spirito A, et al. Mental health and emergency medicine: A research agenda. Acad Emerg Med 2009;16(11):1110–9.
65. Kennedy M, Helfand BKI, Gou RY, et al. Delirium in Older Patients with COVID-19 Presenting to the Emergency Department. JAMA Netw Open 2020;3(11): e2029540.
66. Cole JB, Klein LR, Mullinax SZ, et al. Study Enrollment When “Preconsent” Is Utilized for a Randomized Clinical Trial of Two Treatments for Acute Agitation in the Emergency Department. Acad Emerg Med 2019;26(5):559–66.
67. Mullinax S, Shokraneh F, Wilson MP, et al. Oral Medication for Agitation of Psychiatric Origin: A Scoping Review of Randomized Controlled Trials. J Emerg Med 2017;53(4):524–9.
68. Wilson MP, Pepper D, Currier GW, et al. The psychopharmacology of agitation: Consensus statement of the American Association for emergency psychiatry project BETA psychopharmacology workgroup. West J Emerg Med 2012;13(1): 26–34.
69. Schneider A, Mullinax S, Hall N, et al. Intramuscular medication for treatment of agitation in the emergency department: A systematic review of controlled trials. Am J Emerg Med 2020. https://doi.org/10.1016/j.ajem.2020.07.013.
70. Jovanović N, Campbell J, Priebe S. How to design psychiatric facilities to foster positive social interaction – A systematic review. Eur Psychiatry 2019;60:49–62.
71. Bojdani E, Rajagopalan A, Chen A, et al. COVID-19 Pandemic: Impact on psychiatric care in the United States. Psychiatry Res 2020;289:113069.
72. Unützer J, Kimmel RJ, Snowden M. Psychiatry in the age of COVID-19. World Psychiatry 2020;19(2):130–1.
73. Telepsychiatry program eases patient crowding in the ED, expedites mental health services to patients and providers. Manag 2013;25:121–4.
74. Southard EP, Neufeld JD, Laws S. Telemental health evaluations enhance access and efficiency in a critical access hospital emergency department. Telemed J E Health 2014;20:664–8.

75. Narasimhan M, Druss BG, Hockenberry JM, et al. Impact of a telepsychiatry program at emergency departments statewide on the quality, utilization, and costs of mental health services. Psychiatr Serv 2015;66:1167.
76. Turner Lee N, Karsten J, Roberts J. Removing regulatory barriers to telehealth before and after COVID-19. Brookings John Locke Foundation. 2020. Available at: https://www.brookings.edu/research/removing-regulatory-barriers-to-telehealth-before-and-after-covid-19/. Accessed July 1, 2021.
77. Chen JA, Chung WJ, Young SK, et al. COVID-19 and telepsychiatry: Early outpatient experiences and implications for the future. Gen Hosp Psychiatry 2020;66:89–95.
78. Whiteside T, Kane E, Aljohani B, et al. Redesigning emergency department operations amidst a viral pandemic. Am J Emerg Med 2020;38(7):1448–53.
79. Mohs M. First of Its Kind Mental Health Facility Opens At M Health Southdale Next Week. CBS Minnesota. 2021. Available at: https://minnesota.cbslocal.com/2021/03/24/first-of-its-kind-mental-health-facility-opens-at-m-health-southdale-next-week/. Accessed July 1, 2021.
80. Spectrum Health Community Health Assessment Needs. 2021. Available at: https://www.spectrumhealth.org/-/media/spectrumhealth/documents/community-health-assessment-needs/shgr-2021-implementation-strategy-final.pdf?rev=e024361a92ad4dc8a7d1d970d626bcb6&hash=EFD0474C098D84EE9B60E9D7A37860FE. Accessed June 30, 2021.
81. Zeller S. EmPATH Units as a solution for ED Psychiatric Patient Boarding. Psychiatry Advisor. 2017. Available at: https://www.psychiatryadvisor.com/home/practice-management/empath-units-as-a-solution-for-ed-psychiatric-patient-boarding/. Accessed July 2, 2021.
82. Stamy C, Shane D, Kannedy L, et al. Economic Evaluation of the Emergency Department After Implementation of an Emergency Psychiatric Assessment, Treatment, and Healing Unit. Acad Emerg Med 2021;28:82–91.
83. Joseph A. As the Covid-19 crisis ebbs in the U.S., experts brace for some to experience psychological fallout. STAT News 2021. Available at: https://www.statnews.com/2021/05/07/as-the-covid-19-crisis-ebbs-in-the-u-s-experts-brace-for-a-long-term-impact-on-mental-health/. Accessed July 1, 2021.
84. Whelan R. Americans Seek Urgent Mental-Health Support as Covid-19 Crisis Ebbs. Wall Street J Published June 2021;27. Available at: https://www-wsj-com.cdn.ampproject.org/c/s/www.wsj.com/amp/articles/americans-seek-urgent-mental-health-support-as-covid-19-crisis-ebbs-11624786203. Accessed June 30, 2021.

Coronavirus Disease 2019 and the Impact on Substance Use Disorder Treatments

Osnat C. Melamed, MD, MSc[a,b], Wayne K. deRuiter, PhD[a], Leslie Buckley, MD, MPH[c,d], Peter Selby, MBBS, MHSc[a,b,d,e,*]

KEYWORDS

- COVID-19 • Pandemic • Substance use disorder treatment • Opioid use disorder
- Digital technology • Telemedicine

KEY POINTS

- The societal response to limit the spread of COVID reduced access to in-person care for SUDs.
- In an attempt to keep patients and health care providers safe during the COVID pandemic, many treatment programs for SUDs made a transition from in-person to remote care delivery (ie, telemedicine visits).
- Evidence supports telemedicine's acceptability by patients and providers as well as the need for telemedicine to be complemented by in-person care for those with the greatest need.
- The progress made in the area of telemedicine for the treatment of SUDs should not recede postpandemic.
- Future research is necessary to effectively characterize individuals who are likely to engage and be retained in remote care and in-person care.

INTRODUCTION

The coronavirus disease 2019 (COVID-19) pandemic and the resulting societal response to limit its spread poses a threat to vulnerable groups such as those with substance use disorders (SUDs). The need for social distancing to limit the spread

[a] Nicotine Dependence Service, Centre for Addiction and Mental Health, 1025 Queen Street West, Toronto, Ontario M6J1H4, Canada; [b] Department of Family and Community Medicine, University of Toronto, 500 University Avenue, Toronto, Ontario M5G1V7, Canada; [c] Addictions Division, Centre for Addiction and Mental Health, 1001 Queen Street West, Toronto, Ontario M6J1H4, Canada; [d] Department of Psychiatry, University of Toronto, 250 College Street, Toronto, Ontario M5T1R8, Canada; [e] Dalla Lana School of Public Health, University of Toronto, 155 College Street Room 500, Toronto, Ontario M5T3M7, Canada
* Corresponding author. Nicotine Dependence Service, Centre for Addiction and Mental Health, 1025 Queen Street West, Toronto, Ontario M6J1H4, Canada.
E-mail address: peter.selby@camh.ca

Psychiatr Clin N Am 45 (2022) 95–107
https://doi.org/10.1016/j.psc.2021.11.006 psych.theclinics.com

of the infection disrupted the delivery of care in most specialized SUD treatment programs as well as community-based mutual-aid support groups (eg, Alcoholics Anonymous [AA]). Reduction in access to SUD treatment in general medical settings was further exacerbated by furloughed staff, reduced work hours, and redeployment of primary care and emergency medicine teams to deal with acute COVID infections. Consequently, the treatment gap found among individuals with SUDs before the pandemic was further widened.

Concurrently, the stressors brought about by the pandemic including social isolation, loss of employment, financial concerns, and fear of falling ill with COVID have disproportionally affected individuals with SUDs. An abundance of stressors in the absence of social and institutional support led many individuals to increase their substance consumption as a means of coping with these challenges and may have caused many individuals in recovery to relapse.

Many treatment programs for SUDs made a swift transition from in-person to remote care delivery (ie, telemedicine visits) to keep patients and providers safe from COVID infection. Relaxing of regulatory restrictions on the provision of controlled substances (eg, opioid agonist therapy [OAT]) and payors' coverage of telemedicine visits facilitated the adoption of remote care in the treatment of SUDs during the pandemic. This transition necessitated a considerable organizational effort, and ongoing activities are underway to restore the full breadth of treatment services that were available before the pandemic.

The transition to telemedicine presents both advantages and disadvantages for patients and providers alike, and emerging data acknowledge factors that facilitate or hinder treatment engagement and retention.

This special article used a selective literature review to synthesize emerging evidence regarding changes prompted by the COVID pandemic to the clinical care of individuals with SUDs. We discuss the (1) reduction in availability of care, (2) increase in demand for care, (3) transition to telemedicine use, (4) telemedicine for the treatment of opioid use disorders (OUDs), and (5) considerations for the use of telemedicine in treating SUDs and implications for practice.

REDUCTION IN AVAILABILITY OF TREATMENT OF SUBSTANCE USE DISORDER DURING THE PANDEMIC

Traditionally, in-person care has been the mainstay of treatment of SUDs. In specialized addiction treatment settings, many face-to-face individual and group-based therapies were halted due to reduced hours or partial closures of treatment facilities. In many residential substance rehabilitation programs, patients often sleep, dine, and receive treatment in congregate conditions[1] as part of the recovery milieu. Lack of trained staff in Infection Prevention and Control (IPAC), limited funding, and space limitations made implementing infection control measures a challenge. Specifically, critical activities were affected such as screening for COVID symptoms, access to personal protective equipment (PPE) and quarantine rooms, and the installation of physical barriers.[2] Treatment programs have reported a 20% to 60% reduction in attendance. Consequently, SUD treatment programs have experienced delays in initiating treatment, a reduction in service options, less frequent services, and the prohibition of family visitations.[2] Similarly, public health regulations banned gatherings, which prevented individuals from attending meetings of mutual-aid groups within their communities (eg, AA, SMART recovery); this eliminated much-needed venues of ongoing recovery support.

In general hospital settings, fewer resources were available to treat patients with SUD because of redeployment of clinical staff toward COVID care and preparedness.[3] In particular, the capacity for substance use treatment by emergency medicine staff providers was reduced due to the overwhelming workload created by patients infected by COVID.[4] Furthermore, individuals with SUDs may have been reluctant to approach general hospital care due to fear of infection. However, the percent of hospitalized patients with acute alcohol withdrawal using a Clinical Institute Withdrawal Assessment for Alcohol Scale (CIWA) cutoff of 8 or more was about 34% higher in 2020 compared with the same time in 2019. The peak was at the end of the stay-home orders but continued to be elevated during the reopening phase.[5]

Primary care is another major source of support for individuals with SUDs, providing screening, brief interventions, and medication-assisted therapies.[6] Primary care facilities reported a 21.8% reduction in visit volume during the early days of the COVID pandemic.[7] Many primary care services had reported a decreased capacity for in-person care during the pandemic. Shorter opening hours, staff redeployment, and complete closures were all factors that contributed to a reduction in the availability and accessibility for SUD treatment.

INCREASE IN DEMAND FOR TREATMENT OF SUBSTANCE USE DISORDERS DURING AND POSTPANDEMIC

In the United States, although evidence suggests that more than 20 million individuals are in need of treatment of SUDs, only 1 in 10 have access to care.[8] Accounting for this treatment gap are a lack of skilled providers which creates long wait times, a lack of integration of SUD treatment within general medical settings, stigma, and living in nonurban communities.[9] Concurrently, with the reduction in the availability of treatment of SUDs, the societal response to the pandemic was associated with an increase in the demand for treatment of SUDs. For example, a study looking at medical visits to a large Health Maintenance Organization found a 42% increase in the number of visits for addiction conditions during the first few months of the pandemic when compared with the prepandemic volume visit[10] and a similar increase was also observed in another study conducted in primary care.[11] Specifically, during the pandemic, non-Hispanic whites reported an increase of 10.5% in mental health (MH)/SUD visits.[11] This increased demand for SUD treatment could be attributed to a decline in emotional and psychological well-being of the population. The far-reaching societal responses to limit the spread of COVID-19 led to closures of workplaces, educational institutions, places of worship, and recreational/entertainment community venues. In conjunction with guidance to limit one's interaction to only household members, social isolation, loneliness, and depressive symptoms have been higher than ever.[12,13] Declines in psychological well-being manifested by anxiety or depressive symptoms as well as heightened substance use patterns to cope with such symptoms have been reported by 40% of individuals.[13]

Although infection control measures are necessary to protect the public from the COVID virus, the negative effects are disproportionally borne by vulnerable groups, such as people with SUDs, who tend to have low social capital. Vulnerable groups are also overrepresented in minimum-wage jobs, which saw a greater loss of employment compared with those working in other positions (38% versus 13%) during the first months of the pandemic.[14] Financial stressors and social isolation, especially in the absence of traditional sources of formal and informal addiction support, creates the "perfect storm," which drove many to increase their substance use patterns.[13]

Pandemic-related distress can negatively affect individuals who are in different stages of their SUD illness. Stress is a well-established factor that is involved in relapse to substance use.[15] Stress can induce cravings and preoccupation with substance use that eventually culminates in substance consumption.[16] For example, those who are working toward stabilization of excess substance consumption or those in early remission usually require intensive in-person support, characterized by high frequency of visits (1–2 times per week). The reduction of in-person professional and peer (mutual aid groups) support concomitantly with an increase in pandemic-related concerns (eg, loss of employment) and stressors (eg, loneliness) can potentially trigger a relapse to previous substance use patterns. Moreover, individuals who are in remission from their SUD could experience a relapse due to a new stressor (eg, loneliness) brought about by the pandemic, in the absence of traditional support such as mutual-aid groups (eg, AA meetings). Individuals without SUDs or with subthreshold substance use patterns, such as at-risk drinking, may develop a de novo SUD in response to the changes brought about by the pandemic. Individuals who drank heavily in postwork hours may have a greater opportunity to consume alcohol during their work day when transitioned to work from home. Others may have greater motivation to consume substances to cope with added stressors, such as combining work from home with homeschooling children. Population-based surveys found that approximately 13% or more individuals either started or increased their use of alcohol to cope with stress related to the pandemic.[13,17,18]

It is highly likely that the general increase in alcohol consumption during the pandemic might not return to baseline levels of consumption in the new normal state. The disproportionate increase in drinking especially binge drinking patterns by women, portend a future increase in alcohol-related harms including use disorders in women. The demand for services might increase once people realize they might have developed a problem and cannot stop on their own. It will be important for primary care providers to increase their screening of all their patients and provide effective treatment geared to the severity of use disorder detected.

TELEMEDICINE FOR SUBSTANCE USE DISORDERS: GENERAL CONSIDERATIONS

For many SUD treatment programs, the increased demand for SUD treatment in addition to a reduction in the availability of in-person care during the pandemic led to an adoption of innovative service delivery models, most of which include the use of telemedicine. Recently, the use of telemedicine has been increasing as practitioners attempt to improve their reach and accessibility to care for patients, particularly those in for rural populations.[19] The use of telemedicine provides a solution for health care continuity while keeping patients and providers safe by facilitating stay at home and preserving limited PPE for only those encounters requiring face-to-face visits.[20] By definition, telemedicine includes the use of telecommunications technology to deliver health care services across a distance.[19] The technologies most commonly used are telephone (audio only) and video/Web-conferencing (video conferencing [VC], audio, and visual). Telemedicine can provide care that is similar to in-person delivery with numerous advantages for both the patients and providers. Patients will likely experience a reduction in time and travel commitments for care, increased convenience, a decline in wait time, and reduced stigma.[21,22] Consequently, compared with in-person care, the use of telemedicine suggests greater attendance and a decline in the number of canceled mental health appointments[23] as well as a lower no-show rate (8.3 versus 25.9%) in attendance for treatment of OUDs.[6] Despite these advantages, telemedicine has not been widely adopted in the area of SUD treatment before the pandemic.[24] The most notable barriers among telemedicine providers pertain to regulations imposed by governing bodies and payors. These regulations include a requirement for an in-person assessment for prescribing of controlled substances and a lack of reimbursement for remote visits. Most of these barriers have been removed early in the course of the pandemic, which facilitated a rapid increase in the use of telemedicine in the treatment of SUDs.[25] The patient-level barriers included lack of privacy, access to advanced telecommunication equipment such as smartphones and laptops, poor Internet connections, lack of privacy in their settings, and low levels of digital literacy.[22]

TRANSITION OF SUBSTANCE USE DISORDER TREATMENT PROGRAMS TO TELEMEDICINE DURING THE CORONAVIRUS DISEASE PANDEMIC

At the onset of the pandemic, 43% of mental health treatment facilities in the United States and only 27% of SUD treatment facilities had telehealth capabilities.[26,27] With COVID-19 restrictions preventing in-person care, the number of visits rapidly declined from March 2020, reaching a reduction of 48% by July of 2020 when compared with the previous year.[28] This reduction was more than 2-fold greater than the 21.8% loss of visit volume reported in primary care settings.[7] Primary care settings seemed to demonstrate a greater preparedness and a willingness to adopt remote visits via telemedicine early during the pandemic, which may have limited the number of lost visits.

Both clinicians and patients report encouraging experiences regarding the acceptability of telemedicine. Most providers used a combination of telephone and VC visits. Telephone visits were helpful for patients who lacked digital literacy or computer/Internet access.[22] Most providers thought that telemedicine could provide SUD treatment that was comparable to in-person care.[22] Many practitioners acknowledged the benefits of VC compared with telephone with regard to accurately assessing the patient's condition and learning about the patient's home environment.[29] Other practitioners recognized the need to continue to have in-person visits for new patients or those experiencing substance relapse.[30] For some treatment programs, patient enrollment increased when services were offered remotely, as Langabeer and colleagues[29] found a 2-fold increase in the number of patients attending a peer support recovery group delivered remotely compared with in-person recovery groups. Other services have described an opposite trend in participation rates when transitioning from in-person to remote visits. For example, McKiever and colleagues[31] reported a 46% reduction in attendance when the implementation of a counseling group intended for pregnant women with SUDs transitioned from in-person to remote visits. This finding highlights the need to ensure that adoption of telemedicine services in the treatment of SUDs is evaluated for both accessibility and acceptability to different populations of patients. Future research is needed to elucidate which populations are more likely to benefit from remote versus in-person versus hybrid models of care.

Mutual-aid support groups such as AA, Narcotics Anonymous, and SMART recovery are traditionally delivered in person.[32,33] However, in the context of COVID-19, attendance of mutual support programs via online platforms have flourished.[34] In part, the self-directed nature of mutual aid likely permitted the adoption of existing Web-conferencing platforms, which are low cost or free. Given the global community adoption of mutual aid, online support is essentially available 24/7 across the world. This ease of access partially compensated for the deficits in the availability of SUD treatment programs.[33]

TELEMEDICINE IN THE TREATMENT OF OPIOID USE DISORDERS

During the COVID pandemic, a considerable change occurred in the delivery of treatment of individuals with OUD.[27,35] Traditionally, initiation of OAT such as methadone or buprenorphine for OUD required an in-person assessment as well as frequent follow-up visits until stabilization of substance use patterns and medication dose had been reached. During stabilization visits, a urine drug screen would be performed to verify the presence or absence of misused opioids concurrently with optimization of the OAT dosing. In-person care during the stabilization phase of OUD is considered advantageous because of its ability to provide structured support, close monitoring for OAT side effects, and prevention of diversion of medication, during dose titration (eg, overdose and sedation). Regulators define OAT dose titration schedules, urine drug screen frequency, and the gradual transition process to take-home doses of medication once the individual has stabilized and ceased illicit opioid use.

With the onset of the pandemic, most jurisdictions began to allow for telemedicine visits for the assessment and treatment of OUD, reduced frequency of urine drug screening, and an expedited schedule for take-home doses. In one study of primary care settings, 91.2% of facilities modified their OUD treatment practices, specifically the implementation of medication and behavioral health/counseling visits.[36] Approximately half of the initial and follow-up behavioral health/consulting visits were conducted remotely.[36] This compared with 23.1% and 40.4% of initial and follow-up medication evaluations, respectively, that were conducted virtually,[36] which allowed patients to receive care for OUD while mitigating the risk of contracting or spreading COVID. In some cases, in-person visits were reserved for new patients, patients who relapsed, patients who did not adhere to prescribed medication, patients who lacked proper technology, patients who were homeless, patients requiring injections, and patients who needed a physical examination or testing.[22] To mitigate the risk of COVID, programs may have chosen to offer OAT dropoff at the patient's home or allowing for a family member to pick up their medication in the case the patient was in quarantine.[35,37]

The relaxing of regulations led to fewer disruptions in the delivery of care brought about by the pandemic, and in some cases, provided an opportunity for OUD treatments to have a greater reach than previously occurred.[38,39]

In many cases, OUD treatment programs can successfully transition to the telemedicine platform by using existing provider resources.[29] In one example of an urban center, telemedicine was used to provide comprehensive care for patients including initiation and maintenance of OAT, behavioral counseling, and peer support recovery groups.[29] These remote services reported a greater uptake by patients compared with in-person care. To ensure equity, some programs reported on their efforts to close the "digital divide," when patients could not access telemedicine due to low digital literacy or lack of computer/Internet access. For example, pregnant and postpartum women with SUD were provided with borrowed smartphones and prepaid Internet data, which enabled them to access telemedicine.[40] Technology was used not only for the delivery of telemedicine visits but also for sending patients previsit mental health and substance use screeners for the purpose of informing care.[40]

Given the excess number of deadly opioid overdoses that was observed during the COVID pandemic, certain programs aimed to increase access to OUD treatment.[41] In New England, the availability of OAT via phone visits prompted the use of a treatment "hotline," which provided patients with an opportunity to access buprenorphine treatment while simultaneously removing many of the barriers associated with initiating such treatment.[42] Similarly, in Florida, people attending a needle-exchange site were invited to participate in a telemedicine visit for the initiation of OAT. The latter program was cofacilitated by medical students, which has an added value of reducing stigma against SUDs among future health care providers.[43]

It seems that relaxing regulations to allow for remote OUD treatment and greater flexibility in take-home doses can have several advantages; it improves access to care and is more convenient and less disruptive to patients' lives. Furthermore, based on prepandemic data, most patients reported high levels of satisfaction, simplicity, and comfort with using telemedicine and believed that the quality of virtual care received from practitioners was similar to that of in-person care.[44] However, these benefits need to be balanced with the risk of accidental overdose, misuse, or diversion of OAT, especially during early stabilization periods. Similarly, telemedicine may not provide the structured support that is beneficial to individuals with unstable OUD. In this case, in-person settings could be advantageous.

The advent of monthly injections of buprenorphine as a treatment option in North America also offers a potential solution. By label, the patient had to be on a stable dose of Sub Lingual (SL) buprenorphine greater than 8 mg for at least a week. However, novel models with earlier administration of the injection in emergency rooms after tolerable test doses of SL buprenorphine are being trialed. The monthly in-person visits combined with telemedicine could be a good compromise in providing safe and effective pharmacotherapy and counseling especially during early recovery. Moreover, patients on stable doses of 8 mg or less of buprenorphine could be transitioned to subcutaneous 6-monthly implants to minimize clinic visits.

Although not permitted in the United States, in Canada, Sustained Release Oral Morphine (SROM) has gained acceptance as a suitable form of OAT.[45] In some provinces, supervised injection facilities and injection Opioid Agonist Therapy (iOAT) are also becoming more commonplace. For those patients in quarantine in COVID shelters or hotels, delivery of OAT and/or Supervised Injection Site (SIS) was permitted. Regardless, given the toxic drug supply especially admixture of highly potent illegal benzodiazepines such as etizolam with designer fentanyls including car-fentanyl has led to an increase in opioid-related poisonings and deaths. In British Columbia and Ontario, programs of safe supply have been initiated with access to high-potency prescription opioids such as hydromorphone.

DISCUSSION

The COVID-19 pandemic and the societal response to limit its spread led to regulatory and policy changes that greatly affected the delivery of SUD treatment. SUD treatment programs can now deliver comprehensive care via remote visits, which includes screening, initiation of medication, behavioral counseling, and peer support groups, and this has been a paradigm shift for most SUD treatment facilities that traditionally relied on in-person care. Although this shift was necessary to maintain continuity of care during the pandemic, it may not be suitable for all. Therefore, additional information is needed to characterize which patient populations are likely to benefit from remote care. This information can allow practitioners to dedicate more time and resources, such as frequent in-person care, toward those patients who are more vulnerable.

CONSIDERATIONS REGARDING THE USE OF TELEMEDICINE IN THE TREATMENT OF SUBSTANCE USE DISORDERS

The COVID-19 pandemic provided us with valuable insight regarding the potential advantages and disadvantages of telemedicine use in the treatment of SUDs. Emerging evidence suggests that health care providers find telemedicine to be a venue for care delivery that is comparable with in-person care, but they also identify that remote support may not be enough for patients with severe SUDs, who are struggling.[22,30]

In the early stages of transitioning to remote care, it can become evident that certain groups of the population will derive fewer benefits. Studies indicated that older adults (aged 60+) find the use of telemedicine for SUD treatment challenging. For example, a qualitative study of older adults with alcohol use disorder and their providers found that both patients and providers thought that the quality of remote support was inferior to in-person care.[46] This finding could partially explain the low rates of engagement within remote programs. Similarly, others reported that older adults were disproportionally affected by social isolation during the pandemic. Consequently, for many older adults, remote care may not provide sufficient social support.[47] It was also agreed that many older adults have low digital literacy and limited computer/Internet access that precluded participation.

Studies found that patients with severe SUDs or concurrent psychiatric conditions may also be challenged by remote care leading to poor engagement and retention. Patients who report polysubstance versus single substance use concerns experienced greater disruptions to their care as well as greater difficulty in accessing remote treatment of SUDs.[48] It is likely that remote care does not provide the same level of support that in-person care provides. Similarly, women with OUDs who are pregnant reported a substantial reduction in attending group-based therapy when it was offered remotely.[31] Although this could be attributed to low digital literacy and low digital access (eg, lack of computer, Internet) among vulnerable groups, it also suggests that in-person care is a critical component of care for many individuals.

It is likely that most SUD treatment programs will be able to meet the needs of their patients by allowing for a hybrid model of care that includes a combination of in-person and remote visits.[22] We recognize that in-person and remote care are complementary and that one cannot fully replace the other. The optimal composition of care (remote versus in person) should be tailored to the needs of the individual and agreed upon by patients and providers by shared decision making.

IMPLICATIONS: HOW WILL THESE CHANGES AFFECT FUTURE DELIVERY OF SUBSTANCE USE DISORDER TREATMENTS?

During the pandemic, the use of telemedicine by SUD treatment programs substantially increased and may have partially helped to enhance accessibility and availability of treatment services. As the pandemic evolves, a growing number of SUD treatment programs will continue to acquire telemedicine capacity. Yet, even at this time, a year and a half into the pandemic, the ability of programs to deliver the full breadth of services via remote means is diminished.

SUD programs are now tasked with service planning for years to come with many embracing the use of telemedicine as an integral part of future services. The sustainability of telemedicine postpandemic will be determined by numerous factors. Integrating comprehensive care for SUDs including medication management, behavioral counseling, group-based therapy, and low-intensity care for long-term relapse prevention (ie, aftercare) will be essential. At the same time, the use of telemedicine needs to be balanced with an existing capacity for in-person care for several patient subgroups that are likely to face challenges in engagement and retention via telemedicine care. Investments in infrastructure to expand the reach of telemedicine among practitioners and patients will be necessary, particularly in rural areas.[49] Furthermore, SUD treatment programs will need to train their providers to be proficient in best practices of telemedicine use and provide organizational support for both modalities of care.[49] Programs should offer patients training to improve digital literacy and ensure they have access to computer/smartphone and Internet.[49] To sustain and grow telemedicine use in the post-pandemic era, it will be necessary to extend those policies that allowed for telemedicine visits to occur during the pandemic. Such policies would allow for continued reimbursement to providers for in-person as well as remote care and allow for the provision of care, especially for OUD, without the need for an in-person assessment.

Telemedicine opens up several opportunities to revolutionize SUD treatment by integrating care into general medical settings,[6] offering low access entry to treatment by using phone "hotlines,"[42] using remote screening tools and measurement based-care to inform SUD treatment, and integrating digital health technologies as an adjunct to care delivered by providers.[40,50–52]

SUMMARY

The COVID-19 pandemic is an unprecedented force that has drastically changed our lives. In particular, the pandemic had a negative effect on vulnerable groups such as individuals with SUDs. The societal response to limit the spread of the virus reduced access to in-person care for SUDs but concurrently boosted the adaption of telemedicine for care delivery. Emerging evidence not only supports its acceptability by patients and providers alike but also highlights the need for it to be complemented by in-person care for those with the greatest need. Nevertheless, most agree that gains made in the area of telemedicine for the treatment of SUDs should not be receded postpandemic. Therefore, there is a pressing need for evaluation and participatory research (with patients, families and health care providers) to effectively characterize individuals who are likely to engage and retain in remote care and conversely, those who require in-person care. This information is crucial to inform organizational change in specialized SUD treatment programs and in treatment programs that are integrated into general medical settings.

CLINICS CARE POINTS

- Telemedicine opens up several opportunities to revolutionize SUD treatment by integrating care into general medical settings,[6] offering low access entry to treatment by using phone "hotlines,"[42] using remote screening tools and measurement-based care to inform SUD treatment, and integrating digital health technologies as an adjunct to care delivered by providers.[40,50–52]
- The use of telemedicine needs to be balanced with an existing capacity for in-person care for several patient subgroups that are likely to face challenges in engagement and retention via telemedicine care, such as older adults (aged 60+), people with polysubstance use, and pregnant women with OUD.
- In-person and remote care for the treatment of SUDs are complementary, and a hybrid model of care that includes a combination of both is likely to meet the needs of those seeking care.
- To sustain and grow telemedicine use in the postpandemic era, it will be necessary to extend those policies that allowed for telemedicine visits to occur during the pandemic.
- Higher capacity is needed to treat SUD and increase options for treatment of OUD.

DISCLOSURE

W.K. deRuiter reports receiving grants from the Public Health Agency of Canada and Pfizer. W.K. deRuiter is also a shareholder of Abbott Laboratories. P. Selby reports receiving grants and/or salary and/or research support from the Centre for Addiction and Mental Health, Health Canada, Ontario Ministry of Health and Long-Term Care (MOHLTC), Canadian Institutes of Health Research (CIHR), Canadian Centre on Substance Use and Addiction, Public Health Agency of Canada (PHAC), Ontario Lung Association, Medical Psychiatry Alliance, Extensions for Community Healthcare Outcomes, Canadian Cancer Society Research Institute (CCSRI), Cancer Care Ontario, Ontario Institute for Cancer Research, Ontario Brain Institute, McLaughlin Centre, Academic Health Sciences Centre, Workplace Safety and Insurance Board, National Institutes of Health (NIH), and the Association of Faculties of Medicine of Canada. P. Selby also reports receiving funding and/or honoraria from the following commercial organizations: Pfizer Inc./Canada. Through an open tender process Johnson & Johnson, Novartis, and Pfizer Inc are vendors of record for providing smoking cessation pharmacotherapy, free or discounted, for research studies in which P. Selby is the principal investigator or coinvestigator. The authors O.C. Melamed and L. Buckley have nothing to disclose.

REFERENCES

1. Hanton K, McHugh D, Boris G. A case series: successfully preventing COVID-19 outbreak in a residential community setting at a drug and alcohol addiction treatment center. Healthcare (Basel) 2021;9(1):88.
2. Pagano A, Hosakote S, Kapiteni K, et al. Impacts of COVID-19 on residential treatment programs for substance use disorder. J Subst Abuse Treat 2020;123: 108255.
3. Holland KM, Jones C, Vivolo-Kantor AM, et al. Trends in US Emergency Department visits for mental health, overdose, and violence outcomes before and during the COVID-19 pandemic. JAMA Psychiatry 2021;78(4):372–9.
4. Herring AA, Kalmin M, Speener M, et al. Sharp decline in hospital and emergency department initiated buprenorphine for opioid use disorder during COVID-19 state of emergency in California. J Subst Abuse Treat 2021;123:108260.
5. Sharma RA, Subedi K, Gbadebo BM, et al. Alcohol withdrawal rates in hospitalized patients during the COVID-19 pandemic. JAMA Netw Open 2021;4(3): e210422.
6. O'Gurek DT. Designing and evaluating COVID-19 protocols for an office-based opioid treatment program in an urban underserved setting. J Am Board Fam Med 2021;34(Suppl):S136–40.
7. Stephenson E, O'Neill B, Gronsbell J, et al. Changes in family medicine visits across sociodemographic groups after the onset of the COVID-19 pandemic in Ontario: a retrospective cohort study. CMAJ Open 2021;9(2):E651–8.
8. U.S. Department of Health and Human Services (HHS) and Office of the Surgeon General. Facing addiction in America: the surgeon general's report on alcohol, drugs, and health. Washington, DC: HHS; 2016.
9. Pearlman J. Combatting massachusetts's opioid epidemic: reducing the social stigma of addiction through increased access to voluntary treatment services and expansion of mandatory clinician education programs. Am J Law Med 2016;42(4):835–57.
10. Ridout KK, Alavi M, Ridout SJ, et al. Changes in diagnostic and demographic characteristics of patients seeking mental health care during the early COVID-19 pandemic in a large, community-based health care system. J Clin Psychiatry 2021;82(2). 20m13685.

11. Yang J, Landrum MB, Zhou L, et al. Disparities in outpatient visits for mental health and/or substance use disorders during the COVID surge and partial reopening in Massachusetts. Gen Hosp Psychiatry 2020;67:100–6.
12. Sherman AC, Williams ML, Amick BC, et al. Mental health outcomes associated with the COVID-19 pandemic: Prevalence and risk factors in a southern US state. Psychiatry Res 2020;293:113476.
13. Czeisler ME, Lane RI, Petrosky E, et al. Mental health, substance use, and suicidal ideation during the COVID-19 pandemic - United States, June 24-30, 2020. MMWR Morb Mortal Wkly Rep 2020;69(32):1049–57.
14. Statistics Canada. Labour force survey, may 2020. Ottawa (Ontario): Government of Canada; 2020.
15. Preston KL, Epstein DH. Stress in the daily lives of cocaine and heroin users: relationship to mood, craving, relapse triggers, and cocaine use. Psychopharmacology (Berl) 2011;218(1):29–37.
16. Volkow ND, Koob GF, McLellan AT. Neurobiologic advances from the brain disease model of addiction. N Engl J Med 2016;374(4):363–71.
17. Zajacova A, Jehn A, Stackhouse M, et al. Changes in health behaviours during early COVID-19 and socio-demographic disparities: a cross-sectional analysis. Can J Public Health 2020;111(6):953–62.
18. Centre for Addiction and Mental Health. COVID-19 national survey dashboard 2021. Available at: https://www.camh.ca/en/health-info/mental-health-and-covid-19/covid-19-national-survey. Accessed on Sept 2, 2021.
19. Tuckson RV, Edmunds M, Hodgkins ML. Telehealth. N Engl J Med 2017;377(16): 1585–92.
20. Hollander JE, Carr BG. Virtually Perfect? Telemedicine for Covid-19. N Engl J Med 2020;382(18):1679–81.
21. Lin LA, Casteel D, Shigekawa E, et al. Telemedicine-delivered treatment interventions for substance use disorders: A systematic review. J Subst Abuse Treat 2019;101:38–49.
22. Uscher-Pines L, Sousa J, Raja P, et al. Treatment of opioid use disorder during COVID-19: Experiences of clinicians transitioning to telemedicine. J Subst Abuse Treat 2020;118:108124.
23. Frank HE, Grumbach NM, Conrad SM, et al. Mental health services in primary care: Evidence for the feasibility of telehealth during the COVID-19 pandemic. J Affect Disord Rep 2021;5:100146.
24. Huskamp HA, Busch AB, Souza J, et al. How Is Telemedicine Being Used In Opioid And Other Substance Use Disorder Treatment? Health Aff (Millwood) 2018;37(12):1940–7.
25. Lowey NM. HR 6074-116th Congress (2019-2020): Coronavirus Preparedness and Response Supplemental Appropriations Act2020.
26. Cantor J, Stein BD, Saloner B. Telehealth capability among substance use disorder treatment facilities in counties with high versus low COVID-19 social distancing. J Addict Med 2020;14(6):e366–8.
27. Cantor JH, McBain RK, Kofner A, et al. Availability of Outpatient Telemental Health Services in the United States at the Outset of the COVID-19 Pandemic. Med Care 2021;59(4):319–23.
28. Cantor J, Kravitz D, Sorbero M, et al. Trends in visits to substance use disorder treatment facilities in 2020. J Subst Abuse Treat 2021;127:108462.
29. Langabeer JR 2nd, Yatsco A, Champagne-Langabeer T. Telehealth sustains patient engagement in OUD treatment during COVID-19. J Subst Abuse Treat 2021; 122:108215.

30. Henretty K, Padwa H, Treiman K, et al. Impact of the coronavirus pandemic on substance use disorder treatment: findings from a survey of specialty providers in California. Subst Abuse 2021;15. 11782218211028655.
31. McKiever ME, Cleary EM, Schmauder T, et al. Unintended consequences of the transition to telehealth for pregnancies complicated by opioid use disorder during the coronavirus disease 2019 pandemic. Am J Obstet Gynecol 2020;223(5): 770–2.
32. Substance Abuse and Mental Health Services Administration. Staying connected is important: virtual recovery resources 2021. Available at: https://www.samhsa.gov/sites/default/files/virtual-recovery-resources.pdf. Accessed on July 22, 2021.
33. Kelly JF, Abry A, Ferri M, et al. Alcoholics anonymous and 12-step facilitation treatments for alcohol use disorder: a distillation of a 2020 cochrane review for clinicians and policy makers. Alcohol Alcohol 2020;55(6):641–51.
34. Couto M. Canadians battling addiction in self-isolation turn to online AA meetings. CTV News 2020.
35. Cantor J, Laurito A. The new services that opioid treatment programs have adopted in response to COVID-19. J Subst Abuse Treat 2021;130:108393.
36. Caton L, Cheng H, Garneau HC, et al. COVID-19 adaptations in the care of patients with opioid use disorder: a survey of California primary care clinics. J Gen Intern Med 2021;36(4):998–1005.
37. Dunlop A, Lokuge B, Masters D, et al. Challenges in maintaining treatment services for people who use drugs during the COVID-19 pandemic. Harm Reduct J 2020;17(1):26.
38. U.S. Department of Justice - Drug Enforcement Administration. How to prescribe controlled substances to patients during the COVID-19 public health emergency. Springfield, VA: US Department of Justice -Drug Enforcement Administration; 2020.
39. Lam V, Sankey C, Wyman J, Zhang M. COVID-19 opioid agonist treatment guidance: 2020. Available at: http://www.metaphi.ca/wp-content/uploads/2021/10/COVID19_OpioidAgonistTreatmentGuidance.pdf. Accessed July 21, 2021.
40. Moreland A, Guille C, McCauley JL. Increased availability of telehealth mental health and substance abuse treatment for peripartum and postpartum women: A unique opportunity to increase telehealth treatment. J Subst Abuse Treat 2021;123:108268.
41. Volkow ND. Collision of the COVID-19 and addiction epidemics. Ann Intern Med 2020;173(1):61–2.
42. Samuels EA, Clark SA, Wunsch C, et al. Innovation during COVID-19: improving addiction treatment access. J Addict Med 2020;14(4):e8–9.
43. Castillo M, Conte B, Hinkes S, et al. Implementation of a medical student-run telemedicine program for medications for opioid use disorder during the COVID-19 pandemic. Harm Reduct J 2020;17(1):88.
44. Cole TO, Robinson D, Kelley-Freeman A, et al. Patient satisfaction with medications for opioid use disorder treatment via telemedicine: brief literature review and development of a new assessment. Front Public Health 2021;8:557275.
45. Mielau J, Vogel M, Gutwinski S, et al. New approaches in drug dependence: opioids. Curr Addict Rep 2021;1–8. https://doi.org/10.1007/s40429-021-00373-9.
46. Seddon J, Trevena P, Wadd S, et al. Addressing the needs of older adults receiving alcohol treatment during the COVID-19 pandemic: a qualitative study. Aging Ment Health 2021;1–6. https://doi.org/10.1080/13607863.2021.1910794.

47. Rosen D. Increasing participation in a substance misuse programs: lessons learned for implementing telehealth solutions during the COVID-19 pandemic. Am J Geriatr Psychiatry 2021;29(1):24–6.
48. Mellis AM, Potenza MN, Hulsey JN. COVID-19-related treatment service disruptions among people with single- and polysubstance use concerns. J Subst Abuse Treat 2021;121:108180.
49. Drake C, Yu J, Lurie N, et al. Policies to improve substance use disorder treatment with telehealth during the COVID-19 pandemic and beyond. J Addict Med 2020;14(5):e139–41.
50. Prochaska JJ, Vogel EA, Chieng A, et al. A therapeutic relational agent for reducing problematic substance use (Woebot): development and usability study. J Med Internet Res 2021;23(3):e24850.
51. Marsch LA, Dallery J. Advances in the psychosocial treatment of addiction: the role of technology in the delivery of evidence-based psychosocial treatment. Psychiatr Clin North Am 2012;35(2):481–93.
52. Marsch LA. Digital Health and Addiction. Curr Opin Syst Biol 2020;20:1–7.

Impact of COVID-19 on Mental Health Care Practitioners

Peter Yellowlees, MBBS, MD

KEYWORDS

• Psychiatrist • Telepsychiatry • Hybrid practice • Burnout • Workforce • Well-being

KEY POINTS

- Many mental health practitioners, including psychiatrists, have suffered multiple social and mental health impacts from COVID-19
- A range of actions are described that health care organizations and individuals can take to mitigate these impacts
- There will likely be substantial positive short- and long-term outcomes for psychiatrists individually and as a profession post-COVID-19

Nothing is permanent in this wicked world – not even our troubles

—Charlie Chaplin

INTRODUCTION

COVID-19 has been described as a forced experiment that has had a major impact on mental health practitioners, including psychiatrists, who even before the pandemic were struggling at best with workforce shortages across most of the mental health disciplines. In 2019 approximately half of all patients with significant mental health problems were either not receiving any form of care, or not being treated by a mental health professional of any description. In 2017 future shortages of psychiatrists by 2025 were estimated at between 14,000 and 31,000 following many years of reduced training activities and residency positions, in the setting of an expanding population and increasing needs.[1]

All of these calculations and projections have been changed by COVID-19, which has proven to be a massive disrupter of not just medical and mental health practice, but of the professionals involved in that practice. Future workforce projections are still fluid, but anecdotal reports suggest that it is likely that there will be, and already have been, many more retirements and exits of psychiatrists from psychiatric practice for

Department of Psychiatry and Behavioral Sciences, University of California Davis, 2230 Stockton Boulevard, Sacramento, CA 95817, USA
E-mail address: pmyellowlees@ucdavis.edu
Twitter: @peteryellowlees (P.Y.)

Psychiatr Clin N Am 45 (2022) 109–121
https://doi.org/10.1016/j.psc.2021.11.007
psych.theclinics.com
0193-953X/22/

other reasons than previously predicted, making psychiatry, a workforce shortage discipline before COVID-19, even more so in future.

At first glance it may seem that COVID-19 will have a primarily negative impact on psychiatrists and other mental health professionals. However, there are indications that despite the short-term difficulties related to the individual health and circumstances of all mental health professionals, in the setting of what has been called a "mental health pandemic" of increased numbers of patients, this is not necessarily the case. In fact the disruption that COVID-19 has caused to mental health practice may well have dramatically accelerated numerous structural changes to mental health practice that would have otherwise taken a decade or more to occur, leading to significant improvements and positive impacts on the remaining, and future, generations of mental health professionals.

In this article the focus is on the impact of COVID-19 on mental health care workers, with most of the spotlight on psychiatrists, as the profession that is best described, and where the impact of COVID-19 has probably been greatest. Three major questions are discussed:

- What have been the mental health impacts of COVID-19 on psychiatrists and other mental health professionals?
- What actions can health care organizations and individuals take to mitigate these?
- What are the likely positive short- and long-term outcomes for psychiatrists and other mental health workers post-COVID-19?

All of these questions are examined within the wider context of the pandemic and its' effect on health care workers around the world, many thousands of whom have lost their lives helping their patients often through heroic actions. Although this article, and this issue, focuses mainly on positive outcomes from the pandemic, it is vital to remember that this is occurring on the back of massive sacrifices by many of our colleagues.

WHAT HAVE BEEN THE MENTAL HEALTH IMPACTS OF COVID-19 ON PSYCHIATRISTS AND OTHER MENTAL HEALTH PROFESSIONALS?

COVID-19 has contributed to stress in physicians in many ways.[2] This includes anxiety about family and friends, and of taking the virus home, which most of the author's colleagues have reported as being their number one concern. Also of great importance have been changing policies related to patient care standards, biohazards, and lack of personal protective equipment and a fear of general transmission and contamination. For many there has been increased (or sometimes reduced) physical and emotional work demands, and sometimes anxiety around changed work roles, or possible separation from family members and social supports, and significant economic, work, and social changes. In mental health practice this often meant rapidly transitioning to telehealth approaches with patients which, although most mental health professionals found this straightforward, was still in the context of the need for safety for patients and providers, and to maintain a viable clinical practice. Finally, and especially for those involved clinically, was loss and grief, anger, and frustration at the constant change and uncertainty, and in relation to deaths or illnesses of colleagues or friends.

COVID-19 has also led to a range of moral injuries in physicians and other health care workers. These have been extensively discussed in the literature, including by the National Academy of Medicine.[3] Moral injuries, which have historically been primarily associated with wartime and military scenarios, are most easily defined by the severity and type of the stressor,[4] as in **Box 1**.

Mental health professionals have been affected by several of these moral injury stressors, especially the inability to provide optimal care to patients without COVID in traditional in-person ways via inpatient and outpatient modalities. Certainly, as detailed elsewhere in this issue, the move to telepsychiatry helped, but many patients, especially those with chronic relapsing illnesses, undoubtably suffered through a relative lack of psychiatric care at times. In the United States the politicization of mask wearing and vaccination has caused great distress among many health care workers because large groups within the country have refused public health measures, putting others including health care workers at risk, and themselves. Whether the incidence of moral injuries has increased the vulnerability of health care workers to burnout and a range of psychiatric disorders, especially depression, anxiety, and substance use, is unknown, but likely.

What about the core pre-COVID-19 mental health of physicians in the United States? In terms of general mental health, physicians, including psychiatrists, have the same level of mental health problems as the rest of the community except in relation to four areas as defined in the following clinical care points.[5,6]

Clinical Care Points: Physician Mental Health Differences From the General Population

1. Burnout rates in physicians are known to be at twice the level of other professional groups, mainly caused by organizational dysfunction,[5] because numerous studies have demonstrated that before commencing medical school, physicians are more resilient than equivalent graduate students
2. Female physicians likely have twice the rate of suicide in comparison with community control subjects, and it is possible that male physicians also have increased rates, although the research is not clear[6,7]
3. Although alcohol use rates are similar, physicians tend to abuse prescribed drugs more commonly, and illicit drugs less commonly, than community control subjects
4. A lower prevalence of schizophrenia, which tends to commence before or during the typical years spent at medical school

The other group of physicians affected by COVID-19 in particular are psychiatric residents and other learners. Few studies have been published on the impact on these groups in particular, but there are studies in internal medicine trainees showing

Box 1
Definitions of moral injuries

Severe moral stressors

- Denial of treatment to patients with COVID because of lack of resources
- Inability to provide optimal care to patients without COVID for many reasons
- Concern about passing COVID to loved ones

Moderate moral stressors

- Preventing visitors, especially to dying patients
- Triaging patients for health care services with inadequate information
- Trying to solve the tension between the need for self-preservation and the need to treat

Lower level but common moral challenges, especially in the community

- Seeing others not protecting the community by hoarding food, partying, not social distancing, or not wearing masks

significantly disrupted training, especially with the forced move to see patients using video visits, often from home, where residents typically have less privacy and financial capacity to set up a study area than do more senior physicians. Anecdotal reports of psychiatric residents being required to work beyond the usual scope of their roles on general medical wards, the reduction in important supportive friendships with other residents, and of increased loneliness and reduced opportunities for relationships at an important developmental stage in their lives are other important stressors on this group.

So if one takes these issues into account, and includes in a calculation the effect of moral injuries and immediate pandemic-related traumas that many physicians have suffered, it is reasonable to hypothesize that the overall mental health impact of COVID-19 on physicians, including psychiatrists and other mental health workers, has been at least the same as for the general population, or possibly slightly greater. Although the research on the general population in the United States is still incomplete it seems clear that at least the mental health impacts in **Box 2** have occurred.[2,8,9]

One can assume that, taking these epidemiologic variations into account, physicians should have suffered at least the same, or more, mental health consequences from the impact of the pandemic than the general population. As a consequence it is likely that physicians will be part of what is now being called a mental health shadow pandemic following COVID-19.[8] One cross-sectional study early in the pandemic from Cyprus, a country at the time little affected by COVID-19, showed high rates of depression and post-traumatic stress disorder in physicians and other health care workers, especially nurses,[10] indicating how vulnerable was this group.

Finally, more than 3600 physicians and other health care workers, including several psychiatrists and other mental health care workers, have died from COVID-19 in the United States during the pandemic. "Lost on the Frontline," a project run for a year from April 2020 by Kaiser Health News and the Guardian, is the most complete accounting of US health care worker deaths.[11] The project found that two-thirds of deceased health care workers identified as people of color, revealing the deep inequities tied to race, ethnicity, and economic status in America's health care workforce. Other findings were:

- Lower-paid workers who handled everyday patient care, including nurses, support staff, and nursing home employees, were far more likely to die in the pandemic than physicians
- The median age of health care workers who died was 59, whereas in the general population, the median age of death from COVID was 78

Box 2
Mental health impacts of COVID-19 on the general population

1. Increased incidence of anxiety, depression, and substance use disorders
2. Increased grief and loss in relation to illnesses, deaths, relationships, and missed important life or transitional events
3. Increased rates of trauma-related disorders, especially intimate partner violence, gambling, excess online activities, and possibly abortions and suicides
4. Increased isolation and loneliness, which lead to chronic medical and psychiatric disorders and impaired work performance
5. Increased levels of social division, extremism, and polarization, especially via social media, leading to interpersonal, family, and community division

- More than a third of the health care workers who died were born outside the United States
- Nurses and support staff members died in far higher numbers than physicians
- Twice as many workers died in nursing homes as in hospitals
- The death rate among health care workers has slowed dramatically since COVID vaccines were made available to them in December 2020

It is obvious that support and treatment services for physicians and other health care workers need to be increased and made more available post-COVID-19, and that organizational interventions to prevent physician burnout and distress are even more important postpandemic than previously. This brings us to the second question.

WHAT ACTIONS CAN HEALTH CARE ORGANIZATIONS AND INDIVIDUALS TAKE TO MITIGATE THE IMPACTS OF COVID-19 ON MENTAL HEALTH CARE WORKERS?

A recent guidance document from the American Psychiatric Association[12] describes a range of practical initiatives that all health care organizations could implement to do exactly this. The guidance covers five major themes, discussed next.

Create an Organizational Leadership Structure to Lead Efforts to Address Wellness in the Physician Health Care Workforce

This includes funding the roles of Chief Wellness Officer and support teams, ensuring that leadership training in well-being occurs and that physicians are entrusted to leadership positions throughout the organization so that their voice is heard, and is influential.

Create a Culture of Wellness and Mutual Support Throughout the Organization

This involves developing policies and actions that create a trustworthy team-based medical culture that takes into account a strong focus on diversity, equity, and inclusion and that regularly measures physician burnout and provides widespread mentoring opportunities, especially for physicians at times of career transition. This cultural change also involves transparent bidirectional communication using many differing approaches.

Improve the Clinical Efficiency and Leadership of Physicians and Encourage Team-Based Practice to Reduce Stress and Burnout

Here physicians with innovative ideas should be involved in a mission-driven manner to become part of the larger health system meaning and focus, especially when improving workflows and reducing documentation requirements from the electronic medical record and developing video visits and other electronic ways of improving health outcomes.

Promote and Educate About Individual Self-Care and Resilience Approaches

A large number of effective evidence-based approaches to helping self-care are available and educational programs about self-care and mental health access, all of which support resilience.

Provide Timely Easy Nonstigmatized Access to Emotional Support and Mental Health Care for All Physicians

This includes multiple differing approaches from buddy systems to peer support networks, and self-assessment tools and easy referral to mental health experts.

One example of this wide range of initiatives needed to support physician well-being is transparent and truthful messaging from the leadership of health organizations, not just about the status of the health system and its capacity to cope and plan for the present and the future, but in particular about how health care workers, including physicians, can best be supported. An example of such messaging on the topic of physician well-being is the "Good Stuff" message[13] sent weekly by the author to all UC Davis physicians, and monthly to all staff. During 2020 to 2021 these messages covered a wide range of issues from the importance of gratitude, coping with uncertainty, fostering relationships, psychological first aid and family fun at home to living in a bubble, how to embrace change and overcome anxiety, social connecting, and coping with moral injuries, among many other topics. "Good Stuff" also includes weekly celebrations of positive patient comments about physicians and other health care staff and links to relevant well-being resources and programs. This well-being message became part of the culture of UC Davis Health during COVID-19 and will continue in the postpandemic era as a constant reminder about the importance of well-being for all health care staff, especially physicians.

Looking forward following the pandemic, the National Academy of Medicine[14] has published an important discussion paper examining the lessons learned, and compelling needs going forward, from an impact assessment of COVID-19 on clinicians. The paper summarized the impact on clinicians as follows[14]:

> *Pandemic-era stressors spanning dangers to clinicians' personal safety, to isolation from personal and professional support networks, to the persistent burden of working in understaffed and over-booked care delivery settings, to the role of structural racism in contributing to stark inequities in pandemic outcomes, have all exacerbated pre-pandemic trends of rising burnout, moral distress and deteriorating clinician well-being. COVID-19 has exposed existing challenges for the clinician sector, from the instability of fee-for-service reimbursement to the gaps in clinical capacity for specific specialties (eg, critical care) and populations (eg, rural, safety net), to the inequities embedded into health professionals training and clinical care.*

This article described five priority areas for clinicians generally, not just physicians, for future development as discussed next:

Investing in clinician well-being

Recommendations here included rebuilding trust of clinicians lost during the pandemic and implementing recommendations of prior reports from the Academy, which described how to mitigate burnout, often driven by moral distress, and improve physician leadership opportunities, and to strengthen protections for clinicians to report safety and ethical concerns without fear of retribution or retaliation.

Advancing innovations in clinician practice

Suggestions here included enabling clinicians to be able to work across state lines, while encouraging retention and recruitment strategies to address workforce shortages and standardizing evidence-based protocols more widely, while also investing in infrastructure to achieve more effective health data sharing.

Promoting financial resilience for clinicians

Given that there were multiple failures of the traditional fee-for-service system, with many physician practices failing during the pandemic, the need to develop payment models that support quality, value, and team-based care, while reducing administrative requirements, was promoted, especially long-term coverage of telehealth services.

Transforming education and training
Here a major focus was on reducing inequities in resources, such as structural racism, while addressing financial barriers to student progression in health professions and using more technology and simulation for continuous learning.

Addressing health disparities
The crucial need to develop fair, equitable, and transparent plans for all health care services that do not disadvantage certain groups, and which are constantly surveilled to ensure that unintended consequences are not arising, was a major focus and learning from the pandemic.

Implementing these constructive recommendations within the mental health workforce, and in particular within the psychiatric profession, could lead to positive changes in the future. It may well be that the pandemic will be a tipping point for the profession, giving it the opportunity to change clinical practices extensively, just as it has been a tipping point for telehealth and has led to the widespread rapid implementation and acceptance of video and audio consultations. This leads to possible positive outcomes.

WHAT ARE THE LIKELY POSITIVE SHORT- AND LONG-TERM OUTCOMES FOR PSYCHIATRISTS AND OTHER MENTAL HEALTH WORKERS POST-COVID-19?

The COVID-19 pandemic has been a period of forced experimentation, where several practice changes have occurred much faster than could have ever been predicted. Many of these changes have already started to lead to likely positive outcomes for psychiatrists and other mental health professionals, especially the increased interest in physician well-being across the United States, and the added resources being devoted to assist physicians to receive care, treatment, and support in many health care systems and environments. Such positive outcomes are discussed next.

The Development of Hybrid Care: How Telepsychiatry Will Change and Improve Psychiatric Practice

Psychiatry, unlike many other specialties, was able to change dramatically and take to telehealth early in the pandemic,[15,16] leading to less stress on mental health clinicians than other disciplines, and their continuing ability to manage panels of patients, often better than in the past, and with less "no shows," improved clinical quality, and more continuity of care. A recent report describing the possible future transformation of psychiatry[17] details the history of the use of telepsychiatry and the technological revolution that has affected the profession of psychiatry during the pandemic, noting that digital care is no longer a valuable aid, but an essential need. The authors concluded that psychiatry will: "emerge altered by its new use of technology and by larger societal trends. While this is a time of uncertainty, threat and change, it is also a time of great opportunity to shape and improve access to psychiatric care for the benefit of patients and practitioners."[17]

Before the pandemic new models of hybrid psychiatric care were being developed by blending videoconferencing with other technologies, such as electronic health records, patient portals, and passive data-collection tools on smartphones.[18] Examples of these hybrid approaches included virtual models of integrated care; residential psychiatric care; and asynchronous psychiatry, such as store and forward telepsychiatry e-consultations. This evolution led psychiatrists, and other medical professionals, into a new epoch of "hybrid doctor-patient relationships,"[19] which are now emerging much more commonly postpandemic as groups of patients and psychiatrists start meeting together in person, or continue online, or mix the modalities.

The term "hybrid" describes relationships that are managed through a variety of mediums including in person, videoconferencing, patient portals, telephone, texts, and email. The psychiatrist works to match the most appropriate communication medium based on the patient's diagnosis and needs and social and personal circumstances, with patients also making choices of communication modality depending on their own circumstances and convenience.[18,19] Psychiatrists have had to learn the strengths, weaknesses, clinical adaptations, regulations, and parameters for each of these technologies because these hybrid-relationship models have been radically and rapidly advanced during the pandemic out of necessity, but as a profession have done this extremely well. It is impossible to predict how much traditional psychiatric practice will be affected by this change long-term, but the author has been practicing in this hybrid way for several years and has found that at least 50% of his patients have moved to a hybrid relationship with him.

Reduction of Psychiatrist Workforce Shortages, With Increased Work From Home and More Flexible Work Hours

A side effect of the move to hybrid and virtual care during COVID-19 should be, in the long term, a more efficient use of psychiatrist's time and expertise with more psychiatrists working with increased scheduling and geographic flexibility from home, leading to reduced workforce shortages and reduced burnout levels. This set of outcomes was described in a paper published before the pandemic[20] where the authors reviewed national workforce issues and organizational and individual obstacles for implementing a telepsychiatry workforce based primarily in the home, including administrative, logistical, and clinical considerations. They then offered ideas and resources for how to overcome barriers that may arise in implementing a remote workforce of psychiatrists, as has eventuated during COVID-19. They hypothesized that before the pandemic, burnout was likely a key factor contributing to psychiatrists working less, pursuing less acute cases, and leading to worsened outcomes for patients and the psychiatrists themselves, and then demonstrated evidence that telepsychiatry provides comparable patient and provider satisfaction and equal outcomes when compared with in-person encounters. To support their argument they used several examples of psychiatrists demonstrating successful delivery of care from home in a range of clinic settings and workplace configurations while optimizing their quality of life and reducing their risk of burnout.

There is also widespread publicity about the "mental health pandemic"[8] that is predicted to follow the COVID-19 pandemic. This includes the impact of isolation and loneliness, now viewed as social determinants of disease, and dramatically increased during COVID-19, and the polarization of community views driven by differing perspectives and beliefs about the pandemic and the need, or otherwise, for masking and social distancing public health measures. In this setting it is likely that more attention at a national level will be paid to prior and impending shortages of psychiatrists in future as this second pandemic continues over time, especially in patients with long-haul COVID-19 complications. It is hoped that the need to scale the capacity of the current psychiatric workforce will also include a move away from fee-for-service billing and toward bundled payments models, which should make psychiatrists' work more efficient because they are increasingly paid for care provided over time. A side effect of this change should be a reduction in administrative workloads for many psychiatrists, who not uncommonly spend 10% to 20% of their week on such tasks, especially in private practice environments, as the administrative and financial workflows are improved and more closely parallel the "care as a journey" perspective that many surveys have shown patients prefer.

Psychiatrists' Well-Being Improved With Less Burnout

The increased use of telepsychiatry and working from home is likely to improve psychiatrists' well-being, as is a greater focus on physician needs, as described in an excellent influential 2019 report[21] from the United Kingdom that examined how to meet the "ABC" of physician needs: autonomy, belonging, and competency.

However, there are a series of other positive benefits of telepsychiatry and more flexible working arrangements that will likely improve psychiatrists' overall well-being.[17,18] These include the following:

1. Time saving through seeing patients on video, where it is possible to document notes at the same time as seeing patients, and where there is also time saved with less "no shows" and the lack of time used entering and exiting a physical room during the rooming process. It has been estimated that these time saving elements will average up to 10 minutes of saved time per hour through the average work day, making more than an hour per day available for telephone calls, inbox management, and other administrative matters, which will no longer have to be done after hours.
2. Home visits to patients are cheaper than those in the clinic, especially if the psychiatrist is also working from home. Technology is cheap compared with renting office space, paying for reception staff, and traveling to work. Hybrid relationships are physically and psychologically safer and more intimate, with the extra distance involved in a video visit to a patient in their home enabling the patient to feel more relaxed and confident in their own environment, while at the same time being less intimidated and able to share deeper information with their therapist. Seeing patients at home provides the psychiatrist with more information about their patient, which improves the care they can provide. They get to see the state of the patient's home, a proxy for an extended look at their mental state, and meet other members of the family and pets, and explore the patient's interests and passions via objects and artwork that they can see in the home. The author often asks patients to show him around the house and garden so that he has a better idea of how the patient lives, eats, and relaxes, and looks to connect more closely with his patients by finding mutual interests in art, sport, or cultural events. If privacy does not exist in the home, the car is an excellent alternative therapy room, as long as it is parked in a quiet area and has all the windows shut.
3. Telepsychiatry allows better matching of patients and psychiatrists than is usually possible in a physical clinic. Many psychiatrists like to specialize with the types of patients they see and treat, and this is a significant advantage of using video, where it is possible to see patients with particular disorders who may live far away allowing such psychiatrists to indulge their specific clinical interests in, say, patients with eating disorders or autism. Equally some patients prefer to see particular psychiatrists, perhaps women or those who speak their own language, and this is easier to arrange on video. Equally some patients (**Box 3**) prefer to be seen online than in-person.
4. Language interpretation on video is also highly effective, with several commercial video interpreting groups easily available. The experience for the physician who is talking via the interpreter is often easier online than in-person.
5. Teaching and group work or supervision is often easier on video than in-person. It is possible to bring in larger groups of people or students, and to move people around using breakout video rooms, while taking questions on chat. If seeing patients as part of the teaching, they can be brought in, and then moved to a waiting area while discussion occurs, and then brought back. This can all be done conveniently with a virtual class spread across many different sites.

Box 3
Clinical pearls: patients who prefer being treated online than in-person

- Children
- VIPs (eg, celebrities, physicians, lawyers)
- Individuals who are paranoid, agoraphobic, or who have post-traumatic stress disorder
- Individuals who prefer to be seen from home for any reason (eg, COVID-19)
- Individuals for whom the stigma of attending an office visit is too much
- Individuals who live at a distance, or who cannot easily travel (eg, from nursing homes or correctional institutions)

6. Group therapy has finally, during COVID-19, emerged as something that can commonly be provided online, with several intensive outpatient programs in particular moving their entire group-related activities online successfully, or taking up hybrid approaches. Groups for six to eight people, in particular, seem to work well online with everyone able to see each other and interact easily, leading to an easier role for facilitators.
7. Recording video interviews with patients is becoming more common, and can allow a psychiatrist to replay parts of an interview, for personal learning or supervision purposes, and asynchronous telepsychiatry for clinical care direct to the home has been trialed during COVID-19.[22] With the advent of asynchronous telepsychiatry, where a patient is interviewed and recorded, and the recording sent to a different expert for analysis or a second opinion, a whole new approach to telepsychiatry, asynchronous telepsychiatry, has been developed. Essentially this is a souped-up form of a curbside or e-consultation where, instead of a quick patient summary and a question being sent to an expert, a video of the patient's mental state and a semistructured interview is sent. A recent randomized controlled clinical trial comparing the clinical outcomes of asynchronous and synchronous video consultations in patients with anxiety and depression in primary care showed similar levels of useful clinical improvements in both groups. Although asynchronous telepsychiatry is novel, in future it is likely to become common, and will allow psychiatrists to scale their work more efficiently, doing consultations during clinic "down time."[22] Looking further ahead, the use of video as data allows the implementation of artificial intelligence, machine learning, and voice and facial movement recognition technologies, all of which ultimately should help the psychiatrists of the future.
8. Finally much has been written about the cognitive load required to spend hours on videoconferences leading to what is commonly called "zoom fatigue." Although this may affect some people, if breaks are taken between conferences for 5 to 10 minutes each, especially if they involve some simple exercises or stretches, this seems less of a problem. There is now some evidence that the extra efficiency of videoconferences, with a lack of need to travel between meetings, especially when the agendas for meetings are carefully managed, may actually be less stressful than prior days full of in-person meetings running into each other. Many clinicians and regular users of video visits are now making their consultations and meetings much more structured than previously, and are finding that this not only gives them breaks, but is less stressful overall. In reality the jury is still out in terms of the cognitive load of videoconferences versus the cognitive load of in-person meetings or consultations, and there is probably little difference overall,

because it can certainly be tiring to spend an entire day without breaks in either set of meetings.

Acknowledgment of Psychiatrists and other Health Care Workers As Being Essential Workers, and More Overt Demonstration of their Lived Experience in the Workplace

Early in the pandemic there were numerous examples of communities applauding health care workers as they left work after shifts or returned to their homes. These ranged from groups of grateful people waiting outside hospitals to whole communities living in apartments coming out onto their balconies and applauding. The day-to-day work of health care professionals has traditionally been kept secret from the general public, unless they are patients, because of the need to maintain confidentiality, but in COVID-19 there has been a sudden exposure of many health care worker practices by the media, and usually in a positive or admiring way, especially in emergency departments and intensive care units. Suddenly the potential dangers faced by some health care workers have been understood by the public, and there has been much more open discussion about the lived experience of health care workers.

Has this extended to psychiatrists and the mental health workforce? Likely it has to at least a certain extent, although with less emphasis on the potential personal danger from infection. In many hospitals and inpatient units psychiatrists have been continuing to see patients in-person, wearing full personal protective equipment, as part of a multidisciplinary team. Several have died or become seriously ill, and some were required to work as general physicians when staff shortages occurred. Working in an academic medical center myself, I know that it is difficult to connect with a masked patient while personally also masked and wearing a clear plastic facial guard but many psychiatrists have had to work like this routinely during the pandemic. Given the choice, the author would much rather see a patient on video, with no need for any masking by either person, than in-person with both people masked and in protective equipment.

It will be interesting to see if the positive aspects of being essential workers is sustained postpandemic and is not forgotten. Sadly, in the United States as the pandemic continued on into 2021 there were increasing numbers of reports of people who did not believe in the existence of COVID-19 attacking or abusing health care staff. It is hoped this will not continue. The lesson to be learned from COVID-19, however, is the importance of being transparent about the workforce practices in health care, rather than tending to automatically hide behind the privacy excuse, which only leaves the general public ignorant of the real world of health care, and dependent on overly dramatized television shows for their perception of the lived experience of health care workers.

A Greater Focus on Health Disparities and Structural Racism Throughout the Health Care System

COVID-19 has undoubtably shone a bright light on those in our society who are underserved and disadvantaged, and on the long-term previously poorly acknowledged structural racism that exists within the health care environment, never mind more broadly throughout society, especially in the United States. Much has been written about the increased morbidity and mortality affecting the African American, Hispanic, and Native American communities generally, and which is also seen among the more than 3600 health care workers who have died of COVID-19.[11] Unfortunately, this same problem is seen even when implementing telepsychiatry[18] where such populations as the homeless, the poor, and racially and linguistically diverse groups are less able to receive telepsychiatry services because they cannot afford smartphones with connection plans, or cannot keep them safely, are not technologically literate, or live in inaccessible situations.

A positive bright spot during COVID-19 has been the ability of psychiatrists to do audio-only consultations with patients, which has been shown to be a good way of connecting with patients who have serious mental illness in New York,[23] and in some respects was shown to be a more effective approach than even in-person visits. It is to be hoped that the regulations that were relaxed during the pandemic to allow these consultations will continue permanently. Some states, such as California, are heading in that direction, but at the time of writing it is unclear what will be the federal response to paying for telephony. Returning to the prior regulations restricting geographic use of telehealth and telephony, which have been described as examples of structural racism within the health care system, would seem to be a retrograde step.[24]

SUMMARY

Despite the generally disruptive adverse impact of COVID-19 on the mental health workforce, there are constructive plans being proposed to improve the well-being of clinicians, and several likely positive outcomes from the forced experiment that has been the pandemic. The practice of psychiatry and mental health care has changed significantly and rapidly, and a hybrid approach to care involving the integration of multiple technologies and novel asynchronous approaches into mental health practice is a likely positive consequence. This approach to care should improve the well-being of the mental health workforce, giving practitioners more flexibility and more control over their schedules and their lives, hence reducing the likelihood of burnout and other mental health disorders. It is hoped that the exposure of the lived experience of many practitioners will lead to improved understanding from patients and that in future much more emphasis within mental health care will be placed on providing access and services to those members of society adversely affected by disparities and structural racism.

DISCLOSURE

Dr P. Yellowlees has nothing to disclose.

REFERENCES

1. Satiani A, Niedermier J, Satiani B, et al. Projected Workforce of Psychiatrists in the United States: A Population Analysis Psychiatric Services. 2018. Available at: https://doi.org/10.1176/appi.ps.201700344. Accessed Mar 15 2018.
2. Yellowlees P. Physician well-being: good stuff during COVID-19. Medscape. In Press.
3. Madara J, Miyamoto S, Farley JE, et al. Discussion Paper. Clinicians and Professional Societies COVID-19 Impact Assessment: Lessons Learned and Compelling Needs. National Academy of Medicine; 2021.
4. Yellowlees P. When the only clinical choices are "lose-lose". Medscape. Available at: https://www.medscape.com/viewarticle/938823. Accessed October 8 2020.
5. Yellowlees PM. Physician well-being: cases and solutions. Washington, DC: American Psychiatric Association Press; 2020.
6. Yellowlees PM. Physician suicide: cases and commentaries. Washington, DC: American Psychiatric Association Press; 2019.

7. Ye GY, Davidson JE, Kim K, et al. Physician death by suicide in the United States 2012-16. J Psychiatr Res 2021;134:158–65.
8. Kardaras N. Inside the mental health shadow pandemic caused by COVID-19. New York: New York Post; 2021.
9. Morbidity and Mortality Weekly Report. Mental health, substance use, and suicidal ideation during the COVID-19 pandemic - United States, June 24-30, 2020. CDC; 2020.
10. Chatzittofis A, Karanikola M, Michailidou K. et al. Impact of the COVID-19 pandemic on the mental health of healthcare workers. Int J Environ Res Public Health 2021;18(4):1435.
11. Lost on the Frontline. Kaiser Health News. Available at: https://khn.org/news/lost-on-the-frontline-explore-the-database. Accessed June 17th 2021.
12. American Psychiatric Association. Guidance Document on Actions and Activities that a Healthcare Organization can take to support its Physician Workforce Well-being during COVID-19 and beyond. Available at: www.psychiatry.org. Accessed 11-5-2021.
13. Good Stuff messages 2020-21. UC Davis Health. Available at: https://health.ucdavis.edu/clinician-health-and-well-being/Program/Good-Stuff-Newsletters.html.
14. National Academy of Medicine. Taking action against clinician burnout: a systems approach to professional well-being. A consensus study. 2019. Washington, DC.
15. Ongur D, Perlis R, Goff D. Psychiatry and COVID-19. JAMA 2020;324(12):1149–50.
16. Yellowlees P, Nakagawa K, Pakyurek M, et al. Rapid conversion of an outpatient psychiatric clinic to a 100% virtual telepsychiatry clinic in response to COVID-19. Psychiatr Serv 2020;71(7):749–52.
17. Shore J, Yellowlees P. The COVID-19 pandemic and virtual care: the transformation of psychiatry. Psychiatric News; 20th April 2021. Available at: https://psychnews.psychiatryonline.org/doi/10.1176/appi.pn.2021.5.30. Accessed June 2 2021.
18. Yellowlees P, Shore J. Telepsychiatry and health technologies: a guide for mental health professionals. Washington DC: APPI; 2018.
19. Yellowlees P, Chan SR, Parish M. "The hybrid doctor-patient relationship in the age of technology: telepsychiatry consultations and the use of virtual space." International Review of Psychiatry. Int Rev Psychiatry 2015;27(6):476–89.
20. Gardner JS, Plaven BE, Yellowlees P, et al. Remote telepsychiatry workforce: a solution psychiatry's workforce. Issues Curr Psychiatry Rep 2020;22:8.
21. Caring for Doctors. Caring for Patients. General Medical Council. UK. 2019. Available at: https://www.gmc-uk.org/-/media/documents/caring-for-doctors-caring-for-patients_pdf-80706341.pdf. Accessed June 17th 2021.
22. Yellowlees PM, Parish MB, Gonzalez AD, et al. Clinical outcomes of asynchronous v synchronous telepsychiatry in primary care: a randomized controlled trial. J Med Internet Res 2021. https://doi.org/10.2196/24047.
23. Avalone L, Barron C, King C, et al. Rapid telepsychiatry implementation during COVID-19: increased attendance at the largest health system in the United States. Psychiatr Serv 2021;72(6):708–11.
24. Yellowlees P. Commentary on Avalone et al.: "reimbursement for telepsychiatry: permanent changes are needed. Psychiatr Serv 2021;72(6):724–5.

The Impact of COVID-19 on Brain Stimulation Therapy

Michael Justin Coffey, MD[a,*], Suzanne Kerns, MBBS[b], Sohag Sanghani, MD[c], Lee Wachtel, MD[d]

KEYWORDS

- Electroconvulsive therapy (ECT) • Transcranial magnetic stimulation (TMS)
- Brain stimulation • COVID-19 • Access to care

KEY POINTS

- The COVID-19 pandemic severely restricted access to ECT and all but eliminated access to TMS.
- These changes occurred during a time when the availability of safe and effective psychiatric treatment was vital and, to some degree, may have been avoidable.
- ECT and TMS services have gradually begun to resume operations, but not without significant changes in practice.

INTRODUCTION

Among the far-reaching effects of the COVID-19 pandemic has been restricted access to safe and effective forms of psychiatric treatment. Focusing on electroconvulsive therapy (ECT) and transcranial magnetic stimulation (TMS), we review the pandemic's impact on brain stimulation therapy by asking 3 fundamental questions—Where have we been? How are we doing? And where are we going?

WHERE HAVE WE BEEN?

The onset of the international COVID-19 pandemic in March 2020 taxed health care systems worldwide, and the impact on ECT services was severe. In France and Belgium, for example, half of ECT services suspended operations.[1,2] In the United States, the first 2 months of the pandemic reduced the number of ECT treatments delivered by 74%.[3] Eighty percent of US academic medical centers reported operating at less than half their typical ECT volume.[4] Among these institutions alone, restricted access to ECT care was linked to patient suicide and suicidal behavior.[4]

[a] Geisinger Health System, 100 N Academy Ave, Danville, PA 17822, USA; [b] Medical University of South Carolina, Charleston, SC, USA; [c] Zucker School of Medicine at Hofstra/Northwell, Hempstead, NY, USA; [d] Kennedy Krieger Institute, Baltimore, MD, USA
* Corresponding author.
E-mail address: jcoffey1@geisinger.edu

Psychiatr Clin N Am 45 (2022) 123–131
https://doi.org/10.1016/j.psc.2021.11.008

There were 2 primary drivers of this harsh reality—supply and perception. During an ECT treatment, the need for muscle relaxation necessitates general anesthesia and positive pressure ventilation, thus making ECT an aerosolizing procedure. All such procedures require the use of personal protective equipment (PPE), including N-95 masks, eye protection, isolation gowns, and gloves for each member of the ECT team.[5] When the supply of PPE was limited, hospitals were faced with implementing practices that allowed extended use or limited reuse of PPE beyond that recommended by the CDC for aerosol-generating procedures.[6] Compounding this challenge was the scarce supply of space and anesthesia providers. Anesthesiologists were reassigned to clinical areas where supplemental staff were needed to manage the influx of patients with COVID-19. Hospitals also had to convert spaces such as postanesthesia care units, where ECT treatments are often performed, into hospital or intensive care beds. These factors combined to drastically reduce the number of surgeries and procedures performed. With inadequate PPE, limited COVID-19 testing, conversion of psychiatric beds to medical beds, and reduced availability of space in which to perform ECT safely, many hospitals suspended their ECT services.

The second key driver of restricted access to ECT was the perception of ECT as an "elective" or "nonessential" procedure. During the early phase of the COVID-19 pandemic, the value of such procedures was weighed against the estimated risks to those performing them as well as the "burn rate" of the facility's PPE. Such decisions involve important ethical considerations and are not made in isolation.[7] ECT providers were quick to proclaim that ECT is most certainly not an "elective" procedure, but a lifesaving one. During times of resource scarcity, such as during a pandemic, access to ECT is arguably even more essential. Professional societies reinforced this view[8–12] and implored the medical community to remember the life-saving effects of ECT, particularly for severely ill patients receiving an acute course of ECT, but also for patients receiving maintenance ECT, who are vulnerable to illness recurrence without continued treatment.[2,8] The pediatric population, especially individuals with autism and intellectual disability, were emphasized in such entreaties, especially given the heightened stress associated with loss of structure and programming[13] and increased risk of morbidity and mortality from COVID-19 itself.[14–16]

These advocacy efforts achieved variable success. Even ECT services that were able to continue operating were required to demonstrate exceptional circumstances or obtain formal leadership approval.[17] The following vignette illustrates the impact of delays in ECT care during the pandemic.

Vignette. A previously healthy 15-year-old girl with autism experienced acute onset of catatonia in December 2019. The patient underwent comprehensive serum and cerebrospinal fluid investigations, as well as brain imaging, to rule out any organic etiologies of catatonia, and all results were within normal limits. A lorazepam trial was begun with only mild improvement with dosages up to 14 mg daily. The patient was referred to ECT but was unable to access such for approximately 2 months because of a city-wide waitlist for ECT services resulting from the diversion of both anesthesia services and agents used in anesthesia induction to COVID-19 care settings. This youth required 24-h care including assisted feeding during the wait for ECT, and experienced ongoing psychosocial incapacitation as someone who was previously a diligent high school student and accomplished athlete. The patient demonstrated approximately 85% return to baseline functioning with the introduction of ECT, yet the benefit waned and was lost with cessation of such. When a second ECT course was recommended, there was no timely option for reintroduction of a thrice-weekly acute course of ECT as optimal treatment for catatonia; a maximum of once-weekly therapy was available, and its usage did not confer benefit. Thrice-weekly ECT only became available once again a 3 month wait.

Like its significant effect on ECT services, the onset of the COVID-19 pandemic brought TMS services essentially to a standstill. Barriers to TMS included suspension of "nonessential" procedures, staffing shortages, limited access to PPE and sanitization supplies, and clinics or offices ill-equipped to comply with social distancing recommendations. Both clinical patients and research participants proved difficult to retain because of fears of infection, loss of childcare, transportation difficulties, and a host of other pandemic-related psychosocial stressors. During the same time that access to TMS was reduced, rates of conditions for which TMS is indicated, including depression and cigarette consumption, were observed to climb.[18,19] To further compound patient burden, these psychiatric conditions have been associated with worse COVID-19 outcomes, including higher mortality rates.[18,20]

HOW ARE WE DOING?

As the supply of PPE and COVID-19 tests improved, and as the scientific community learned more about the new SARS-CoV-2 virus responsible for the pandemic, opportunity emerged for brain stimulation services to begin gradually resuming operations. By June 2020, half of the 20 academic medical centers belonging to the National Network of Depression Centers had ramped up to 75% of their typical ECT patient volumes.[4] In addition, case reports emerged of patients receiving ECT safely while also suffering from diagnosed COVID-19 illness.[2,21,22]

The resumption of ECT services was not universal and brought with it significant changes in practice, not only in the United States[23–26] but also in Belgium,[2] Brazil,[27] Canada,[17] France,[28] India,[29] Ireland,[30] Singapore,[31] and Spain.[32] These changes continue to evolve and vary geographically, but the focus remains on infection prevention and control (**Box 1**). Ongoing efforts to ensure access to ECT care are vital, particularly as data indicate a 44% relapse rate at 6 months among patients whose maintenance ECT was discontinued because of the pandemic. Of these individuals, 86% had to restart an acute course of ECT.[33] The following vignette illustrates the challenges of providing optimal ECT care to a patient with COVID-19 illness.

Vignette. A woman in her late 30s suffered from bipolar disorder and had a history of suicide attempts, episodes of catatonia, and multiple psychiatric hospitalizations. She also had obesity and received a kidney transplant in January 2020. She was domiciled with her husband and 6 children. Her bipolar disorder had stabilized with pharmacotherapy and ECT, and she was receiving continuation ECT after a recent psychiatric hospitalization. Her treatment interval was just being extended to every 3 weeks when the COVID-19 pandemic hit. As the pandemic was unfolding, and in the absence of diagnostic testing, shortage of PPE and even surgical masks and given patient's immunocompromised status, the ECT team classified her in a category where the treatment interval should first be extended and, if her symptoms remained stable, suspension of ECT could be considered. However, in the week before her scheduled appointment, she suffered a relapse of major depression with suicidal ideation and despite her immunocompromised status, required hospitalization, placing her at increased COVID-19 risk in the inpatient environment. She received 6 ECT treatments following a 3 times per week schedule, and her symptoms remitted. She was discharged home with continuation/maintenance ECT as an outpatient, which was provided without COVID-19 testing until June 2020 because of testing shortages. When testing became more widely available, she was tested within 3 days of each treatment. In September 2020, she tested positive for COVID-19 during routine

Box 1
Sample of changes in ECT practice due to COVID-19

Environment and scheduling
- Waiting areas restructured to allow social distancing. Families asked to wait in their car.
- Mandatory mask requirements for staff members, patients, and visitors.
- No visitors in the treatment/recovery areas.
- Plexiglass barriers at registration desk, recovery spaces, pre-ECT evaluation areas.
- Limited number of staff members inside the treatment room.
- Regular cleaning according to the institution's infection control guidelines.
- Patients scheduled in "batches," that is, patients from one location treated in the same batch.
- Staff scheduled in "pods" to keep the same staff working together as much as possible.
- Increase in the number of clinic days to accommodate for reduced operational efficiency.

Treatment rooms
- Relocation and/or modification of the treatment room (eg, negative pressure).
- Enough time is allowed for aerosol to be cleared from the treatment room before bringing in the next patient.
- Air purification systems with high-efficiency particulate air (HEPA) filters can be installed in an individual treatment room to achieve higher air exchange rate and thereby lower air-exchange wait time between treatments.

PPE
- Extended use, selective use, and reuse of N95 masks.
- Reduced number of staff inside the treatment room.
- Face shield or eye protection, disposable gown, and gloves.

Anesthesia provision
- HEPA filter between the mask and tubing of the anesthesia circuit.
- Modifications in technique to reduce risks from aerosolization: supraglottic airway,[43] airway box,[32] preoxygenation and avoiding ventilation,[26] use of a plastic cover on the patient's head at the initiation of bag-mask ventilation,[23] use of hydrogen peroxide mouthwash and povidone-iodine nasal swabs to each nostril,[25] and apneic ventilation.[44]

Testing
- Frequently evolving requirements and approaches to preprocedure COVID-19 screening and testing, including the difficulty providers and patients experienced meeting such requirements for a procedure scheduled multiple times each week.

screening. She had denied symptoms or exposure at the time of testing but later admitted to having mild symptoms and being exposed to her infected son, who had returned sick from school. Her symptoms were limited to mild fatigue and muscle aches. Her course of ECT was suspended for 21 days. Upon reinitiation of ECT, she continued to test positive for COVID-19 during most of her visits for the subsequent 4 months and was considered "persistently positive." For that duration, she was scheduled as the last patient of the day or as the last patient of the shift, followed by terminal cleaning of the room. She continues to receive maintenance ECT every 2 weeks and at times has required rescue ECT treatments. She has received both doses of COVID-19 vaccine and plans to continue her course of maintenance ECT.

For TMS services, resuming operations was again like that of ECT. The Clinical TMS Society posted a rough outline of recommendations for how to continue operating clinical services under pandemic conditions, and a more formal framework for continuing clinical and research TMS was published a month later by an international group of experts.[34,35] **Box 2** lists modifications for continuing clinical and research TMS during the COVID-19 pandemic that were based on the aforementioned literature, Centers for Disease Control and Prevention (CDC) recommendations, and the

Box 2
Sample of changes in TMS practice due to COVID-19

Patient selection

- Patients triaged for suitability by weighing the risks of withholding TMS with the risks of potential SARS-CoV-2 infection.
- If treatment paused or withheld, referrals made to ensure continuity of care.
- Daily screening measures include a COVID-19 symptom checklist and exposure inquiry.
- COVID-19 testing, or documentation of COVID-19 vaccination before commencing any acute TMS course.
- CDC guidelines on quarantine and testing after COVID-19 exposure or symptom emergence for both patients and staff followed.

Distancing and PPE

- Waiting areas restructured to allow social distancing. Where possible, patients asked to wait in their car until called up for appointment and other visitors prohibited.
- Mandatory mask requirements for staff members, patients, and visitors.
- Plexiglass barriers between staff and patient at registration desk and other locations.
- Number of staff members inside the treatment room limited.
- Consultation and follow-up appointments performed via telemedicine whenever possible.
- Staff shifted to remote work where possible.
- In academic settings, number of students and trainees limited.
- Use of intermittent theta-burst stimulation to minimize in-person contact time.

Sanitization

- Regular cleaning according to the institution's infection control guidelines.
- Increased attention to hand sanitization before and after any patient/participant interaction.
- Use of disposable gloves considered when applying treatment coil.
- Sanitization supplies kept more readily accessible throughout clinics.
- Items touched by patients or research participants sanitized thoroughly between patients.
- Device-specific sanitization protocols followed per manufacturer's instructions.

Research

- Encourage telecollaboration across institutions for all meetings, conferences, and trainings.
- Review changes to study protocols or consents with the institutional review board.
- Modify budgets to allow for additional participants secondary to increased dropouts, additional costs associated with mitigating SARS-CoV-2 transmission.
- Ensure researchers working remotely have required access to appropriate hardware, software, secure databases, study forms, or any other sensitive or specialized tools.
- Mentoring and social support for researchers who may be negatively impacted by social isolation or lack of support during the pandemic.

clinical and research experience of the Brain Stimulation Service and Brain Stimulation Laboratory at the Medical University of South Carolina (MUSC).

WHERE ARE WE GOING?

The COVID-19 pandemic has had a devastating effect on mental health worldwide. The magnitude of the challenge ahead is already apparent in the pediatric population, with escalating mental health emergencies and suicide attempts in the context of a medical system struggling to provide acutely needed pediatric mental health care.[36] As it becomes apparent that COVID-19 will not come to an abrupt and definite end, it will be necessary for mental health care providers to continue to adapt and advocate. A vital component of such efforts will be to ensure that brain stimulation therapy is safely, readily, and reliably accessible.

In the case of TMS, there was already enthusiastic interest in accelerated TMS protocols for depression before the emergence of COVID-19. During a pandemic, potential reductions in time to response, treatment time, and overall days of treatment with accelerated intermittent theta-burst stimulation (aiTBS), in comparison to standard TMS protocols, may have exciting implications for mitigating viral transmission risk as well as for increasing treatment accessibility. To date, one small, open-label study found that 18 of 22 patients suffering from severe TRD met remission criteria with 50 high dose aiTBS sessions over 5 consecutive days.[37] Building on this work, Konstantinou and colleagues describe case reports of 2 patients with TRD whose symptom severity warranted ECT, but who instead received, and achieved remission from depression with aiTBS.[38,39] These cases along with the following vignette highlight the need for more research into the use of aiTBS as an alternative to ECT in cases where ECT is necessary but maybe unsafe or unavailable, such as during the early days of the COVID-19 Pandemic.

Vignette. A 40-year-old woman presented with a history of severe and recurrent major depressive disorder, rheumatoid arthritis, and migraines. Her medication history included adequate trials of citalopram, sertraline, fluoxetine, vortioxetine, desvenlafaxine, bupropion, aripiprazole, cariprazine, and dextroamphetamine. She had completed a standard course of rTMS treatments in October of 2019 and was considered a responder to that course of treatment. Despite medication changes, she experienced a relapse in depressive symptoms and returned to TMS in May of 2020. She completed an extended course of 50 TMS treatments with an FDA-cleared protocol, but this time did not respond to TMS treatment. Her outpatient psychiatrist started her on lithium, but she continued to struggle with worsening suicidal ideation. ECT was the next reasonable step in care, but the patient was not interested in pursuing ECT. A few months prior, ECT would not have been a treatment option because of a COVID-related hospital policy that restricted ECT to only immediately life-threatening cases. Two weeks after lithium was titrated to a therapeutic dose, in an attempt to avoid hospitalization, a course of aiTBS was proposed. Over 5 consecutive days, the patient received 50 aiTBS sessions in total. She had 10 sessions per day with 50-min intersession intervals, 1800 pulses per session in triplet 50 Hz bursts repeated at 5 Hz, train duration of 2 seconds, and an intertrain interval of 8 seconds, at 120% of the resting motor threshold over the left dorsolateral prefrontal cortex (DLPFC), localized with the modified BeamF3 method.[40] Her depression was monitored using the patient health questionnaire 9 (PHQ-9).[41] Her PHQ-9 ratings decreased from 19 on day 1 to 16 on day 5, and her affect appeared to improve. She reported a PHQ-9 of 15 1 week after her last treatment and 13 2 weeks after her last treatment. She reported stable and euthymic mood with full remission within a month of her last aiTBS session. She remained in reported remission for 6 months in the absence of any further medication changes. She tolerated treatments well with no reported side effects or adverse events. The patient's remission following a 5-day aiTBS protocol may have been multifactorial in nature, but her case does highlight the need for further research into aiTBS. The literature supporting aiTBS is limited, and there are still many questions to be answered regarding coil placement, dosing, optimal schedule, and durability.

How can brain stimulation services be allocated in unprecedented times? What is the acceptable threshold for clinical suffering? What can be done when treatments such as ECT are needed immediately, but simply not accessible? In some ways, this is not a new issue in the field of brain stimulation. In 2004, Ottoson and Fink found that ECT met all principles of medical ethics except for justice, as it was not universally and equally available to all in need.[42] Perhaps the experience of the COVID-19 pandemic offers a unique opportunity to consider solutions to remove barriers to access that have existed for decades.

DISCLOSURES

Dr M.J. Coffey has no relevant conflicts of interest to disclose; he reports receiving author royalties from UpToDate and MedLink Neurology. Drs S. Kerns, S. Sanghani, and L. Wachtel have no relevant conflicts of interest to disclose.

REFERENCES

1. Amad A, Magnat M, Quilès C, et al. Evolution of electro-convulsive therapy activity in France since the beginning of the COVID-19 pandemic. Encephale 2020; 46(3S):S40–2.
2. Sienaert P, Lambrichts S, Popleu L, et al. Electroconvulsive Therapy During COVID-19-Times: Our Patients Cannot Wait. Am J Geriatr Psychiatry 2020; 28(7):772–5.
3. Francis A, Mormando C. Electroconvulsive therapy during early COVID-19: national data. Presented at the Annual Meeting of the International Society for ECT and Neurostimulation, April 25, 2021.
4. Maixner DF, Weiner R, Reti IM, et al. Electroconvulsive therapy is an essential procedure. Am J Psychiatry 2021;178(5):381–2.
5. Centers for Disease Control and Prevention. Interim Infection Prevention and Control Recommendations for Healthcare Personnel During the Coronavirus Disease 2019 (COVID-19) Pandemic. Secondary Interim Infection Prevention and Control Recommendations for Healthcare Personnel During the Coronavirus Disease 2019 (COVID-19) Pandemic. Feb 23, 2021 2021. Available at: https://www.cdc.gov/coronavirus/2019-ncov/hcp/infection-control-recommendations.html. Accessed June 30, 2021.
6. Centers for Disease Control and Prevention. Strategies for optimizing the supply of COVID-19 respirators. Secondary Strategies for optimizing the supply of COVID-19 respirators. April 9, 2021 2021. Available at: https://www.cdc.gov/coronavirus/2019-ncov/hcp/respirators-strategy/index.html#crisis. Accessed June 30, 2021.
7. Robertson J, Flint AJ, Blumberger D, et al. Ethical Considerations in Providing Electroconvulsive Therapy during the COVID-19 Pandemic. Can J Psychiatry 2021. https://doi.org/10.1177/0706743721993617. 706743721993617.
8. Espinoza RT, Kellner CH, McCall WV. Electroconvulsive Therapy During COVID-19: An Essential Medical Procedure-Maintaining Service Viability and Accessibility. J ECT 2020;36(2):78–9.
9. (APA) APA. Electroconvulsive therapy as an essential procedure. Secondary Electroconvulsive therapy as an essential procedure. 2020. Available at: https://www.psychiatry.org/file%20library/psychiatrists/apa-guidance-ect-covid-19.pdf. Accessed June 30, 2021.
10. (ISEN) ISoEaN. COVID-19 and ECT. Letter to ISEN members and others in the ECT profession. Secondary COVID-19 and ECT. Letter to ISEN members and others in the ECT profession. April 2, 2020 2020. Available at: https://www.isen-ect.org/sites/default/files/ISEN.COVID19.letter.pdf.
11. (ISEN) ISoEaN. Position Statement on ECT as an Essential Procedure during COVID-19. Secondary Position Statement on ECT as an Essential Procedure during COVID-19. December 8, 2020 2020. Available at: https://www.isen-ect.org/covid-19-essential-procedure.
12. (NNDC) NNoDC. NNDC Urges Medical Officials to Consider ECT an Essential Medical Service. . Secondary NNDC Urges Medical Officials to Consider ECT an Essential Medical Service. April 21, 2020 2020. Available at: https://nndc.

org/nndc-urges-medical-officials-to-consider-ect-an-essential-medical-service/. Accessed June 30, 2021.

13. Wachtel LE. Far From an Elective Procedure: Electroconvulsive Therapy and Autism in the Era of COVID-19. J ECT 2021;37(1):10–2.
14. Shapiro, J. Covid-19 infections and deaths are higher among those with intellectual disabilities. 2020. Available at: https://www.npr.org/2020/06/09/872401607/covid-19-infections-and-deaths-are-higher-among-those-with-intellectual-disabili.
15. Turk MA, Landes SD, Formica MK, et al. Intellectual and developmental disability and COVID-19 case-fatality trends: TriNetX analysis. Disabil Health J 2020;13: 100942.
16. Gleason, J., et al., The devastating impact of covid-19 on individuals with intellectual disabilities in the United States. NEJM Catalyst, 2021.
17. Tenenbeim M EM, Haberman C. COVID-19 Guidelines for ECT in Shared Health. Secondary COVID-19 Guidelines for ECT in Shared Health 2020 April 7. Available at: https://umanitoba.ca/faculties/health_sciences/medicine/units/anesthesia/media/ECT-COVID19_Guidelines_April_9_2020.pdf. Accessed June 30, 2021.
18. Umnuaypornlert A, Kanchanasurakit S, Lucero-Prisno DEI, et al. Smoking and risk of negative outcomes among COVID-19 patients: A systematic review and meta-analysis. Tob Induc Dis 2021;19:09.
19. Maloney J. Cigarette smoking makes comeback during coronavirus pandemic. Wall Street J 2020;2020.
20. Wang Q, Xu R, Volkow ND. Increased risk of COVID-19 infection and mortality in people with mental disorders: analysis from electronic health records in the United States. World Psychiatry 2021;20(1):124–30.
21. Braithwaite R, McKeown HL, Lawrence VJ, et al. Successful electroconvulsive therapy in a patient with confirmed, symptomatic COVID-19. J ECT 2020;36(3): 222–3.
22. Kashaninasab F, Panahi Dashdebi R, Ghalehbandi MF. Comorbidity of Coronavirus disease (COVID-19) and the first episode of bipolar disorder and its treatment challenges: A case report. Med J Islam Repub Iran 2020;34:103.
23. Bryson EO, Aloysi AS. A strategy for management of electroconvulsive therapy patients during the COVID-19 pandemic. J ECT 2020;36(3):149–51.
24. Lapid MI, Seiner S, Heintz H, et al. Electroconvulsive therapy practice changes in older individuals due to COVID-19: expert consensus statement. Am J Geriatr Psychiatry 2020;28(11):1133–45.
25. Limoncelli J, Marino T, Smetana R, et al. General anesthesia recommendations for electroconvulsive therapy during the coronavirus disease 2019 pandemic. J ect 2020;36(3):152–5.
26. Luccarelli J, Fernandez-Robles C, Fernandez-Robles C, et al. Modified anesthesia protocol for electroconvulsive therapy permits reduction in aerosol-generating bag-mask ventilation during the COVID-19 Pandemic. Psychother Psychosom 2020;89(5):314–9.
27. Bellini H, Cretaz E, Rigonatti LF, et al. Electroconvulsive therapy practice during the COVID-19 pandemic. Clinics (Sao Paulo) 2020;75:e2056.
28. Sauvaget A, Dumont R, Bukowski N, et al. [Recommendations for a gradual and controlled resumption of electroconvulsive therapy in France during the period of lifting of the containment and of the COVID-19 pandemic linked to SARS-CoV-2]. Encephale 2020;46(3s):S119–22.
29. Yeole S, Kapri P, Karia S, et al. Electroconvulsive therapy administered during the COVID-19 Pandemic. J ECT 2021;37(1):e2–3.

30. Colbert SA, McCarron S, Ryan G, et al. Immediate impact of coronavirus disease 2019 on electroconvulsive therapy practice. J ECT 2020;36(2):86–7.
31. Tor PC, Phu AHH, Koh DSH, et al. Electroconvulsive therapy in a time of coronavirus disease. J ECT 2020;36(2):80–5.
32. Gil-Badenes J, Valero R, Valentí M, et al. Electroconvulsive therapy protocol adaptation during the COVID-19 pandemic. J Affect Disord 2020;276:241–8.
33. Abrupt discontinuation of M-ECT during the COVID-19 Pandemic. A 6- month prospective cohort study. ISEN 30th Annual meeting; 2021 April 24-25.
34. Kinback K. Doing TMS Safely in a Covid World, A Paradigm Shift. Clinical TMS Society; 4/27/2020 2020.
35. Bikson M, Hanlon CA, Woods AJ, et al. Guidelines for TMS/tES clinical services and research through the COVID-19 pandemic. Brain Stimul 2020;13(4):1124–49.
36. de Figueiredo CS, Sandre PC, Portugal LCL, et al. COVID-19 pandemic impact on children and adolescents' mental health: Biological, environmental, and social factors. Prog Neuropsychopharmacol Biol Psychiatry 2021;106:110171.
37. Cole EJ, Stimpson KH, Bentzley BS, et al. Stanford accelerated intelligent neuromodulation therapy for treatment-resistant depression. Am J Psychiatry 2020; 177(8):716–26.
38. Konstantinou GN, Downar J, Daskalakis ZJ, et al. Accelerated intermittent theta burst stimulation in late-life depression: a possible option for older depressed adults in need of ECT During the COVID-19 Pandemic. Am J Geriatr Psychiatry 2020;28(10):1025–9.
39. Konstantinou GN, Trevizol AP, Goldbloom D, et al. Successful treatment of depression with psychotic features using accelerated intermittent theta burst stimulation. J Affect Disord 2021;279:17–9.
40. Mir-Moghtadaei A, Caballero R, Fried P, et al. Concordance between BeamF3 and MRI-neuronavigated target sites for repetitive transcranial magnetic stimulation of the left dorsolateral prefrontal cortex. Brain Stimul 2015;8(5):965–73.
41. Kroenke K, Spitzer RL, Williams JB. The PHQ-9: validity of a brief depression severity measure. J Gen Intern Med 2001;16(9):606–13.
42. Ottosson J-O, Fink M. Ethics of electroconvulsive therapy. New York: Brunner-Routledge; 2004.
43. Thiruvenkatarajan V, Dharmalingam A, Armstrong-Brown A, et al. Uninterrupted anesthesia support and technique adaptations for patients presenting for electroconvulsive therapy during the COVID-19 Era. J ECT 2020;36(3):156–7.
44. Flexman AM, Abcejo AS, Avitsian R, et al. Neuroanesthesia practice during the COVID-19 pandemic: recommendations from Society for Neuroscience in Anesthesiology and Critical Care (SNACC). J Neurosurg Anesthesiol 2020;32:202–9.

Impact on Child Psychiatry

Shireen F. Cama, MD, Brigitta E. Miyamoto, MD,
Sandra M. DeJong, MD, MSc*

KEYWORDS

• COVID-19 • Pandemic • Child • Adolescent • Psychiatry • Mental health • Parent

KEY POINTS

- The mental health system for youth was already in crisis before the COVID-19 pandemic struck.
- The pandemic has affected all youth, and its sequelae are expected to play out over time as children move through the developmental stages.
- Those youth who were most at risk prepandemic (those with preexisting mental health, substance use, and developmental disorders or adverse childhood experiences) are also expected to suffer the greatest fallout from the pandemic.
- Improvements in the mental health care workforce, financial and technical support for innovations to improve access, and ongoing community recovery and resilience efforts will be vital in mobilizing protective factors and promoting the health and well-being of youth and their families.

INTRODUCTION

The mental health of children and adolescents has been a cause for serious concern worldwide even before the start of the COVID-19 pandemic. Pediatric systems of mental health care have long-standing, significant gaps including shortages of inpatient beds and lack of outpatient services covered through insurance plans. Such gaps are even larger for racial and ethnic minorities and rural populations.[1]

The global coronavirus pandemic exacerbated the mental health crisis across age-groups. For youth, the pandemic led to an unprecedented and abrupt cessation of structure and normalcy in daily life, a loss compounded by death and bereavement for many. Those with the most risk factors are expected to be disproportionately impacted, including youth with preexisting trauma and mental illness[2] and those facing health disparities and unmet needs.[3]

Cambridge Health Alliance, Harvard Medical School, 1493 Cambridge Street, Macht 317B, Cambridge, MA 02139, USA
* Corresponding author.
E-mail address: sdejong@cha.harvard.edu

Psychiatr Clin N Am 45 (2022) 133–146
https://doi.org/10.1016/j.psc.2021.11.009
0193-953X/22/
psych.theclinics.com

Information on the immediate mental health effects of the pandemic is emerging, but long-term sequelae are also a major concern. The potential negative impacts of adverse childhood experiences across the lifespan have long been recognized, including increased risk of physical and mental health conditions and early death.[4] Pandemic stressors may change the developmental course of youth and cause epigenetic changes to their DNA that will have ramifications for years to come.[5]

This paper examines emerging data about ways COVID-19 has affected youth mental health and development, mediated in part by such factors as social isolation, school closures, family functioning, and modifications in health care delivery systems. Changes resulting from the pandemic in how child psychiatry is practiced and taught are also addressed. Suggestions for the future for mitigating long-term negative outcomes and optimizing new opportunities are offered.

IMPACT OF THE PANDEMIC ON YOUTH MENTAL HEALTH AND DEVELOPMENT

Social Isolation During the Pandemic and Its Effects on Child Development

The pandemic profoundly altered youth development by dismantling social contact across all ages. Young children learn about themselves, the perspectives of others, and the world around them by engaging in play and exploration with similarly aged peers. Play is the work of the child, offering a training ground for developing skills in fine and gross motor, speech and language, cognition, social-emotional regulation, and moral reasoning. During latency (6–12 years) the growing presence of peer groups and friendships help children further develop their capacities for perspective-taking and resolving conflict. During adolescence, youth naturally turn toward peer relationships to develop a sense of individual and communal identity.

With the abrupt closing of daycare centers and schools and the cessation of playdates and spontaneous social time, the COVID-19 pandemic severely disrupted normal social-emotional learning. Decreased access to safe and trusted adults, such as teachers and extended family, also limited youth's ability to be closely observed, share their true selves, and receive reflective, positive feedback. For many, the resultant social isolation has led to the experience of high levels of loneliness. Loneliness, especially for long time periods, is associated with future mental health problems in youth, including increased social anxiety and depression,[6] with children who were quarantined having a higher likelihood of experiencing trauma- and grief-related disorders than those who were not.[7]

Worsened Mental Health for Youth During the Pandemic

The combined stressors of the pandemic have challenged the mental health of youth with and without prior mental health concerns. Although some youth, such as those with social anxiety, may have experienced short-term improvement in mental health symptoms because of a relative reduction in anxiety-provoking interactions with peers,[8] most of the mounting evidence points to the deleterious cumulative effects of the pandemic on mental health across ages.

In a Canadian study, two-thirds of youth reported worsening mental health several months after enforced lockdown, even in the absence of significant COVID-19 disease exposure or economic concerns.[9] Youth without prior mental health concerns reported increased rates of anxiety-related symptoms.[10] In the adolescent age group, health insurance claims during 2020 for generalized anxiety disorder, major depressive disorder, and adjustment disorder all increased by about 90% as a percentage of all medical claims compared with similar months during 2019.[11] With emphasis in the media around the importance of handwashing and respiratory spread of the virus, youth with obsessive-compulsive disorder perceived even more threat from contamination, and studies noted an increase in obsessions about contamination, cleaning-centered compulsions, and avoidance behaviors.[12]

Behavioral problems also increased in children. Abrupt cessation of supports, such as in-home behavioral and therapeutic services, and the closure of schools and residential placements resulted in less structure to help children regulate their behaviors. Children with autism spectrum disorder and their families suffered from sudden reduction in occupational, speech, and behavioral therapy services and respite care. Many families of children with autism spectrum disorder noted an increase in behavioral problems, adding more challenges to already stressed family systems.[13]

Eating disorders also rose during the pandemic. With disruption of routine activities, and an increase in sedentary behaviors, screen time, and social media use,[14] clinic visits and hospitalizations for eating disorders and calls to the National Eating Disorder Association's hotline surged across all age groups. Delays in diagnosis caused by reduced pediatric checkups may have resulted in a more serious course of illness.

Although research has suggested that the pandemic's stressors have increased many forms of substance use in adults, the data for youth may be more positive. Reduced peer interactions and disruptions in supply from commercial sources of drugs may be a mitigating factor in youth. A national survey of more than 2000 teenagers and young adults found that nearly 70% noted that they had reduced or quit their use of e-cigarettes, in part because of inability to purchase products.[15]

Influence of Social Media on Mental Health of Youth During the Pandemic

In a world where youth already heavily relied on screens and smart phones for communication, the pandemic was associated with a spike in social media use. Technology may have helped mitigate feelings of isolation and loneliness through use of online apps and "face-to-face" interactions across the screen.[16] In a nationally representative survey of teenagers and young adults conducted nearly a year into the pandemic, most noted that social media played an important and positive role in helping them stay connected with family and friends, and several used health-specific apps meant to promote positive coping skills.[17]

However, recent research has also suggested harmful effects of social media on mental health including depression, self-harm, negative body image, and self-esteem.[18,19] These negative sequelae of social media use may have been exacerbated by the pandemic, and several groups have reported an increase in cyberbullying and use of online pornography among youth during this time.[20]

IMPACT OF THE PANDEMIC ON SCHOOLS AND EDUCATION

In response to the public health emergency of the COVID-19 pandemic, communities across the world rapidly closed schools and shifted to home-based distance-learning models. In the United States, almost all 55 million students from kindergarten through twelfth grade were affected by these closures starting in March 2020. In addition to academics, American schools provide physical education and sports, nutrition, mental health services, monitoring for abuse and neglect, and a social focal point for communities. The full impact of these closures and the resulting loss of resources is yet to be learned; however, early data are concerning.

School Lunch/Food Insecurity

Schools provide lunches for more than 30 million students in the United States, where 35 million children live in poverty.[21] Although schools tried creative ways to continue providing children with food during the pandemic's school closures, this effort met with limited success. Within months, the pandemic brought increased reports of food insecurity.[22]

Learning: Access and Other Inequities

School closures resulted in a massive shift to digital platforms for learning, which presented significant challenges and resulting inequities.[23] Families faced digital obstacles, such as doing schoolwork on cell phones, relying on public Wi-Fi to complete schoolwork because of unreliable Internet connection at home, and being unable to fully participate in their work and learning because of lack of computer access at home.[24] Lower income parents and those from minority communities reported a higher likelihood of these obstacles. Even before the pandemic, 25% of Black students reported struggling to complete schoolwork because they lacked a computer at home.[25] Non-English speakers found attempts to assist their children's remote learning and communicate with teachers to be particularly challenging.[26]

Educational Achievement

Educational achievement and growth have also been impacted by school closures and remote learning. Multiple surveys document that most teachers were unprepared to teach virtually and taught less new material, particularly in lower-income communities. Many students did not consistently log on for virtual classes and the summer 2020 makeup time was variably used, exacerbating the problem of "summer learning loss."[27] Studies documented declines in educational achievement, particularly in mathematics.[28] The loss of services provided through individualized education plans was particularly challenging, and students with neurodevelopmental, sensory, and learning disorders seem to be at increased risk for the pandemic's negative impacts on learning.[29] The poorest performing students prepandemic also had the largest declines in academic achievement and school attendance during 2020.[28]

School Mental Health Services

Schools are also a critical site for mental health evaluation and treatment of youth.[30] Approximately 35% of adolescents who receive any mental health services receive them only in school settings. This percentage disproportionately includes youth from racial and ethnic minorities, lower family income, and those with public health insurance.[31] With the rapid institution of fully remote and later hybrid models of schooling during the pandemic, the ability of teachers and school counselors to provide therapeutic interventions or meet regularly with students was limited. Therapeutic schools that relied on the entire school milieu as being part of a child's treatment plan were handicapped by the virtual modality, leaving parents with the challenge of structuring a child's day or managing significant behavioral outbursts.[32,33]

IMPACT OF THE PANDEMIC ON PARENTS AND FAMILIES

The COVID-19 pandemic impacted families directly through illness and bereavement, and through detrimental effects on mental health, financial and employment uncertainty, and increased pressures on work-life balance.

Parental Mental Health Effects

Parents' mental health is a key determinant of the mental health of their children. Although some families reported more positive effects of pandemic-induced changes in family life, such as increased time spent with children,[34] most evidence suggests a decline in parental and family mental health during the pandemic. Young children, who are particularly vulnerable to distress in their caregivers, displayed increased clinginess, worrying, inattention, restlessness, and irritability.[35] A survey of economically vulnerable families of preschool children found a strong association between parental job and income loss with a parent's symptoms of depression, stress, decreased sense of hope, and negative parent-child interactions; families who experienced several simultaneous hardships during the pandemic reported a worsened mental health than those who experienced fewer.[36]

Shifting Landscape of Work and Childcare

As the pandemic continued, families experienced a significant reshifting in their work and childcare responsibilities. With abrupt closures of schools, businesses, and childcare services at the start of the pandemic, many Americans, especially low-wage workers in the service industry, experienced a drastic reduction in work hours and an increase in layoffs, resulting in increased financial stress.

Parents were often unable to work because of the lack of childcare. In a June 2020 national survey, 48% of those families who reported worsening mental health early in the pandemic noted that they had lost childcare. The mental health effects were noted to be greater in mothers and single parents.[22] Stress and difficulty balancing work and family responsibilities ensued, with most changes seeming to fall on mothers.[37] Latina and Black mothers, who are more likely to be single or have a partner working outside the home, were twice as likely to take on all childcare and housework once COVID-19 struck.[38]

Parental Stress and Child Maltreatment

Classic risk factors for childhood maltreatment, including poverty, economic instability, and employment insecurity, were exacerbated by the COVID-19 crisis, increasing concerns about the safety of children. In general, levels of cumulative parental stress, such as those experienced during the pandemic, have been linked to increased likelihood of engaging in harsh parenting practices and increased risk of childhood maltreatment and intimate partner violence.[39] Data from previous pandemics suggest that risk of violence for children increases with school closure associated with public health emergencies.[40] Rising rates of parental substance abuse and job loss during the pandemic are believed to be associated with this phenomenon.[39] In families where parents worked out of the home, sparse childcare options may have also resulted in less than ideal caretaking arrangements.

Despite these, risks, official reports to child protective agencies and total number of emergency room visits related to suspected child abuse and neglect decreased starting in March 2020 when compared with the corresponding times from the previous year.[41] This decrease is thought to be caused by the markedly limited interaction of children with mandated reporters, such as physicians, teachers, and childcare workers. This concern was one of the key factors leading national organizations, such as the American Academy of Pediatrics, to support returning to in-person schooling.[42]

IMPACT OF THE PANDEMIC ON MENTAL HEALTH SERVICE DELIVERY FOR YOUTH

The implementation of the public health emergency in March 2020 led to a rapid transformation of the mental health delivery system and unanticipated changes that have affected virtually all service domains. Simultaneously, the pandemic's negative impact on parent and child mental health described previously led to an increase in demand for mental health services in an already underresourced system. In the May 2021 American Psychiatric Association survey, 26% of parents reported seeking professional mental health help for their children and nearly half of parents reported seeking such help for themselves. However, with waitlists increasing, more than one in five parents reported having difficulty scheduling an appointment for their child with a mental health professional.[43]

Wraparound Services

Therapists in community agencies before the pandemic were often able to achieve rapport and buy-in for treatment through their ability to meet patients and families in their homes and offer in-the-moment parenting guidance and in vivo crisis stabilization. This home-based care, a critical element of "wraparound services," often mitigated the need for acute levels of care. With the pandemic, most of these services either ceased or converted to telephone and/or video platforms, which diminished their in-person benefits.

Emergency Room Visits

Although the child mental health system of care in the United States was already in crisis before the pandemic, COVID-19 exacerbated the problem of children "boarding" in emergency rooms awaiting psychiatric beds.[44] Early in the pandemic, all pediatric emergency room visits decreased largely because of fear of contracting the virus; however, the proportion of total emergency room visits for mental health concerns simultaneously rose. According to data from the Centers for Disease Control and Prevention, the proportion of children's mental health–related visits to emergency rooms across the country between April 2020 and October 2020 increased by between 24% and 31% for children aged 5 to 17 when compared with data from the same months in 2019.[45] Several studies noted a relative increase in the number of emergency room presentations related to self-harm and suicidal ideation.[46,47] Some evidence indicates that the height of these visits corresponded with times of peak community concern and efforts to curb the spread of the virus through increased restrictions and lockdowns. This suggests that youth may have experienced heightened levels of distress during this time related to stressors in their home environment and increased isolation from peers and supports.[46] Across the country, news reports documented the experience of children spending days to weeks in emergency rooms waiting for psychiatric admission.[48] As of the writing of this paper, this crisis is still ongoing.

Inpatient Hospitalizations

On inpatient units, the pandemic required implementation of infection control measures, such as mask-wearing and remote-contact mobile devices, a reduction or cessation in milieu-based treatment approaches, and reduced family and social visits.[49–51] Family-based and parent-centered treatment became more challenging to provide. The loss of therapeutic groups and alteration in the therapeutic milieu may have made the provision of care less optimal.[50,51] Children and adolescents on inpatient units who required discharge to other treatment programs, such as residential facilities or partial hospitalization, may have had their stays extended or, alternatively, their discharge to home hastened because of the limitations on availability and quality of services. These care facilities were subject to the same requirements in securing personal protective equipment and preventing outbreaks as all other health care facilities, with often less access to supplies and experience in these procedures, meaning that many of them were unable to accommodate the number of patients needing that level of care.[52]

Outpatient Services

Outpatient clinicians also had to adjust the treatment they offered. To continue providing outpatient care safely, health care systems rushed to implement telepsychiatry platforms that yielded benefits and concerns for the provision of health care for children and families. A major benefit was increased access to services and decrease in no-show rates because of elimination of barriers, such as long commute times, parking fees, and patient preference for virtual care.[52–54] However, many believe that the rapid reliance on telepsychiatry may have also inadvertently worsened mental health disparities for families with limited English proficiency and without Internet or computer access.[55]

Televisits in people's homes afforded clinicians unprecedented and valuable glimpses into a child's environment and family functioning.[56] However, they also required clinicians and patients to adapt their interactions to the virtual space. Clinicians had to be more intentional about addressing aspects of an evaluation often taken for granted during in-person visits, such as assessing a child's play or ensuring privacy for sensitive conversations.[56] In situations of safety concern, clinicians had to preemptively consider the best way to access emergency services for patients in the virtual context. Trauma-focused therapy, psychological first aid,[57] and disaster response strategies became more salient[52] modes of treatment. The rapid rise in anxiety and depression symptoms required a more nuanced distinction between a "normal" reaction to pandemic stress and pathologic anxiety.[58] The frame of the encounter also shifted, with the adolescent or family having far more control over where the appointment took place and how engaged they chose to be during a visit. Appointments regularly occurred while patients were driving in cars; shopping in stores; or otherwise distracted by video games, television, or social media.[56] Professional organizations rapidly promulgated new and existing guidelines on telepsychiatry professionalism, billing, and technological concerns to help anticipate and navigate potential challenges.[59,60]

Training Considerations

Child and adolescent psychiatry fellowship training directors also had to strike a balance between safety of their fellows and providing high-quality training. Learning to provide telepsychiatry became an unanticipated focus of training programs. A 2020 national survey of child psychiatry training directors found an increase from 12% to 90% in reported "direct-to-consumer" visits in outpatient training services when contrasting pre-COVID-onset and post-COVID-onset telehealth services.[61] More care was delivered to patients via telepsychiatry in their homes and much more teaching, training, and supervising was done virtually. Educators are concerned that certain learning objectives, such as those significantly benefitting from in-person interaction (eg, play therapy), have suffered because of virtual care. To get around difficulties in assessing younger patients, some institutions asked parents to video their young children playing or interacting in their natural setting.[62] The extent to which the state of emergency waivers continue or are modified as the pandemic progresses is likely to affect mental health care for children and families and, secondarily, how fellows are trained.

SUMMARY

The COVID-19 pandemic's impact on the mental health and development of children and adolescents will be a topic of study for years to come. As the pandemic evolved, child psychiatry experts formulated a research agenda to better understand the short-

and long-term effects of the pandemic on the mental health of children, families, and society.[63] The loss of social contact and schooling and effects of illness and bereavement will continue to have lasting foreseen and unforeseen consequences. The impact is expected to be greatest on those youth already at risk because of such factors as economic hardship, unsafe neighborhoods, poor educational and health care services, prepandemic mental illness or neurodevelopmental disorders, and family dysfunction including abuse and neglect. Minority groups, disproportionately affected by COVID-19 through social determinants of health and the effects of systemic racism,[64] may suffer more from the travesties of the pandemic. Those youth with protective factors, such as sufficient resources for daily needs, community connections, academic competence, strong self-regulation skills, and close relationships with caretaking adults, may prove most resilient against the fallout.

As the pandemic evolves and society builds a "new normal," the needs of those most vulnerable must be kept at the forefront, although all youth will be processing this experience over and over as they move through each developmental stage. Despite overall improvements in society's response to the pandemic, the reality remains that the mental health needs of youth are still at a crisis point, as emphasized in a joint statement of the American Academy of Child and Adolescent Psychiatrists, the American Academy of Pediatrics, and the Children's Hospital Association released in October 2021 that declared a National State of Emergency in Children's Mental Health and called on policymakers to do the same. Among other recommendations, the organizations called for increased funding for the mental health needs of youth to support initiatives that address regulatory challenges, expand on sustainable models of school-based and integrated care, and address ongoing challenges of acute care needs.[65]

To serve the needs of youth in the postpandemic world, the prepandemic health, socioeconomic, and racial inequities in systems and institutions that the pandemic highlighted must be addressed. For children and families, this means addressing:

- The well-established shortage of child/adolescent psychiatrists, psychologists, social workers, school counselors and other mental health professionals trained to address the complex mental health needs of children and families
- Financial and technical support for innovations that helped promote mental health access during the pandemic, such as telepsychiatry
- Social determinants of health and structural inequities, such as through efforts to promote housing security, end systemic forms of racism, and close the "digital divide"

Proposed improvements include comprehensive screening for social determinants of health; flexible, inclusive, and coproduced models of care; potential redefinition of what constitutes an "essential" service, such as in-person provision of care in some situations; and fostering community-led initiatives, which may promote resilience through positive and protective experiences.[66]

In shaping the future of youth mental health care, pandemic "lessons" include the need for increased emphasis on community engagement, empowerment of patients and families in their own treatment,[2,67] and adaptation of existing services to include a trauma-informed approach. Child psychiatry training needs to address what may have been lost during the pandemic (eg, training in dynamic play therapy) and embrace positive changes (eg, increased telepsychiatry experience). The pandemic-induced rapid adoption of digital technology and videoconferencing may lead to positive innovations in personal-professional balance for working parents, hybrid educational models that better meet the individual needs of students, and health care services that improve the lack of access to pediatric mental health care across the country and even the world. It is hoped that vulnerable youth, who were so adversely impacted by the pandemic, will be in a position to gain from such improvements in the future.

CLINICS CARE POINTS

- The mental health system for youth was already in crisis before the COVID-19 pandemic struck.
- The pandemic has affected all youth, and its sequelae are expected to play out over time as children move through the developmental stages.
- Those youth who were most at risk prepandemic are also expected to suffer the greatest fallout from the pandemic. These include youth with preexisting mental health, substance use, and neurodevelopmental problems and those facing social determinants that adversely affect mental health: poverty, racism, health inequities, poor education, and lack of a close relationship with a caretaking adult.
- Improvements in the mental health care workforce, financial and technical support for innovations to improve access, and ongoing community recovery and resilience efforts will be vital in mobilizing protective factors and promoting the health and well-being of youth and their families.

DISCLOSURE

The authors have nothing to disclose.

REFERENCES

1. Cook BL, Barry CL, Busch SH. Racial/ethnic disparity trends in children's mental health care access and expenditures from 2002 to 2007. Health Serv Res 2013; 48(1):129–49. https://doi.org/10.1111/j.1475-6773.2012.01439.x.
2. Waddell C, Schwartz C, Barican J, et al. COVID-19 and the impact on children's mental health. Burnaby, BC, Canada: Child Heal Policy Centre, Simon Fraser Univ; 2020. p. 1–28.
3. Loeb TB, Ebor MT, Smith AM, et al. How mental health professionals can address disparities in the context of the COVID-19 pandemic. Traumatology (Tallahassee Fla) 2020;27(1):60–9. https://doi.org/10.1037/trm0000292.
4. Shonkoff JP, Garner AS, Siegel BS, et al. The lifelong effects of early childhood adversity and toxic stress. Pediatrics 2012;129(1). https://doi.org/10.1542/peds.2011-2663.
5. Odgers C, Schmidt K, et al. The long-term biological effects of COVID-19 stress on kids' future health and development. Waltham, MA: The Conversation; 2020. Available at: https://theconversation.com/the-long-term-biological-effects-of-covid-19-stress-on-kids-future-health-and-development-140533. [Accessed 6 December 2021].
6. Loades ME, Chatburn E, Higson-Sweeney N, et al. Rapid systematic review: the impact of social isolation adolescents in the context of COVID-19. J Am Acad Child Adolesc Psychiatry 2020;59(11):1218–39. Available at: www.jaacap.org.
7. Sprang G, Silman M. Posttraumatic stress disorder in parents and youth after health-related disasters. Disaster Med Public Health Prep 2013;7(1):105–10. https://doi.org/10.1017/dmp.2013.22.

8. Bruining H, Bartels M, Polderman TJC, et al. COVID-19 and child and adolescent psychiatry: an unexpected blessing for part of our population? Eur Child Adolesc Psychiatry 2020. https://doi.org/10.1007/s00787-020-01578-5.
9. Cost KT, Crosbie J, Anagnostou E, et al. Mostly worse, occasionally better: impact of COVID-19 pandemic on the mental health of Canadian children and adolescents. Eur Child Adolesc Psychiatry 2021. https://doi.org/10.1007/s00787-021-01744-3.
10. Smirni P, Lavanco G, Smirni D. Anxiety in older adolescents at the time of COVID-19. J Clin Med 2020;9(10):3064. https://doi.org/10.3390/jcm9103064.
11. FAIR Health. WHITE paper. The impact of COVID-19 on pediatric mental health; a study of private healthcare claims. New York, NY: Fair Health, Inc; 2021.
12. Tanir Y, Karayagmurlu A, Kaya İ, et al. Exacerbation of obsessive compulsive disorder symptoms in children and adolescents during COVID-19 pandemic. Psychiatry Res 2020;293:3–7. https://doi.org/10.1016/j.psychres.2020.113363.
13. Eshraghi AA, Li C, Alessandri M, et al. COVID-19: overcoming the challenges faced by individuals with autism and their families. Lancet Psychiatry 2020; 7(6):481–3. https://doi.org/10.1016/S2215-0366(20)30197-8.
14. Jones C. Eating disorders among teens surging during the pandemic. Oakland, CA: EdSource; 2021. Available at: https://edsource.org/2021/eating-disorders-among-teens-surging-during-the-pandemic/650882. [Accessed 6 December 2021].
15. Gaiha SM, Lempert LK, Halpern-Felsher B. Underage youth and young adult e-cigarette use and access before and during the coronavirus disease 2019 pandemic. JAMA Netw Open 2020;3(12):1–16. https://doi.org/10.1001/jamanetworkopen.2020.27572.
16. Biernesser C, Montano G, Miller E, et al. Social media use and monitoring for adolescents with depression and implications for the COVID-19 pandemic: qualitative study of parent and child perspectives. JMIR Pediatr Parent 2020;3(2). https://doi.org/10.2196/21644.
17. Rideout V, Fox S, Peebles A, et al. Coping with COVID-19: how young people use digital media to manage their mental health. San Francisco, CA: Common Sense and Hopelab; 2021.
18. Hill D, Ameenuddin N, Chassiakos YR, et al. Media and young minds. Pediatrics 2016;138(5). https://doi.org/10.1542/peds.2016-2591.
19. Twenge JM, Joiner TE, Rogers ML, et al. Increases in depressive symptoms, suicide-related outcomes, and suicide rates among U.S. Adolescents after 2010 and links to increased new media screen time. Clin Psychol Sci 2018; 6(1):3–17. https://doi.org/10.1177/2167702617723376.
20. Tummala P, Muhammad T. Conclusion for special issue on COVID-19: how can we better protect the mental health of children in this current global environment? Child Abus Negl 2020;110(P2):104808. https://doi.org/10.1016/j.chiabu.2020.104808.
21. USDA Food and Nutrition Service. The National School Lunch Program Fact Sheet. Washington, DC: USDA Food and Nutrition Service; 2017. Available at: https://fns-prod.azureedge.net/sites/default/files/resource-files/NSLPFactSheet.pdf. [Accessed 7 December 2021].
22. Patrick SW, Henkhaus LE, Zickafoose JS, et al. Well-being of parents and children during the COVID-19 pandemic: a national survey. Pediatrics 2020;146(4). https://doi.org/10.1542/peds.2020-016824. e2020016824.

23. Pokhrel S, Chhetri R. A literature review on impact of COVID-19 pandemic on teaching and learning. High Educ Futur 2021;8(1):133–41. https://doi.org/10.1177/2347631120983481.
24. Ogels EA. 59% of U.S. parents with lower incomes say their child may face digital obstacles in schoolwork. Washington, DC: Pew Research Center; 2020. Available at: https://www.pewresearch.org/fact-tank/2020/09/10/59-of-u-s-parents-with-lower-incomes-say-their-child-may-face-digital-obstacles-in-schoolwork/. [Accessed 7 December 2021].
25. Anderson M, Perrin A. Nearly one-in-five teens can't always finish their homework because of the digital divide. Washington, DC: Pew Research Center; 2018. Available at: https://www.pewresearch.org/fact-tank/2018/10/26/nearly-one-in-five-teens-cant-always-finish-their-homework-because-of-the-digital-divide/#:~:text=Nearly one-in-five teens,because of the digital divide&text=Some15%25ofU.S.households. [Accessed 7 December 2021].
26. Sadeque S. These immigrant mothers had to help their children remote learn - in a language they don't speak. Washington, DC: The Lily; 2021. Available at: https://www.thelily.com/these-immigrant-mothers-had-to-help-their-children-remote-learn-in-a-language-they-dont-speak/. [Accessed 7 December 2021].
27. Middleton KV. The longer-term impact of COVID-19 on K–12 student learning and assessment. Educ Meas 2020;39(3):41–4.
28. Kuhfeld M, Soland J, Tarasawa B, et al. How is COVID-19 affecting student learning? Washington DC: Brown Center Chalkboard, Brookings Institution; 2020. Available at: https://www.brookings.edu/blog/brown-center-chalkboard/2020/12/03/how-is-covid-19-affecting-student-learning/. [Accessed 7 December 2021].
29. Anderson G. Accessibility suffers during pandemic. Washington, DC: Inside Higher Education; 2020. Available at: https://www.insidehighered.com/news/2020/04/06/remote-learning-shift-leaves-students-disabilities-behind. [Accessed 7 December 2021].
30. Burns BJ, Costello EJ, Angold A, et al. Children's mental health service use across service sectors. Health Aff 1995;14(3):147–59.
31. Ali MM, West K, Teich JL, et al. Utilization of mental health services in educational setting by adolescents in the United States. J Sch Health 2019;89(5):393–401. https://doi.org/10.1111/josh.12753.
32. Koushik NS. A population mental health perspective on the impact of COVID-19. Psychol Trauma 2020;12(5):529–30. https://doi.org/10.1037/tra0000737.
33. Fegert JM, Vitiello B, Plener PL, et al. Challenges and burden of the Coronavirus 2019 (COVID-19) pandemic for child and adolescent mental health: a narrative review to highlight clinical and research needs in the acute phase and the long return to normality. Child Adolesc Psychiatry Ment Health 2020;14(1):1–11. https://doi.org/10.1186/s13034-020-00329-3.
34. Kalil A, Mayer S, Shah R. Impact of the COVID-19 crisis on family dynamics in economically vulnerable Households. Chicago, IL: Beck Friedman Institute for Economics at Univeristy of Chicago; 2020. https://doi.org/10.2139/ssrn.3706339.
35. Jiao WY, Wang LN, Liu J, et al. Behavioral and emotional disorders in children during the COVID-19 epidemic. J Pediatr 2020;221:264–6.e1. https://doi.org/10.1016/j.jpeds.2020.03.013.
36. Gassman-Pines A, Ananat EO, Fitz-Henley, et al. COVID-19 and parent-child psychological well-being. Pediatrics 2020;146(4). https://doi.org/10.1542/peds.2020-007294.

37. Igielnik R. A rising share of working parents in the U.S. say it's been difficult to handle child care during the pandemic. Washington, DC: Pew Research Center; 2021. Available at: https://www.pewresearch.org/fact-tank/2021/01/26/a-rising-share-of-working-parents-in-the-u-s-say-its-been-difficult-to-handle-child-care-during-the-pandemic/. [Accessed 7 December 2021].
38. Take your child to work (every) day: how the pandemic has upended the lives of working parents. The Economist; 2021. Available at: https://www.economist.com/international/2021/05/22/how-the-pandemic-has-upended-the-lives-of-working-parents.
39. Lawson M, Piel MH, Simon M. Child maltreatment during the COVID-19 pandemic: consequences of parental job loss on psychological and physical abuse towards children. Child Abus Negl 2020;110(P2):104709. https://doi.org/10.1016/j.chiabu.2020.104709.
40. COVID-19: children at heightened risk of abuse, neglect, exploitation and violence amidst intensifying containment measures. UNICEF; 2020. Available at: https://www.unicef.org/press-releases/covid-19-children-heightened-risk-abuse-neglect-exploitation-and-violence-amidst. [Accessed 7 December 2021].
41. Swedo E, Idaikkadar N, Leemis R, et al. Trends in U.S. emergency department visits related to suspected or confirmed child abuse and neglect among children and adolescents aged <18 years before and during the COVID-19 pandemic—United States, January 2019–September 2020. MMWR Morb Mortal Wkly Rep 2020;69(49):1841–7. https://doi.org/10.15585/mmwr.mm6949a1.
42. Masonbrink AR, Hurley E. Advocating for children during the COVID-19 school closures. Pediatrics 2020;146(3). https://doi.org/10.1542/PEDS.2020-1440.
43. New APA Poll Shows Sustained Anxiety Among Americans. More than half of parents are concerned about the mental well-being of their children. Washington, DC: American Psychiatric Association: News Releases; 2021. Available at: https://www.psychiatry.org/newsroom/news-releases/new-apa-poll-shows-sustained-anxiety-among-americans-more-than-half-of-parents-are-concerned-about-the-mental-well-being-of-their-children. [Accessed 7 December 2021].
44. McEnany FB, Ojugbele O, Doherty JR, et al. Pediatric mental health boarding. Pediatrics 2020;146(4). https://doi.org/10.1542/peds.2020-1174.
45. Leeb RT, Bitsko RH, Radhakrishnan L, et al. Mental health–related emergency department visits among children aged <18 years during the COVID-19 pandemic—United States, January 1–October 17, 2020. MMWR Morb Mortal Wkly Rep 2020;69(45):1675–80. https://doi.org/10.15585/mmwr.mm6945a3.
46. Hill RM, Rufino K, Kurian S, et al. Suicide ideation and attempts in a pediatric emergency department before and during COVID-19. Pediatrics 2021;147(3). https://doi.org/10.1542/PEDS.2020-029280.
47. Ougrin D, Wong BH, Vaezinejad M, et al. Pandemic-related emergency psychiatric presentations for self-harm of children and adolescents in 10 countries (PREP-kids): a retrospective international cohort study. Eur Child Adolesc Psychiatry 2021. https://doi.org/10.1007/s00787-021-01741-6.
48. Caron C. A mental health crisis flares among young children. New York, NY: The New York Times; 2021. Available at: https://www.nytimes.com/2021/06/28/well/mind/mental-health-kids-suicide.html?referringSource=articleShare. [Accessed 7 December 2021].
49. Clemens V, Deschamps P, Fegert JM, et al. Potential effects of "social" distancing measures and school lockdown on child and adolescent mental health. Eur Child Adolesc Psychiatry 2020;29(6):739–42. https://doi.org/10.1007/s00787-020-01549-w.

50. Ozbaran NB, Kose S, Barankoglu I, et al. A new challenge for child psychiatrists: inpatient care management during coronavirus pandemic. Asian J Psychiatr 2020;54. https://doi.org/10.1016/j.ajp.2020.102303.
51. Lazar M. A firsthand look at life in a psychiatric ward during a pandemic. Issues Ment Health Nurs 2020;41(8):665–6. https://doi.org/10.1080/01612840.2020.1773737.
52. Pinals DA, Hepburn B, Parks J, et al. The behavioral health system and its response to covid-19: a snapshot perspective. Psychiatr Serv 2020;71(10):1070–4. https://doi.org/10.1176/APPI.PS.202000264.
53. Rosic T, Lubert S, Samaan Z. Virtual psychiatric care fast-tracked: reflections inspired by the COVID-19 pandemic. Bjpsych Bull 2020;1–4. https://doi.org/10.1192/bjb.2020.97.
54. Boydell KM, Hodgins M, Pignatiello A, et al. Using technology to deliver mental health services to children and youth: a scoping review. J Can Acad Child Adolesc Psychiatry 2014;23(2):87–99.
55. Smith-East M, Starks S. COVID-19 and mental health care delivery: a digital divide exists for youth with inadequate access to the Internet. J Am Acad Child Adolesc Psychiatry 2021;60(7):798–800. https://doi.org/10.1016/j.jaac.2021.04.006.
56. Mitrani P, Cain S, Khan S, et al. An expert panel discussion on the current and future state of telepsychiatry for children and adolescents. J Child Adolesc Psychopharmacol 2021;31(2):137–43. https://doi.org/10.1089/cap.2021.29195.pm.
57. Stark AM, White AE, Rotter NS, et al. Shifting from survival to supporting resilience in children and families in the COVID-19 pandemic: lessons for informing U.S. mental health priorities. Psychol Trauma 2020;12:S133–5. https://doi.org/10.1037/tra0000781.
58. Goldberg JF. Psychiatry's niche role in the COVID-19 pandemic. J Clin Psychiatry 2020;81(3). https://doi.org/10.4088/JCP.20com13363.
59. Telepsychiatry Guidelines and Policies. American Academy of Child & Adolescent Psychiatry. Available at: https://www.aacap.org/AACAP/Clinical_Practice_Center/Business_of_Practice/Telepsychiatry/Telepsychiatry_Guide_and_Pol.aspx. Accessed on 7 December 2021.
60. Telepsychiatry. American Psychiatric Association. Available at: https://www.psychiatry.org/psychiatrists/practice/telepsychiatry/toolkit/practice-guidelines. Accessed on 7 December 2021.
61. DeJong S, Brooks D, Khan S, et al. The Impact of COVID-19 on Pediatric Telepsychiatry Training in Child and Adolescent Psychiatry Fellowships. *Acad Psychiatry.* Published online 02 December 2021. https://doi.org/10.1007/s40596-021-01563-3
62. Kaku SM, Moscoso A, Sibeoni J, et al. Transformative learning in early-career child and adolescent psychiatry in the pandemic. Lancet Psychiatry 2021;8(2):e5. https://doi.org/10.1016/S2215-0366(20)30524-1.
63. Novins DK, Stoddard J, Althoff RR, et al. Editors' note and special communication: research priorities in child and adolescent mental health emerging from the COVID-19 pandemic. J Am Acad Child Adolesc Psychiatry 2021;60(5):544–54.e8. https://doi.org/10.1016/j.jaac.2021.03.005.
64. Farquharson WH, Thornton CJ. Debate: exposing the most serious infirmity – racism's impact on health in the era of COVID-19. Child Adolesc Ment Health 2020;25(3):182–3. https://doi.org/10.1111/camh.12407.
65. AAP-AACAP-CHA declaration of a national emergency in child and adolescent mental health. American Academy of Pediatrics; 2021. Available at: https://

www.aap.org/en/advocacy/child-and-adolescent-healthy-mental-development/aap-aacap-cha-declaration-of-a-national-emergency-in-child-and-adolescent-mental-health/.

66. Suleman S, Ratnani Y, Stockley K, et al. Supporting children and youth during the COVID-19 pandemic and beyond: a rights-centred approach. Paediatr Child Heal 2020;25(6):333–6. https://doi.org/10.1093/pch/pxaa086.
67. Moreno C, Wykes T, Galderisi S, et al. How mental health care should change as a consequence of the COVID-19 pandemic. Lancet Psychiatry 2020;7(9):813–24. https://doi.org/10.1016/S2215-0366(20)30307-2.

Impact of Coronavirus Disease 2019 on Geriatric Psychiatry

Azziza Bankole, MD

KEYWORDS

• COVID-19 • Geriatrics • Mental health • Loneliness • Social isolation

KEY POINTS

- Social isolation has a significant negative impact on the both physical and mental mealth of older adults.
- Pre-existing health disparities and inequities in our communities were severely exacerbated by the pandemic.
- Physical inactivity in older adults led to worse physical and mental health outcomes.

INTRODUCTION

The twenty-first century has seen a resurgence of infectious diseases causing epidemics and pandemics. Initially seen as a regional disease, the coronavirus disease 2019 (COVID-19), caused by the severe acute respiratory syndrome coronavirus 2 (SARS-CoV-2), quickly and relentlessly spread across the globe. Unlike other recent viral diseases, COVID-19 was not circumscribed to a particular population or region. It affected everyone and caused unprecedented changes in day-to-day life for the entire world. As a new disease, it also brought with it a tremendous amount of uncertainty about how it spreads, who is more susceptible, and the possible harms it could cause.

Much has been learned about the virus since it first appeared in 2019. According to the World Health Organization (WHO), there have been more than 200 million confirmed cased of COVID-19 and more than 5 million deaths from the disease.[1] According to the Centers for Disease Control and Prevention (CDC), the United States has had almost 40 million cases and more than 600,000 deaths.[2] Older adults and those with comorbid medical disorders have higher mortalities. As older adults tend to have more chronic illnesses than younger adults, they have been significantly

The author has no commercial or financial conflicts of interest.
Virginia Tech Carilion School of Medicine, Carilion Center for Healthy Aging, 2001 Crystal Spring Avenue, Roanoke, VA 24014, USA
E-mail address: aobankole@carilionclinic.org

Psychiatr Clin N Am 45 (2022) 147–159
https://doi.org/10.1016/j.psc.2021.11.010
0193-953X/22/

impacted by COVID-19. Eight out of 10 deaths from COVID-19 in the United States occurred in adults aged 65 years and older.[3]

Meeting the mental health needs of older adults has always been challenging, and coupled with the pandemic, it became very difficult. Previously sound and clinically impactful recommendations for mental and physical well-being, such as regular socialization, group exercises, adult day programs, and so forth, were no longer available and placed this population at increased risk of infection. Telepsychiatry was adopted as a way of maintaining treatment relationships with patients. However, this supposes that older adults have access to an Internet-capable device (eg, computer, tablet, or smartphone), live in an area with reliable broadband connectivity and are able to afford it, and that they are able to navigate the different telehealth services used by their providers. The challenge moving forward is to continually adapt to the changing landscape of care while simultaneously providing quality care for patients and support for their loved ones.

EPIDEMIOLOGY

Age has been shown to be the strongest risk factor for severe COVID-19 disease. Data from the CDC show that older adults have significantly higher rates of hospitalization and death when compared with children and younger adults even if the risk of infection is about the same.[3] Hospitalization rates range from 40× in those 65 to 74 years old to 65× in those 75 to 84 years old, to 95× in those older than 85 years. The calculated mortalities are even more astounding at 1300× (65–74 years old), to 3200× (75–84 years old), to 8700× (>85 years). More than 80% of COVID-19 deaths occurred in people older than 65 years of age.[4,5]

Long-term care facility residents were an exceptionally vulnerable population. They had a disproportionate number of cases spurred on by their communal nature, high percentage of residents with chronic illnesses, as well as the close proximity required for many of their care needs. Long-term care facilities had high rates of severe cases, hospitalization, and death. This population makes up less than 1% of the US population but accounted for more than 35% of all COVID-19 deaths.[6,7]

SOCIAL ISOLATION

One of the most notable changes during the COVID-19 pandemic for the older adult population with or without preexisting mental health problems has been the significant increase in social isolation. Social isolation relates to the lack or deficits seen in the objective characteristics of an individual's social network or relationships,[8] whereas loneliness refers to the negative feeling derived from the discrepancy between the desired and actual social network or relationships.[9]

For many older adults, social isolation happened swiftly with little or no warning as countries suddenly implemented nationwide lockdowns. Because older adults experienced worse COVID-19 morbidity and mortality outcomes, national disease control centers focused much of their education and messaging on the importance of establishing and maintaining physical distance from others. As a result, unless they lived in the same household as other family members, older adults were separated from their families and friends for long periods of time regardless of whether they lived in their own homes or in a long-term care facility. Before the pandemic, certain underserved older adult populations (black, indigenous, and other people of color; those living in poverty; those being homebound; and those living in rural communities) were at higher risk of social isolation with the impact only worsening with the pandemic.[10]

Social connectedness plays an important role in maintaining health and quality of life and has been shown to help reduce both morbidity and mortality.[11]

A meta-analysis completed by Holt-Lunstad and colleagues[12] revealed a 50% increased likelihood of survival in individuals with strong social relationships and remained steady across several variables, including age, sex, and health status (odds ratio [OR] = 1.5). The association was found to be higher with more complex measures of relationships (OR = 1.9) than with binary measures of social relationships (OR = 1.19). The investigators conclude that the effects of social relationships on mortality are comparable to the effects seen on well-established risk factors for mortality, such as smoking and alcohol use, and more than is seen with lack of physical activity and obesity.

In an ongoing study started before the pandemic, Rolandi and colleagues[13] assessed baseline use of social networks. Those in the intervention group received training in social network sites use, including smartphone use, Facebook and WhatsApp use, privacy rules, and fraud risk prevention using Facebook. Participants 81 to 85 years old were contacted during the pandemic, a year following the initial post-evaluation assessments. Participants that had received social network site training had higher usage of such sites, had fewer feelings of being left out, and had a smaller reduction in their social network contacts. This provides evidence of the benefits of training older adults in the use of available and new technologies and continually combating ageism related to such trainings.

Other helpful strategies to combat social isolation and loneliness include old-fashioned letter writing, phone calls, video calls, pet therapy, and self-guided or clinician-guided remote psychological interventions, including cognitive behavioral therapy, problem-solving therapy, and life review.[14–17] It is important to keep in mind that the technological limitations discussed earlier will affect the feasibility and quality of implementing some of these interventions.

MENTAL HEALTH

The proportion of older adults worldwide is increasing and doing so rapidly. According to the WHO, the population of people 60 years of age and older is estimated to increase from 12% in 2015 to 22% by 2050.[18] More than 20% of people 60 years of age and older suffer from a mental or neurologic disorder, whereas 6.6% of all disability in this age group is due to these disorders.[18] Depression and dementia are the most common disorders affecting 7% and 5% of the population, respectively.[18] Anxiety affected 3.8% and substance use disorders affected 1%.[18] Of suicide deaths worldwide, 25% was in people 60 years of age and older.[18]

Social isolation has been associated with increased risk of depression and anxiety in older adults.[19] However, many studies showed a more significant impact on the mental health of younger people (<35 years), on women, on those with low income, and in the unemployed than in older adults.[20–22] These studies were carried out earlier during the pandemic and involved completing online surveys. Surveys completed during the later stages of the pandemic showed significant negative impact on mental health, highlighting the difference in impact of acute versus chronic stress on older adults.[23] One multinational study involving 33 countries showed that being separated from family and close friends predicted depression and anxiety.[24] Having conflicts with other adults in the home was the largest predictor of anxiety and the second largest predictor for depression. Living in a higher-income country was the biggest predictor of depression and the second biggest predictor of anxiety. Geographic differences emerged, with Europe and Central Asia having the highest levels of depression followed by North America, Sub-Saharan Africa, East Asia and Pacific, and Latin America and the Caribbean. For anxiety, the top 3 regions remained the same as seen in depression, but Latin America and the Caribbean had higher levels than East Asia and the Pacific.

Not having a partner and receiving treatment for COVD-19 were positively associated with depression, whereas increased workload responsibility was negatively associated with depression. Other factors associated with depression and anxiety include prolonged separation from social networks, female gender, trans/nonbinary identification, and difficulty with work transition.

The COVID-19 Coping Study[25] showed a high prevalence of anxiety, depression, and loneliness when compared with prepandemic levels. There were strong associations between these 3 and increased alcohol consumption in the past week when compared with prepandemic levels.

According to the National Poll on Healthy Aging,[26] most of the respondents (59%) had no changes in their alcohol consumption, whereas 27% reported a reduction in alcohol consumption when compared with prepandemic levels. Those who reported lack of companions were more likely to have increased their alcohol consumption during the pandemic (19% vs 12%) as were those who reported feeling isolated compared with those who did not (19% vs 10%).

Suicide is a major public health issue. There has been an increase in suicide ideation, attempts, and death in at-risk populations in time of crises.[27] Loneliness is a known risk factor for suicide and has been associated with worse health outcomes.[12]

Hobfoll and colleagues[28] identified empirically supported strategies that could be used for mass trauma intervention and management. They recommend promoting a sense of safety, calming, a sense of self and community efficacy, connectedness, and hope. Many studies emphasize the importance of finding new ways to establish and maintain connections with a great deal of focus on telehealth. Telephone and video-based interventions have been shown to be effective in the management of depression, anxiety, posttraumatic stress disorder (PTSD), and adjustment disorder.[29]

PHYSICAL HEALTH

National and local lockdowns put in place as a result of the COVID-19 pandemic negatively affected the physical health of older adults in multiple ways. The lockdowns imposed a significant restriction on what, when, where, and how much physical activity older adults could do. In older adults, physical inactivity has been found to contribute significantly to disability and is the fourth highest risk factor for mortality in this age group.[30,31]

Reduced physical activity increases the risk of falls and all its ensuing complications. Maintaining physical activity is important in preserving independence, mental health, and physical health in older adults.[32] Researchers have found significant decline in physical activity in older adults during this pandemic. Older adults who were hospitalized during the pandemic, either with COVID-19 or for other reasons, had even more severe physical effects.[32,33]

Researchers have recommended walking, exercise games on video game consoles, interactive rehabilitation technologies, or exercise DVDs that require no Internet connection but do require a DVD player.[34,35] A major concern has been the ability of older adults to complete these exercises safely while unsupervised by a health care provider, which is pertinent during this pandemic. The Preventing Loss of Autonomy by Treatment Post-Hospitalization tool, a home-based intervention, can be individually tailored based on a person's balance and strength profile and has been shown to be safe and efficient in older adults after hospitalization.[36]

Malnutrition is commonly found in older adults, especially when hospitalized.[37] There was increased concern about malnutrition in older adults during the pandemic, especially in those who had little or no support systems. This concern was worsened by increased food insecurity with the economic impact of the pandemic, food supply issues, and shortages especially at the beginning of the pandemic, and changing eating habits.[38,39] The effect of malnutrition on older adults hospitalized with COVID-19 was even worse. Malnutrition impairs the immune system and increases risk of infections along with its associated increased risks of morbidity and mortality.[40] Infections themselves can also worsen malnutrition, creating a vicious cycle in which cause and effect become difficult to differentiate.

Another way that lockdowns have affected physical health is in delay of treatment of physical ailments especially if there were preexisting medical conditions that put them at higher risk of infection of the virus.[39] Anxiety about being infected with COVID-19 led many to avoid hospitals entirely. Routine surveillance for chronic disorders, cancers, and such was delayed; routine vaccinations were skipped.

COVID-19 affected sleep in older adults. The National Poll on Aging found that 64% of people aged 50 to 80 years old had difficulty falling or staying asleep at least once the previous week. This was double the percentage of a 2017 poll conducted in a comparable group of older adults.[41] Impaired sleep can have a negative impact on cognition, including attention, working memory, long-term memory, and decision making.[42]

COGNITIVE IMPACT OF CORONAVIRUS DISEASE 2019

COVID-19 is associated with neurologic disorders, including encephalopathy and anosmia. Greater than 80% of those infected have some form of neurologic manifestation.[43] The neurologic symptoms observed included cerebrovascular accidents (ischemic and hemorrhagic), delirium, encephalopathy, agitation, and seizures.[43] Patients with more severe neurologic disease as a result of infection tended to be older.[44]

People with dementia are vulnerable to infection because of they may be unable to understand the significance or impact of the disease and thus are less able to comply with public health recommendations for minimizing spread, such as wearing masks and maintaining distance from others. Dementia patients who require assistance with activities of daily living are limited in their ability to minimize their social contacts, thus increasing risk. A significant proportion of persons with dementia reside in long-term care facilities, which had high rates of severe cases, hospitalization, and death from COVID-19 and accounted for more than 35% of all COVID-19 deaths.[6,7] There are data to suggest that increased mortality is associated with dementia, cerebrovascular accidents,[45,46] and ApoE4 homozygosity.[47]

HEALTH CARE DISPARITIES

As with other patient populations, the COVID-19 pandemic highlighted chronic racial and ethnic health care disparities. One's ZIP code has been shown to have a greater effect on health than genetics.[48,49] Nursing homes with higher nonwhite residents experienced 3.3-fold higher death rates when compared with those with the highest percentages of white residents and were associated with larger nursing home size and the local COVID-19 prevalence rates.[50,51]

Health care disparities between rural and urban populations persisted. Rural populations tend to have reduced access to health care, lower capacities in health care facilities with greater distances to travel to these facilities, a higher percentage of older adults, more chronic illnesses, lower access to reliable broadband technology, lower use of smartphones and so forth, and fewer economic resources.[52] Geographic distance initially spared rural populations from the full brunt of the pandemic when compared with high-density urban areas. However, once the virus was detected in the community, the toll was just as severe.[53]

Rural areas with higher proportions of ethnic minorities, including black and indigenous peoples, experienced higher rates of severe illness and death from COVID-19.[54–56] Older adults living in long-term care facilities had the worst outcomes from COVID-19, and this was found in numerous studies across the globe. They accounted for most of the mortality associated with the disease, with mortalities ranging from 19% to 72% of all deaths.[57]

ELDER ABUSE

The pandemic caused significant social, interpersonal, and financial distress that cut across the entire population. Caregiving is associated with worse mental and physical health outcomes.[58] The added stress from the pandemic has led to reports of increased rates of abuse.[59–61] The social isolation engendered by the pandemic meant that avenues that caregivers would have used to help alleviate stress were no longer available to them or there was very limited availability. At the same time, the isolation meant that any older adult being abused was less likely to be noticed by an outside person or agency, such as Adult Protective Services. Other ways the pandemic could increase risk include increased demand on caregiver resources, such as time and money, increased caregiver substance use, and increased purchase of weapons.[62]

Elder abuse can be physical, psychological, sexual, or financial. Before the pandemic, the estimated yearly prevalence of people 60 years and older who had experienced some form of abuse was 10%.[63] In the pandemic era, Chang and Levy[64] found the overall prevalence of elder abuse to be 21.3%, an 83.6% increase when compared with prepandemic levels. The rate of reported physical abuse went from 1.6% to 5.4%, an astounding increase of 237.5%, and financial abuse increased from 3.5% to 7.5%, an increase of 114.3%. The study did not find significant increase in verbal abuse (9% vs 9.2%, an increase of 0.02%). Of note, this study did not include older adults with poor health conditions and limited resources, including those living with dementia. It is, therefore, possible that these estimates lean on the more conservative side. Societal connectedness and stronger sense of community were associated with reduced risk.

To help mitigate elder abuse, increased awareness is key. Screening for elder abuse should be a regular part of the assessment of older adults regardless of the specialty and will require appropriate education and training of everyone involved in caring for older adults. Telemedicine can play an important role, as videos can provide the clinician with an insight into the patient's home and living situation. Changes on the individual level will likely not be enough for long-term changes and will require societal and structural changes, including providing more resources for at-risk older adults and their families, for example, for housing, food, reliable broadband access, providing Adult Protective Services with adequate funding.[64,65]

IMPACT OF CORONAVIRUS DISEASE 2019 ON GERIATRIC PSYCHIATRY WORKFORCE

Older patients were not the only ones affected by the COVID-19 pandemic. The pandemic affected everyone everywhere in one way or another. There was uncertainty about this new virus, the overwhelming number of deaths, fear of contracting the virus; shortages of hospital beds, ventilators and other equipment, and personal protective equipment (PPE); and lack of knowledge about which PPE were appropriate to use and when. Coupled with the seemingly shifting recommendations from national health bodies that were working with incomplete knowledge of the virus, these circumstances created an environment rife with uncertainty and anxiety.

In epidemics, such as the severe acute respiratory syndrome, Middle East respiratory syndrome, Ebola, and H1N1 epidemic, health care workers have been shown to have high prevalence rates of anxiety (45%), depression (38%), acute stress disorder (31%), burnout (29%), and PTSD (19%) during and after the epidemics.[66,67] These significant negative mental health outcomes were found to be associated with female gender, younger age, nurses, less job security, and frontline work.

Results from cross-sectional surveys completed during the current COVID-19 pandemic show worse outcomes in nurses and physician trainees with more impact on their mental health.[68,69]

Physicians and nurses are more often exposed to traumatic events in the course of their work and in prepandemic times have been shown to have higher rates of PTSD than non–health care workers (14.8%[70] and 18%,[71] respectively, vs 7%–8%[72]). Long-term care facility workers also experienced substantial negative outcomes during the COVID-19 pandemic. There was inadequate staff education about infection control, inadequate access to PPE, significant staff turnover rates owing to safety concerns, staff COVID infections, and burnout.[73]

A survey of 653 health care workers conducted by Bassi and colleagues[69] in the early days of the pandemic in the hardest hit region in Italy showed that 39.8% of the respondents met the criteria for provisional PTSD. They posit that taking preemptive action to train and protect vulnerable health care worker categories as well as promoting positive mental health may help reduce the negative mental health impact of this pandemic and serve as a roadmap in allaying these effects in future disaster events.

TELEMEDICINE AND CORONAVIRUS DISEASE 2019

There were swift shifts to telemedicine in many health care systems with the announcements of lockdowns. Nonemergent procedures were canceled, and staff was diverted to frontline work when possible. Telemedicine was one of the bigger health care shifts during this pandemic.

Before the pandemic, Psychiatry was among the medical specialties that used telemedicine the most.[74] Changes in Centers for Medicare and Medicaid Services[75] regarding reimbursement and certain easing or waivers of legal restrictions allowed physicians in the United States to bill for telemedicine services on par with in-person visits. State health departments provided temporary licensing or waivers to physicians in nearby states to provide telemedicine services.

Geriatric psychiatrists and other geriatric clinicians were able to provide care while minimizing viral exposure to this particularly affected group of patients. Medical care was also possible for patients who were in quarantine via telemedicine services.

It should be noted that telemedicine is not a universal remedy. Other previously identified barriers to telemedicine, such as technological challenges for health care staff and patients, older age, rural setting, lack of equipment or outdated equipment, inadequate broadband services, and computer literacy, persisted.[76] Telemedicine has the potential to promote health equity and reduce health disparities but only if the current barriers are removed. It is telling that most of the research on telemedicine in older adults has been conducted in high-income countries.[77] The quick uptake in telemedicine usage in the United States during the COVID-19 pandemic was facilitated by policy changes on state and federal levels. In order to maintain the benefits we have seen from using telemedicine during the pandemic, long-term policy decisions and careful implementation that takes into account everyone involved are essential.

SUMMARY

The COVID-19 pandemic led to numerous changes in health care. As a newly defined disease, it brought with it a significant amount of apprehension about all the unknowns regarding its origin, infectivity, transmission, susceptibility, as well as the long- and short-term outcomes associated with it. It has been learned that older adults and those with comorbid medical disorders, of which older adults also form a majority, have significantly higher morbidities and mortalities.[3] This was especially true in long-term care facilities that were shown to have high rates of severe cases, hospitalization, and death.[6,7]

Social isolation increased in the older adult population as a direct result of the mitigation strategies recommended by national disease control centers to help reduce infectivity rates. Social connectedness is important in maintaining health, improving quality of life, and reducing morbidity and mortality in older adults[11]; with older adults accounting a quarter of all suicide deaths worldwide,[18] implementing strategies that reduce social isolation will promote positive health outcomes. Studies looking at potential strategies for mass trauma interventions have recommended interventions that promote a sense of safety, calming, a sense of self and community efficacy, connectedness, and hope with many focusing on telehealth.[27] As with other health outcomes, the impact of social isolation during the COVID-19 pandemic has been worse in underserved older adult communities.

Physical inactivity resulting from lockdowns and other social distancing measures and malnutrition has directly contributed to an increase in disability in older adults. Anxiety about contracting the virus led many older adults to postpone routine screenings for chronic disorders or cancers, resulting in worse health outcomes. Older adults have also reported worse sleep[14] and are more likely to have severe neurologic sequelae of the disease.[44]

The increased caregiver stress during the pandemic resulted in an increase in physical and financial elder abuse.[64] Regrettably, this may be an underestimation of the true prevalence, as older adults with poor health conditions and limited resources were not included in the study.

Protecting the geriatric workforce is also an important part of caring for the older adult population. Health care workers have higher exposure to traumatic events with subsequently worse mental health outcomes.[70,71] Reducing these negative outcomes requires protecting vulnerable health care worker categories, providing appropriate training for all health care workers, and promoting positive mental health.[69]

The COVID-19 pandemic presented the health care field with the challenge of continuously adapting to the changing health care landscape while ensuring the provision of needed quality care for patients and support for the loved ones in their lives. In the United States, the rapid and widespread adoption of telemedicine was encouraged by key regulatory changes at federal and state levels.[75] Access to care remained inequitable, was exacerbated by the pandemic, and highlighted the already present and long-standing health disparities seen in racial, ethnic, and gender minority populations as well as in rural communities. Individual and systemic changes in addition to innovations in strategy and implementation will be critical in meeting the current and future mental health needs of all older adults.

CLINICAL PEARLS

- Long-term care facilities had high rates of severity and hospitalizations and accounted for more than 35% of deaths in the United States[6,7] and 19% to 72% of deaths worldwide.[57]
- Social connectedness is important in helping older adults maintain good health, improve quality of life, and reduce morbidity and mortality.[11]
- There is a higher prevalence of anxiety, depression, and loneliness in older adults when compared with prepandemic levels.[25]

- Older adults who reported social isolation were more likely to report increased alcohol consumption.[26]
- Physical inactivity contributes significantly to disability and is the fourth highest risk factor for mortality in older adults.[29,30]
- Older adults had significant decline in physical activity, and those that were hospitalized for any reason had even more severe physical effects.[32,33]
- The postponement of routine surveillance for chronic disorders or cancers resulted in worse health outcome.
- Patients with more severe neurologic disease were more likely to be older.[44]
- The COVID-19 pandemic highlighted chronic racial, ethnic, rural health care disparities.
- There was an 83.6% increase in elder abuse when compared with prepandemic levels.[64]
- Health care workers had worse mental health outcomes in prepandemic times and only worsened with the pandemic.[69–73]
- State and federal regulatory changes helped spur on the use of telemedicine during the pandemic.[75]

RECOMMENDED INTERVENTIONS

Social Isolation: training in the use of available and new technologies[13] as well as low-tech strategies, such as letter writing, phone calls, pet therapy.[14–17]

Mental Health: telephone and video-based interventions are effective in the management of depression, anxiety, PTSD, and adjustment disorder.[28]

Physical Health: walking, exercise games on video game consoles, interactive rehabilitation technologies, or exercise DVDs that require no Internet connection but do require a DVD player.[32,34]

Elder Abuse: increased awareness and screening should be a regular part of the assessment of older adults in any health care setting.

Health Care Workers: training and protecting vulnerable health care worker categories and promoting positive mental health may help reduce negative mental health outcomes.[69]

Systemic and Structural Changes: societal and structural changes, including providing more resources for at risk older adults and their families, policy updates and changes, infrastructure development.

REFERENCES

1. WHO coronavirus (COVID-19) dashboard. Available at: https://covid19.who.int/. August 14, 2021.
2. United States COVID-19 Cases. Deaths, and laboratory testing (NAATs) by state, territory, and jurisdiction. Available at: https://covid.cdc.gov/covid-data-tracker/#cases_casesper100klast7days. August 14, 2021.
3. Increased risk of hospitalization or death. Available at: https://www.cdc.gov/coronavirus/2019-ncov/need-extra-precautions/older-adults.html. June 5, 2021.
4. Cronin AM, Railey S, Fortune D, et al. Notes from the field: effects of the COVID-19 response on tuberculosis prevention and control efforts—United States, March–April 2020. MMWR Morb Mortal Wkly Rep 2020;69(29):971–2.
5. Centers for Disease Control and Prevention COVID-19 Response Team. Severe outcomes among patients with coronavirus disease 2019 (COVID-19)—United States, February 12–March 16, 2020. MMWR Morb Mortal Wkly Rep 2020; 69(12):343–6.

6. Grabowski DC, Mor V. Nursing home care in crisis in the wake of COVID-19. J Am Med Assoc 2020;324(1):23–4.
7. Yourish K, Lai KKR, Ivory D, et al. One-third of all U.S. coronavirus deaths are nursing home residents or workers. Available at: https://www.nytimes.com/interactive/2020/us/coronavirus-nursing-homes.html. June 13, 2021.
8. de Jong-Gierveld J, van Tilburg TG, Dykstra PA. Loneliness and social isolation. In: Perlman D, Vangelisti A, editors. The Cambridge handbook of personal relationships. Cambridge University Press; 2006. p. 485–500.
9. Peplau LA, Perlman D. Perspectives on loneliness. In: Peplau LA, Perlman D, editors. Loneliness. New York: Wiley; 1982. p. 1–18.
10. A national survey of adults 45 and older: loneliness and social connections. Available at: https://www.aarp.org/content/dam/aarp/research/surveys_statistics/life-leisure/2018/loneliness-social-connections-2018.doi.10.26419-2Fres.00246.001.pdf. June 13, 2021.
11. Steptoe A, Shankar A, Demakakos P, et al. Social isolation, loneliness, and all-cause mortality in older men and women. Proc Natl Acad Sci U S A 2013;110(15):5797–801.
12. Holt-Lunstad J, Smith TB, Layton JB. Social relationships and mortality risk: a meta-analytic review. PLoS Med 2010;7(7):e1000316.
13. Rolandi E, Vaccaro R, Abbondanza S, et al. Loneliness and social engagement in older adults based in Lombardy during the COVID-19 lockdown: the long-term effects of a course on social networking sites use. Int J Environ Res Public Health 2020;17(21):7912.
14. Smith M, Steinman L, Casey EA. Combating social isolation among older adults in a time of physical distancing: the COVID-19 social connectivity paradox. Front Public Health 2020;8:403.
15. Gorenko J, Moran C, Flynn M, et al. Social isolation and psychological distress among older adults related to COVID-19: a narrative review of remotely-delivered interventions and recommendations. J Appl Gerontol 2021;40(1):3–13.
16. Jarvis M, Padmanabhanunni A, Balakrishna Y, et al. The effectiveness of interventions addressing loneliness in older persons: an umbrella review. International Journal of Africa Nursing Sciences, 12, Article 100177, 2020.
17. Gardiner C, Geldenhuys G, Gott M. Interventions to reduce social isolation and loneliness among older people: an integrative review. Health Soc Care Community 2018;26(2):147–57.
18. World Health Organization. Mental health of older adults. 2017. Available at: https://www.who.int/en/news-room/fact-sheets/detail/mental-health-of-older-adults. June 15, 2021.
19. Santini ZI, Jose PE, Cornwell EY, et al. Social disconnectedness, perceived isolation, and symptoms of depression and anxiety among older Americans (NSHAP): a longitudinal mediation analysis. Lancet Public Health 2020;5(1):e62–70.
20. Pieh C, Budimir S, Probst T. The effect of age, gender, income, work, and physical activity on mental health during coronavirus disease (COVID-19) lockdown in Austria. J Psychosom Res 2020;136:110186.
21. Czeisler MÉ, Lane RI, Petrosky E, et al. Mental health, substance use, and suicidal ideation during the COVID-19 pandemic — United States, June 24–30, 2020. MMWR Morb Mortal Wkly Rep 2020;69:1049–57.
22. González-Sanguino C, Ausín B, Castellanos M, et al. Mental health consequences during the initial stage of the 2020 coronavirus pandemic (COVID-19) in Spain. Brain Behav Immun 2020;87:172–6.

23. De Pue S, Gillebert C, Dierckx E, et al. The impact of the COVID-19 pandemic on wellbeing and cognitive functioning of older adults. Sci Rep 2021;11:4636.
24. Tyler CM, McKee GB, Alzueta E, et al. A study of older adults' mental health across 33 countries during the COVID-19 pandemic. Int J Environ Res Public Health 2021;18(10):5090.
25. Eastman M, Finlay J, Kobayashi L. Alcohol use and mental health among older American adults during the early months of the COVID-19 pandemic. Int J Environ Res Public Health 2021;18(8):4222.
26. Fernandez A, Kullgren J, Malani P, et al. Alcohol use among older adults. University of Michigan National Poll on Healthy Aging; 2021. Available at: 10.7302/1328. Accessed June 16, 2021.
27. Cheung YT, Chau PH, Yip PS. A revisit on older adults suicides and severe acute respiratory syndrome (SARS) epidemic in Hong Kong. Int J Geriatr Psychiatry 2008;23(12):1231–8.
28. Hobfoll SE, Watson P, Bell CC, et al. Five essential elements of immediate and mid-term mass trauma intervention: empirical evidence. Psychiatry Interpersonal Biol Process 2007;70(4):283–315.
29. Varker T, Brand RM, Ward J, et al. Efficacy of synchronous telepsychology interventions for people with anxiety, depression, posttraumatic stress disorder, and adjustment disorder: a rapid evidence assessment. Psychol Serv 2019;16(4): 621–35.
30. World Health Organization . WHO; Geneva: 2010. Global Recommendations on Physical Activity for Health. chap. 2.1.
31. Gomes M, Figueiredo D, Teixeira L, et al. Physical inactivity among older adults across Europe based on the SHARE database. Age Ageing 2017;46(1):71–7.
32. Goethals L, Barth N, Guyot J, et al. Impact of home quarantine on physical activity among older adults living at home during the COVID-19 pandemic: qualitative interview study. JMIR Aging 2020;3(1):e19007.
33. Yamada M, Kimura Y, Ishiyama D, et al. Effect of the COVID-19 epidemic on physical activity in community-dwelling older adults in Japan: a cross-sectional online survey. J Nutr Health Aging 2020;24(9):948–50.
34. Ortiz-Alonso J, Bustamante-Ara N, Valenzuela PL. Effect of a simple exercise programme on hospitalisation-associated disability in older patients: a randomised controlled trial. J Am Med Dir Assoc 2020;21:531–7.e1.
35. Barbosa Neves B, Franz R, Judges R. Can digital technology enhance social connectedness among older adults? A feasibility study. J Appl Gerontol 2019; 38:49–72.
36. Carvalho LP, Kergoat MJ, Bolduc A, et al. A systematic approach for prescribing posthospitalization home-based physical activity for mobility in older adults: the PATH Study. J Am Med Dir Assoc 2019;20:1287–93.
37. Cerri AP, Bellelli G, Mazzone A, et al. Sarcopenia and malnutrition in acutely ill hospitalized elderly: prevalence and outcomes. Clin Nutr 2015;34:745–51.
38. Niles MT, Bertmann F, Belarmino EH, et al. The early food insecurity impacts of COVID-19. Nutrients 2020;12:2096.
39. Batsis JA, Daniel K, Eckstrom E, et al. Promoting healthy aging during COVID-19. J Am Geriatr Soc 2021;69(3):572–80.
40. Zabetakis I, Lordan R, Norton C, et al. COVID-19: the inflammation link and the role of nutrition in potential mitigation. Nutrients 2020;12. https://doi.org/10.3390/nu12051466.

41. Gerlach L, Solway E, Singer D, et al. Mental health among older adults before and during the COVID-19 pandemic. University of Michigan National Poll on Healthy Aging; 2021. Available at: 10.7302/983. Accessed June 16, 2021.
42. Alhola P, Polo-Kantola P. Sleep deprivation: impact on cognitive performance. Neuropsychiatr Dis Treat 2007;3:553–67.
43. Liotta EM, Batra A, Clark JR, et al. Frequent neurologic manifestations and encephalopathy-associated morbidity in Covid-19 patients. Ann Clin Transl Neurol 2020;7:2221–30.
44. Mao L, Jin H, Wang M, et al. Neurologic manifestations of hospitalized patients with coronavirus disease 2019 in Wuhan, China. JAMA Neurol 2020;77(6):1-9.
45. Williamson E, Walker AJ, Bhaskaran KJ, et al. OpenSAFELY: factors associated with COVID-19-related hospital death in the linked electronic health records of 17 million adult NHS patients. medRxiv 2020;2020. 05.06.20092999.
46. Atkins JL, Masoli JA, Delgado J, et al. Preexisting comorbidities predicting severe COVID-19 in older adults in the UK biobank community cohort. medRxiv 2020;2020. 05.06.20092700.
47. Kuo CL, Pilling LC, Atkins JL, et al. APOE e4 genotype predicts severe COVID-19 in the UK biobank community cohort. J Gerontol A Biol Sci Med Sci 2020;75(11): 2231–2.
48. Graham G. Why your ZIP code matters more than your genetic code: promoting healthy outcomes from mother to child. Breastfeed Med 2016;11:396–7.
49. Sloggett A, Joshi H. Deprivation indicators as predictors of life events 1981-1992 based on the UK ONS Longitudinal Study. J Epidemiol Community Health 1998; 52(4):228–33.
50. Gorges RJ, Konetzka RT. Staffing levels and COVID-19 cases and outbreaks in U.S. nursing homes. J Am Geriatr Soc 2020;68(11):2462–6.
51. Weech-Maldonado R, Lord J, Davlyatov G, et al. High-minority nursing homes disproportionately affected by COVID-19 deaths. Front Public Health 2021;9: 606364.
52. Henning-Smith C. The unique impact of COVID-19 on older adults in rural areas. J Aging Soc Policy 2020;32(4–5):396–402.
53. Paul R, Arif A, Adeyemi O, et al. Progression of COVID-19 from urban to rural areas in the United States: a spatiotemporal analysis of prevalence rates. J Rural Health 2020;36(4):591–601.
54. Melvin S, Wiggins C, Burse N, et al. The role of public health in COVID-19 emergency response efforts from a rural health perspective. Prev Chronic Dis 2020; 17:E70.
55. Huyser K, Yang T, Yellow Horse A. Indigenous peoples, concentrated disadvantage, and income inequality in New Mexico: a ZIP code-level investigation of spatially varying associations between socioeconomic disadvantages and confirmed COVID-19 cases. J Epidemiol Community Health 2021;75(11):1044–9.
56. Schiff R, Buccieri K, Schiff JW, et al. COVID-19 and pandemic planning in the context of rural and remote homelessness. Can J Public Health 2020;111(6):967–70.
57. Thompson D, Barbu M, Beiu C, et al. The impact of COVID-19 pandemic on long-term care facilities worldwide: an overview on international issues. Biomed Res Int 2020;2020:8870249.
58. Schulz R, Sherwood P. Physical and mental health effects of family caregiving. Am J Nurs 2008;108(9 Suppl):23–7.
59. Taub A. A new COVID-19 crisis: domestic abuse rises worldwide. The New York Times; 2020. Available at: https://www.nytimes.com/2020/04/06/world/coronavirus-domestic-violence.html. June 14, 2021.

60. Sserwanja Q, Kawuki J, Kim J. Increased child abuse in Uganda amidst COVID-19 pandemic. J Paediatr Child Health 2021;57:188–91.
61. Mazza M, Marano G, Lai C, et al. Danger in danger: interpersonal violence during COVID-19 quarantine. Psychiatry Res 2020;289.
62. Makaroun L, Bachrach R, Rosland A. Elder abuse in the time of COVID-19—increased risks for older adults and their caregivers. Am J Geriatr Psychiatry 2020;28(8):876–80.
63. Pillemer K, Burnes D, Riffin C, et al. Elder abuse: global situation, risk factors, and prevention strategies. Gerontologist 2016;56(Suppl. 2):S194–205.
64. Chang E, Levy R. High prevalence of elder abuse during the COVID-19 pandemic: risk and resilience factors. Am J Geriatr Psychiatry 2021;29(11):1152–9.
65. Elman A, Breckman R, Clark S, et al. Effects of the COVID-19 outbreak on elder mistreatment and response in New York City: initial lessons. J Appl Gerontol 2020;39(7):690–9.
66. Ricci-Cabello I, Meneses-Echavez JF, Serrano-Ripoll MJ, et al. Impact of viral epidemic outbreaks on mental health of healthcare workers: a rapid systematic review. medRxiv 2020. https://doi.org/10.1101/2020.04.02.20048892.
67. Maunder RG, Lancee WJ, Balderson KE, et al. Long-term psychological and occupational effects of providing hospital healthcare during SARS outbreak. Emerg Infect Dis 2006;12:1924–32.
68. García-Fernández L, Romero-Ferreiro V, López-Roldán PV, et al. Mental health impact of COVID-19 pandemic on Spanish healthcare workers. Psychol Med 2020;1–6. https://doi.org/10.1017/S0033291720002019.
69. Bassi M, Negri L, Delle Fave A, et al. The relationship between post-traumatic stress and positive mental health symptoms among health workers during COVID-19 pandemic in Lombardy, Italy. J Affect Disord 2021;280(Pt B):1–6.
70. Sendler DJ, Rutkowska A, Makara-Studzinska M. How the exposure to trauma has hindered physicians' capacity to heal: prevalence of PTSD among healthcare workers. Eur J Psychiat 2016;30:321–34.
71. Mealer M, Burnham EL, Goode CJ, et al. The prevalence and impact of post traumatic stress disorder and burnout syndrome in nurses. Depress Anxiety 2009;26: 1118–26.
72. Kessler RC, Berglund P, Demier O, et al. Lifetime prevalence and age-of-onset distributions of DSM-IV disorders in the National Comorbidity Survey Replication. Arch Gen Psychiatry 2005;62:593–602.
73. Ouslander JG, Grabowski DC. COVID-19 in nursing homes: calming the perfect storm. J Am Geriatr Soc 2020;68(10):2153–62.
74. Robeznieks A. Which medical specialties use telemedicine the most? American Medical Association; 2019. Available at: https://www.ama-assn.org/practice-management/digital/which-medical-specialties-use-telemedicine-most. June 22, 2021.
75. Services CfMaM state Medicaid and CHIP telehealth toolkit - policy considerations for states expanding use of telehealth COVID-19 version. 2019. Available at: https://www.medicaid.gov/medicaid/benefits/downloads/medicaid-chip-telehealth-toolkit.pdf. June 22, 2021.
76. Scott Kruse C, Karem P, Shifflett K, et al. Evaluating barriers to adopting telemedicine worldwide: a systematic review. J Telemed Telecare 2018;24(1):4–12.
77. Doraiswamy S, Jithesh A, Mamtani R, et al. Telehealth use in geriatrics care during the COVID-19 pandemic—a scoping review and evidence synthesis. Int J Environ Res Public Health 2021;18(4):1755.

The Impact of COVID-19 on Financing of Psychiatric Services

Laurence H. Miller, MD[a,*], Joseph Parks, MD[b], Rebecca Yowell, BS[c]

KEYWORDS

• COVID • Financing • Waiver • Telehealth • Psychiatric services • Lessons learned

KEY POINTS

- The financial impacts owing to the COVID-19 crisis have varied based on 3 major variables: time since the onset of the epidemic, payment methodology and financing, and type of psychiatric service.
- Initial impact was severe service and revenue loss. Subsequent service and revenue recovery was surprisingly swift but has not yet been restored to prepandemic levels.
- Lasting benefits will be expansion of and payments for virtual services
- Epidemic exposed the weakness and lack of flexibility in fee-for-service payment methodologies
- Swift governmental intervention can have a significant impact on the financial viability of clinical sites

INTRODUCTION

The onset of the COVID-19 pandemic in early 2020 had a significant impact on the delivery of behavioral health services which, in turn, has had significant short-term and long-range consequences. Intertwined with the delivery of services has been the financial ramifications of the pandemic which have varied based on 3 major variables: time phases since the onset of the epidemic, payment methodology and financing, and type of psychiatric service.

[a] Division of Medical Services, Arkansas Department of Human Services, Department of Psychiatry, University of Arkansas for Medical Sciences, 700 Main Street Suite 415, Little Rock, AR 72201, USA; [b] Practice Improvement & Consulting, National Council for Mental Wellbeing, 1400 K Street Northwest, Suite 400, Washington, DC 20005, USA; [c] Reimbursement Policy and Quality, American Psychiatric Association, 800 Maine Avenue Southwest, Suite 900, Washington, DC 20024, USA

* Corresponding author.

E-mail address: Laurence.miller@dhs.arkansas.gov

Psychiatr Clin N Am 45 (2022) 161–177

https://doi.org/10.1016/j.psc.2021.11.014

Abbreviations	
AMA	American Medical Association
CARES	Coronavirus Aid, Relief, and Economic Security Act
CMS	Centers for Medicare and Medicaid Services
PACE	Program for All-Inclusive Care for the Elderly
PHE	public health emergency

DISCUSSION

Time Since the Onset of the Pandemic

For any particular location the impact on financing and access to services has fallen into 3 broad phases.

First, the initial closure of services and subsequent loss of revenue occurred mostly during late February and throughout March 2020. Between March 12 and April 6, all US states and territories issued advisory or mandatory stay-at-home orders, with the exception of Iowa.[1] This resulted in the cessation of the majority of nonemergency psychiatric services. In this early phase, even the majority of virtual services were curtailed because, in most cases, the originating site had to be in a clinic setting and not in the community to be billable.

The second phase was the 60- to 90-day lag between the closure of services and the implementation of waivers that allowed billing for virtual services, including federal COVID-19 relief measures, various Medicaid and state interim payment arrangements, and commercial payer flexibilities. The federal actions to allow expanded and alternate payments occurred promptly. However, providers required time to reorganize service delivery and put in place the virtual service delivery infrastructure. States implemented changes to Medicaid plans through the use of 1115 and 1135 waivers (**Box 1**).

Authorization was given for hardship or supplemental payments to incentivize, stabilize, and retain clinicians who were experiencing disruptions to their revenue streams (North Carolina, Oregon, and Washington); states waived requirements that tied payment to a minimum number of hours or contacts to address limitations owing to social distancing mandates (California and New York). Commercial plans expanded in a patchwork way; and some like Anthem made a national decision, whereas others like Centene varied plan by plan.

- Medicare expanded telehealth coverage to all beneficiaries regardless of location on March 6 and on March 17 specifically included mental health counseling and outpatient visits.
- On March 24, Medicare announced it would not prevent health insurance companies from making policy changes to increase telehealth coverage, including decreases in cost-sharing requirements for telehealth to ensure access to care.

Box 1
Federal Medicaid waivers

The i115 Waivers give the Secretary of Health and Human Services the authority to approve multiyear pilot or demonstration projects requested by the states that are likely to promote the objectives of the Medicaid program.

The 1135 Waivers may be granted once a public health emergency has been declared by the Secretary of Health and Human Services. It enables the secretary to temporarily waive or modify certain Medicare, Medicaid, and Children's Health Insurance Program (CHIP) requirements to ensure necessary services are available during the period of the emergency and to allow clinicians providing care in good faith to be paid for services and exempt from sanctions (absent a determination of fraud or abuse).

- On March 30, the Centers for Medicare and Medicaid Services (CMS) added an additional 85 services to the list of Medicare telehealth services and expanded coverage of specific services by audio only.[2]

Individual state Medicaid programs and commercial insurers showed wide variation in how promptly they allowed expanded billing for virtual care. By June, most payers were reimbursing for virtual services by video or audio only at the same rates they had previously reimbursed for in-person services. The implementation of alternative payment methodologies was not widely or promptly done and varied based on type of service. Habilitation and personal care serviced were paid based on historic prospective payment amounts, mitigating the impact of any service interruptions. Some states authorized an interim payment based on historic payments for other services that was then subject to reconciliation and repayment if the service volume was not maintained. Other states implemented retroactive rate changes to help practices stay afloat.

The National Council for Behavioral Health, representing more than 3200 providers of treatment for addiction and mental illness, conducted an online survey of 880 behavioral health organizations across the country in April 2020 to quantify the impact of COVID-19 on patients, employment, safety, and financial viability. At that time,

- 62.1% of behavioral health organizations reported that they could only survive financially for 3 months or less under the COVID-19 conditions in place at that time;
- Only 9.4% of organizations reported they could survive 1 year or more;
- 46.7% of behavioral health organizations had to, or planned to, lay off or furlough employees as a result of COVID-19;
- Organizations canceled, rescheduled, or turned away 31.0% of patients;
- 61.8% closed at least 1 program; and
- Nearly all (92.6%) had reduced their operations.

The financial impact was more severe for smaller organizations (serving 2000 patients or less annually) who canceled, rescheduled, or turned away 36.1% of patients (National Council Behavioral Health, April 2020).[3] Congress, through legislative action, authorized a number of mechanisms (**Table 1**) to provide financial support to clinicians and entities providing mental health and substance use disorder services.

Although the Paycheck Protection Program was initiated as part of the Coronavirus Aid, Relief, and Economic Security Act (CARES), allocating $349 billion in forgivable loans for businesses to maintain employment at pre-COVID levels, a second online survey done in early June by the National Council for Behavioral Health found that:

- 31% of behavioral health organizations had not received any relief funding and among those who did receive funding, 39% got less than $50,000;
- On average, behavioral health organizations reported having lost 24.3% of their revenue during COVID-19; and
- 71% reported having to cancel, reschedule, or turn away patients over the previous 3 months.[4]

The third phase, since mid-2020, has seen the stabilization of operations with a new mix of virtual services and payments in an environment of ongoing uncertainty regarding how long the expanded billable services for virtual care would remain in place. A third National Council for Behavioral Health poll of 343 members conducted during the last 2 weeks of August found that:

- 26% of organizations had laid off employees, 24% had furloughed employees, and 43% had decreased the hours for staff;

Table 1
Breakdown of COVID supplemental bills, 2020 to 2021

	CARES Act, March 2020	COVID Supplemental, December 2020	FY2021 SAMHSA appropriations	American Rescue Plan, March 2021
SAPT block grant	—	$1.65 billion	$1.858 billion	$1.5 billion
Mental health block grant	—	$1.65 billion (half to providers)	$757 million (5% crisis set aside)	$1.5 billion
CCBHC expansion grants	$250 million	$600 million	$250 million	$420 million
Project AWARE	—	$50 million	$107 million	$30 million
Suicide prevention	$50 million	$50 million	$66 million (multiple programs)	$20 million (youth suicide)

Adapted from Parks, J. Impact of COVID on Demand for and Access to Behavioral Healthcare. National Council for Behavioral Health. 2020, with permission

- On average, organizations lost 22.6% of their revenue over the past 3 months during COVID-19;
- 39% believed they could only survive 6 months or less;
- Although 52% of organizations reported an increased demand for services, 62% reported that they had to cancel, reschedule, or turn away patients over the past 3 months;
- 48% of organizations reported telehealth services were providing an equal amount of revenue as previously received for in-person services. However, of those (52%) who said telehealth was not providing the same revenue on average as in-person services, they reported a 28% decrease in revenue; and
- 32% reported not receiving any funding from the CARES Act, with smaller organizations more often reporting they did not receive any stimulus funding or provider relief funds.[5]

As reflected in **Fig. 1** (changes in clinical practice), international respondents of the Global Clinical Practice Network reported changes in the number of services provided within their clinical practice. Slightly less than one-half of the respondents were providing less frequent diagnostic, psychological assessments, or psychotherapy services since the pandemic began, although only 37% of the respondents indicated they were providing psychopharmacology less frequently than before the pandemic.

Payment Methodology and Financial Impact

Overall, the predominant fee-for-service payment methodology has proven the least resilient and adaptive payment methodology during the pandemic. Limiting payment to a narrow list of individual services with specific requirements often involving face-to-face care has required many more administrative changes, including a rapid transition to telehealth and limited rapid innovation to the new pandemic conditions. In general, those operating under a capitated or prospective payment system fared better given the existing flexibilities inherent in the structure of the payment. Adjusting rates applied to individual services or expanding coverage as in a fee-for-service environment is much more administratively complex.

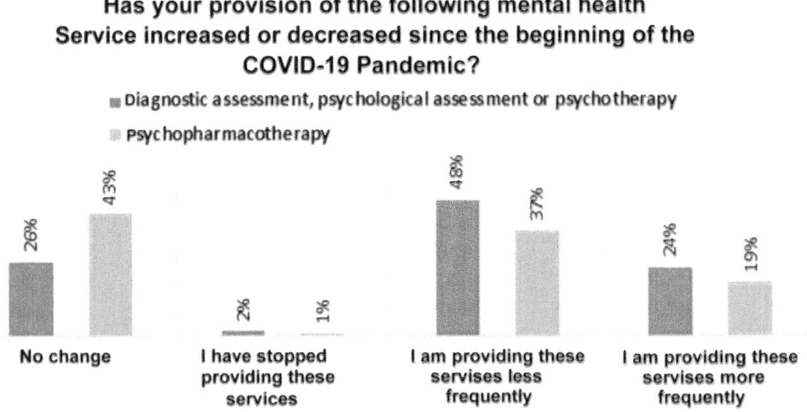

Fig. 1. Changes in the provision of mental health services. (*From* Parks J. Impact of COVID on Demand for and Access to Behavioral Healthcare. National Council for Behavioral Health. 2020)

The best performing payment methodologies have been in full capitation arrangements providing that the payment adjustment flows through the administrative bodies to the direct service providers and in grant-based funding, where agencies receive a periodic lump sum of money for a broadly defined set of services to a defined population. These payments were immediately adaptable at the provider level in response to the pandemic. Prospective payment methodologies such as those used for funding certified community behavioral health centers and federally qualified health centers, afforded immediate operational adaptability and provider financial resilience. CMS telehealth flexibilities enabled these entities to continue to provide services while receiving the same historic payment amounts.

Medicare, Medicaid, and the Children's Health Insurance Program were hampered by not having the same statutory authority for behavioral health clinicians as they do in the case of community habilitation services to persons with developmental disabilities to issue an 1135 waiver allowing interim alternative payments based on prior historic payments for all behavioral health services. As a result, community habilitation and personal care services were able to maintain their revenue stream owing to the stability in the payment methodology. In a number of cases, states instead resorted to temporary rate increases to avoid providers going out of business and programs closing. In some cases, the rate increases were done retroactively.

The pandemic significantly impacted physician livelihood and outlook. A survey conducted in April 2020 of 842 physicians revealed that 21% had recently been furloughed or experienced a pay cut, 14% planned to change practice settings as a result of COVID-19, and 18% planned to retire, temporarily close their practices, or opt out of patient care.[6] According to a yearly report published in October 2020, average physician compensation seemed to increase by 1.5%, but this was lower than increases in previous years and, when taking account the rate of inflation, actually represented a decrease in real income.[7] A similar pattern held for psychiatrists—a survey published in May 2021 had 22% reporting some decrease in compensation over the year prior.[8] The same group, however, was optimistic, with 83% expecting an eventual return to pre–COVID-19 income levels. Because labor costs typically make up the highest portion of practice expenses, it follows that pandemic-related decreases in patient volume, and thus revenue, led practices to reevaluate employee contracts accordingly.

A recent American Medical Association (AMA) analysis of Medicare Physician Fee Schedule[a] spending (spending is the allowed Medicare charge and includes both what Medicare pays and beneficiary deductible) for all physicians reflects a decrease in payments from Medicare during the first months of the pandemic, before rebounding and leveling off in the fall of 2020 (**Fig. 2**). The AMA found that overall spending decreased by 57% before leveling off at a roughly 8% below expected spending September 2020. The AMA estimates that the cumulative reduction for all clinicians during the first 9 months of 2020 is $11.5 billion.

The AMA estimates that the cumulative decrease in Medicare physician fee schedule spending from January to September 2020 for psychiatry was 9%, $702 million in spending down from the expected $773 million. Psychologists spending was down by 11% ($549 million, down from $614 million), and social workers

[a] *Reflects Medicare Physician Fee Schedule spending, which is one component of the category classified as Part B spending which also includes outpatient hospital, DME, lab, ambulance; Part A (inpatient services) spending is not included.

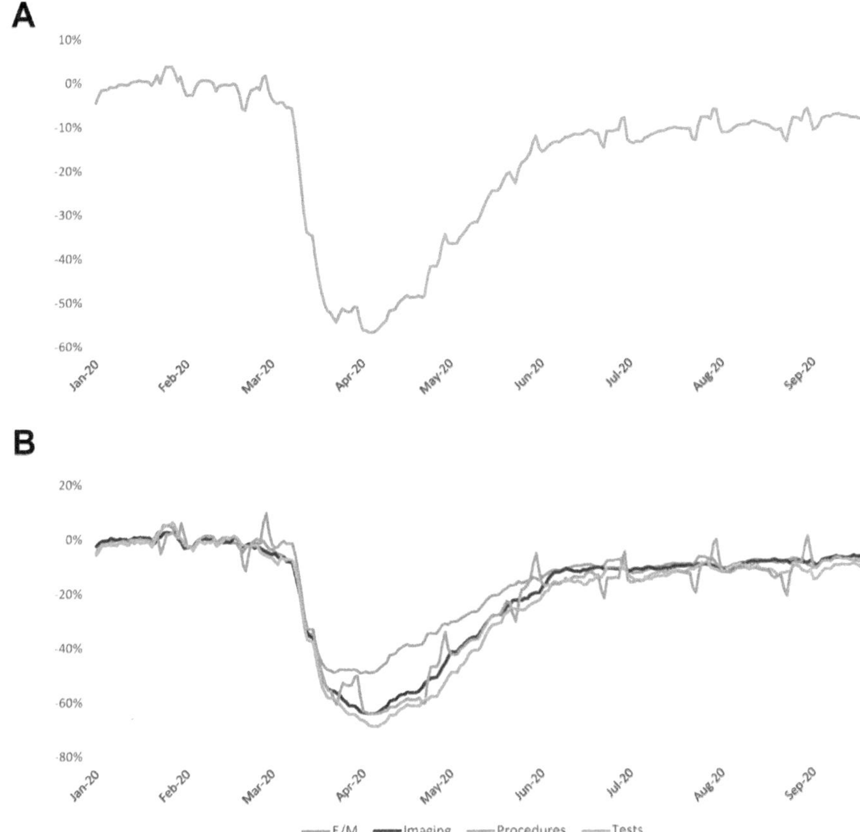

Fig. 2. *A*) Overall Medicare physician fee schedule spending January to September 2020 as compared with expected spending. (*B*) Medicare physician fee schedule spending by place of service as compared with expected spending. Evaluation/Management (E/M). (*From* Economic and Health Policy Research, American Medical Association with permission.)

spending was down by 9% ($447 million, down from $494 million). The decrease in payments to mental health clinicians was less than for some of the other medical specialties, in part because of the ability to provide care via telehealth.

Type of Psychiatric Service

Financial impact by type of psychiatric service varied depending on the payment methodology in place, but a review of the publicly available data reflects that payments for services overall were less in 2020.

Preliminary data from CMS about Medicaid, the largest payer for mental health and substance use disorder services, and the Children's Health Insurance Program shows a significant decrease in services provided to the Medicaid population over the course of the public health emergency (PHE) for all sites of service. As reflected in the tables, services for children under 19 years of age decreased by 34% between March 2020 and October 2020 when compared with the same period in 2019; mental health services for adults decreased by 22% during the same timeframe; and services for patients with substance use disorders declined by 13% when compared with services provided in 2019. As reflected in **Fig. 3**, services continue to remain below levels in 2018 and 2019.[9]

Outpatient and office-based services

Disruptions in care occurred in the outpatient office setting during the initial months of the PHE as clinicians shifted from seeing patients in person to providing care virtually. A survey of members of the American Psychiatric Association found that 64% of respondents were not using telehealth as a mode of care at all before the implementation of the PHE; 2 months into the PHE, this number shifted dramatically to 85% of respondents seeing more than three-fourths or all of their patients via telehealth.

Some behavioral health clinicians and organizations have reported an increase in revenue for these services owing to a decrease in the rate of patients not keeping appointments for virtual care compared with in-person care. There is continued uncertainty and concern that commercial payers will decrease rates for virtual care at some point in the future or discontinue coverage for audio-only services.

Inpatient and residential care

Inpatient and residential treatment programs continue to operate at substantial losses unless they are paid through alternative interim payment methodologies such as temporary rate increases (see case example in **Box 2**). Social distancing and masking have required them to operate at reduced census while maintaining the pre-COVID level of staffing requirements, maintenance of clinical services such as group therapy (reduction in group size but not frequency) as well as one-to-one observation standards. Many have reported having to intermittently further limit capacity owing to shortages of personal protective equipment. Unexpected expenditures for personal protective equipment, testing kits, and technology used to implement telemedicine have likely had an impact on the traditionally thin margins under which psychiatric inpatient units operate.[10]

Partial hospitalization programs and intensive outpatient programs

Initially partial hospitalization and intensive outpatient programs were decreased or closed as facilities, including community mental health centers, adapted care during the COVID-19 PHE. The closure of services resulted in a loss of revenue that was primarily dependent on the transition time needed to implement telepsychiatry. The CMS eventually extended emergency waivers, retroactive to March 1, 2020, allowing community mental health centers and other facilities to provide certain partial hospitalization services in temporary expansion locations (ie, patient's homes) through the use of telehealth.[11] CMS also waived the requirement that a community mental health center provide at least 40% of its services to patients who are not eligible for Medicare benefits, enabling the provision of services to proceed without regard to payer.[12] Private payers followed suit and began to provide coverage to patients from their homes via telehealth. A recent study indicated that patient satisfaction was as high with telehealth partial hospital treatment as with in-person treatment in a general adult program.[13] However, some specialized PHPs or IOPs faced specific monitoring challenges like obtaining weights or blood pressures in patients enrolled in eating disorders programming. As the PHE has continued, some programs have shifted to a hybrid model of care that includes group sessions that includes patients joining the sessions either virtually or in person (see **Box 2**).

Long-term care

A 2020 World Health Organization survey described disruptions in mental health services for children and adolescents, older adults and peripartum women in 130

A

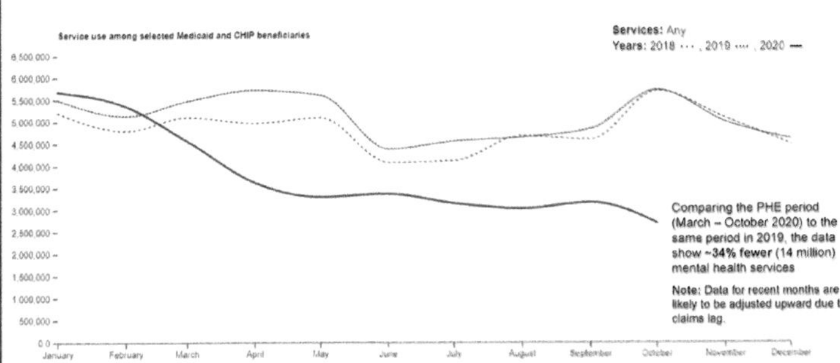
Service use among selected Medicaid and CHIP beneficiaries
Services: Any
Years: 2018 ···, 2019 ····, 2020 —
Comparing the PHE period (March – October 2020) to the same period in 2019, the data show ~34% fewer (14 million) mental health services
Note: Data for recent months are likely to be adjusted upward due to claims lag.
January
February
March
April
May
June
July
August
September
October
November
December

B

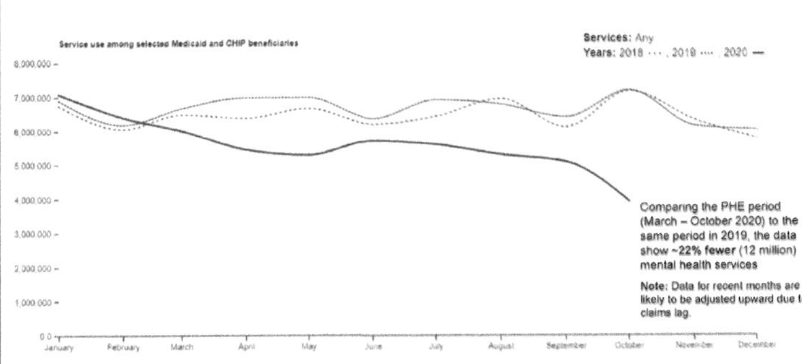
Service use among selected Medicaid and CHIP beneficiaries
Services: Any
Years: 2018 ···, 2019 ····, 2020 —
8,000,000
7,000,000
6,000,000
5,000,000
4,000,000
3,000,000
2,000,000
1,000,000
0.0
Comparing the PHE period (March – October 2020) to the same period in 2019, the data show ~22% fewer (12 million) mental health services
Note: Data for recent months are likely to be adjusted upward due to claims lag.
January
February
March
April
May
June
July
August
September
October
November
December

C

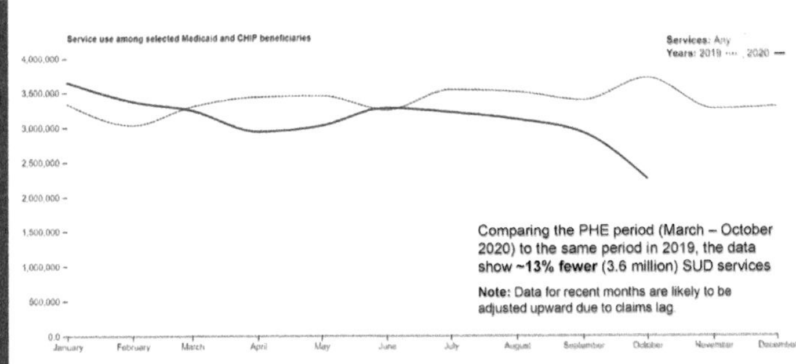
Service use among selected Medicaid and CHIP beneficiaries
Services: Any
Years: 2019 ····, 2020 —
4,000,000
3,500,000
3,000,000
2,500,000
2,000,000
1,500,000
1,000,000
500,000
0.0
Comparing the PHE period (March – October 2020) to the same period in 2019, the data show ~13% fewer (3.6 million) SUD services
Note: Data for recent months are likely to be adjusted upward due to claims lag.
January
February
March
April
May
June
July
August
September
October
November
December

countries. More than 60% of respondents reported disruptions in counseling and psychotherapy, harm reduction services and opioid agonist therapy. More than one-third of countries reported disruptions in emergency services for mental health crises. Closer to home, disruptions in mental health services were reported in all levels of behavioral health care, as outlined elsewhere in this article.[16]

Older individuals with behavioral health conditions confront the risk of COVID-19 on 3 key fronts. First, estimates of mental health condition prevalence in older adults is more than 20%, and near 50% in long-term care settings.[17,18] Second, individuals with behavioral health conditions experience a higher prevalence of high risk chronic conditions associated with high COVID-19 morbidity and mortality.[19,20] Third, individuals with behavioral health conditions often reside in settings with elevated risk of COVID-19 exposure, such as shared or congregant housing settings, including

Fig. 3. *A*) Mental health services for children under age 19 during COVID-19. Preliminary 202 data show that mental health services for children under age 19 decreased starting in March and continue to be substantially below prior years' levels through October. Mental health services among children under 19 years decreased from 145 per 1000 in February to a low of 72 per 1000 beneficiaries in October 2020. *Note*: These data are preliminary Data are sourced from the T-MSIS Analytic Files v4 in AREMAC, using final action claims. They are based on December T-MSIS submissions with services through the end of November. Recent dates of service have very little time for claims runout and we expect large changes in the results after each monthly update. Because data for November are incomplete, results are only presented through October 31, 2020. (*B*) Mental health services for adults during COVID-19. Preliminary 2020 data show mental health services for adults ages 19 to 64 decreased through May and have not rebounded to prior years' levels through October. Mental health services among adults ages 19 to 64 decreased from 176 per 1000 beneficiaries in February 2020 to a low of 100 per 1000 beneficiaries in October 2020. *Notes*: These data are preliminary. Data are sourced from the T-MSIS Analytic Files v4 in AREMAC, using final action claims. They are based on December T-MSIS submissions with services through the end of November. Recent dates of service have very little time for claims runout and we expect large changes in the results after each monthly update. Because data for November are incomplete, results are only presented through October 31, 2020. (*C*) Substance use disorder services for adults during COVID-19. Preliminary 2020 data show SUD services for adults age 19 to 64 decreased starting in March, increased in June, and are still below 2019 levels through October. *Notes*: These data are preliminary. Data are sourced from the T-MSIS Analytic Files v4 in AREMAC, using final action claims. They are based on December T-MSIS submissions with services through the end of November. Recent dates of service have very little time for claims runout and we expect large changes in the results after each monthly update. Because data for November are incomplete, results are only presented through October 31, 2020. We compare SUD service use in 2020 with 2019 only. Coverage of SUD treatment services has increased dramatically over the past 3 years with the implementation of several 1115 demonstrations. As a result, we do not compare treatment rates in 2020 to treatment rates in 2018 and 2017, when coverage of services was generally lower. Additionally, as of January 1, 2020, Medicare Part B pays Opioid Treatment Programs through bundled payments for opioid use disorder. This change in coverage may impact results for dually eligible beneficiaries. SUD services for adults ages 19 to 64 decreased from about 92 per 1000 beneficiaries in February 2020 to a low of 57 per 1000 beneficiaries in October 2020. (*Data from* CMS, Medicaid & CHIP and the COVID-19 to 19 Public Health Emergency: Preliminary Medicaid & CHIP Data Snapshot, Services through October 31, 2020. 2021. Available at: DOI: https://www.medicaid.gov/state-resource-center/downloads/COVID-19-19-medicaid-data-snapshot.pdf. Published May 14, 2021. Accessed May 15, 2021.)

Box 2
Case example: University of North Carolina Hospitals emergency department and inpatient

At the most basic level, the physician coding is a factor of the volume multiplied by relative value units, so to maximize billing physicians would desire maximum volume at the highest relative value units (highly acute patients moving quickly through the emergency department/inpatient areas). In March of 2020, at the beginning of the COVID-19 epidemic in the United States, most emergency rooms across the United States initially saw a marked decrease in the total number of emergency department visits. The decrease in volume has been theorized to be a reaction to the stay-at-home order and the public's attempt to delay care to minimize exposure to coronavirus infection. A recent study highlighted the overall decrease in total number of emergency room encounters in 2020 as compared with 2019. However, that same study indicated the total number of visits for mental health conditions, suicide attempts, and drug and opioid overdose all increased in the study time period (weeks 1–41 of 2020) as compared with the same time period in 2019.[14] The University of North Carolina saw an initial decrease in overall psychiatric visits in March 2020 (40% decrease) and April 2020 (49% decrease) before returning to expected prepandemic levels by late summer (September 2020).

At the University of North Carolina Hospitals, the coronavirus exacerbated inpatient psychiatry services by several factors that contributed to reduced inpatient capacity during the pandemic. First, following infection prevention guidance, the total number of inpatient psychiatric beds at the Chapel Hill campus was decreased by necessity to convert semiprivate rooms to private rooms to allow for appropriate physical distancing between beds. Second, several nurses either retired or resigned early in the year as the stress of the pandemic hit. This factor impacted the ability to fully staff inpatient units and operate at full volume. Finally, the need to have a designated inpatient psychiatric COVID-positive unit decreased inpatient capacity. The University of North Carolina hospital converted a subsection of a unit to a 3-bed COVID-positive unit for patients in need of inpatient psychiatric care, but medically asymptomatic or mildly symptomatic. Patients who tested positive in the emergency room or converted to positive on the inpatient psychiatric units would be transferred to these beds. Although this action was necessary to meet the needs of the greater system, it frequently was empty and never reached full capacity, leaving unfilled beds. The impact of these changes was increasing the length of stay for psychiatric patients boarding in the emergency room.

During the height of the COVID-19 pandemic, the number of main campus inpatient beds decreased from 76 (before COVID) to 52 (during COVID). At the same time, some of the traditional dispositions for discharging patients (housing shelters, group homes, state psychiatric hospitals, and long-term care facilities) greatly tightened admission criteria or delayed referrals altogether. A recent article described a range of discharge delays between 7 and 47 days owing to reluctance of congregate care facilities to accept COVID-19 patients back into the community.[15] The 2 inpatient units most impacted by these restrictions were the geropsychiatry unit and the psychotic disorders unit. The crisis stabilization unit, child and adolescent units, and eating disorder units all experienced relatively minor increases in their average length of stays (ALOS) and total number of discharges but were less disrupted than the geropsychiatry and psychotic disorders units.

- In the pre-COVID year (March 2019 to February 2020), the ALOS on the psychotic disorder unit (**Fig. 4**) was 15.2 days and the total number of discharges was 400.
- During COVID (March 2020 to February 2021), the ALOS was 20.8 days and the total number of discharges 238 for that psychotic disorder unit (see **Fig. 4**; **Figs. 5** and **6**).
- In the pre-COVID year (March 2019 to February 2020), the ALOS was 17.7 days and the total number of discharges was 163 on the geropsychiatry unit.
- During COVID (March 2020 to February 2021), the ALOS was 30.6 days and the total number of discharges 78 for that geropsychiatry unit (see **Figs. 4** and **5**).
- The overall financial impact on the psychotic disorders unit was a 14% decrease in physician charges from March 1, 2020, to February 28, 2021, as compared with March 1, 2019, to February 28, 2019.

- The overall financial impact on the geropsychiatry unit was a 37% decrease in physician charges from March 1, 2020, to February 28, 2021, as compared with March 1, 2019, to February 28, 2019.
- Inpatient units were operating at a decreased volume and patient discharges were delayed, decreasing relative value units (volume and level), which decreased overall physician charges.

What cannot be adequately depicted in charts and graphs is the emotional toll and burnout that decimated staff in the emergency departments and inpatient psychiatric units. The time and mental energy that was spent in contingency planning was unfathomable: (a) infection prevention (screening, rescreening, personal protective equipment distribution, and disinfection), (b) restrictions of visitors and minimization of overcrowding, (c) staff workforce planning and redeployment, (d) operational adjustments (telepsychiatry protocols, revising admission criteria, and designing a COVID-positive unit), and (e) group therapy changes (limiting number of participants, practicing physical distancing). Although the height of the pandemic looks to have past most for emergency and inpatient facilities, the emotional impact remains ever present.

long-term care facilities such as assisted living facilities and skilled nursing facilities that house frail and elderly adults in need of 24/7 supervision and progressive levels of skilled needs.[21,22] Finally, the November 20, 2020, Morbidity Mortality Weekly Report noted:

> *As of October 15, 2020, an average of one death occurred among every five Assisted Living Facility residents with COVID-19, compared with one death among every 40 persons in the general population with COVID-19 in states with available data.*[23]

Furthermore, long-standing racial and ethnic disparities in the quality of care in long-term care, compound overall quality of care issues seen in the behavioral health population.[24]

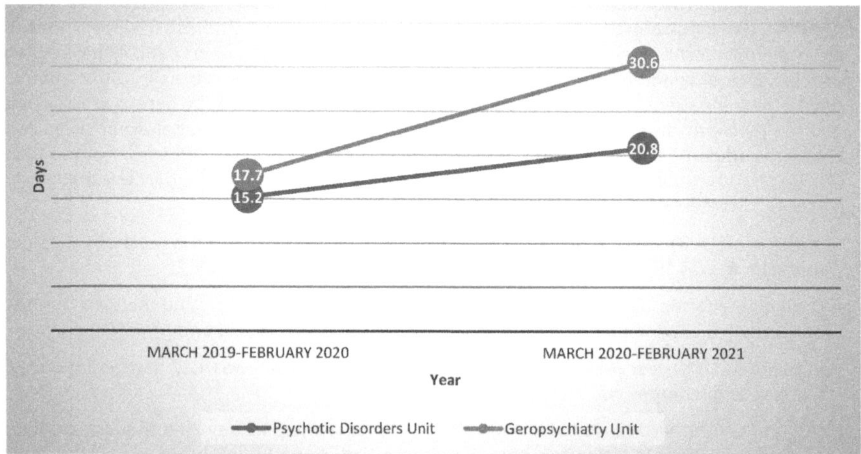

Fig. 4. Comparison of average lengths of stay before COVID-19 and during COVID-19. (*Data from* Millard H, Wilson C, Fortunati F, Li L. COVID-19 to 19 psychiatric patients: Impact of variability in testing on length of hospital stay and disposition back to congregate care settings. Psychiatry Res. 2020 Oct;292:113324. https://doi.org/10.1016/j.psychres.2020.113324. Epub 2020 Jul 24. PMID: 32736265; PMCID: PMC7380225)

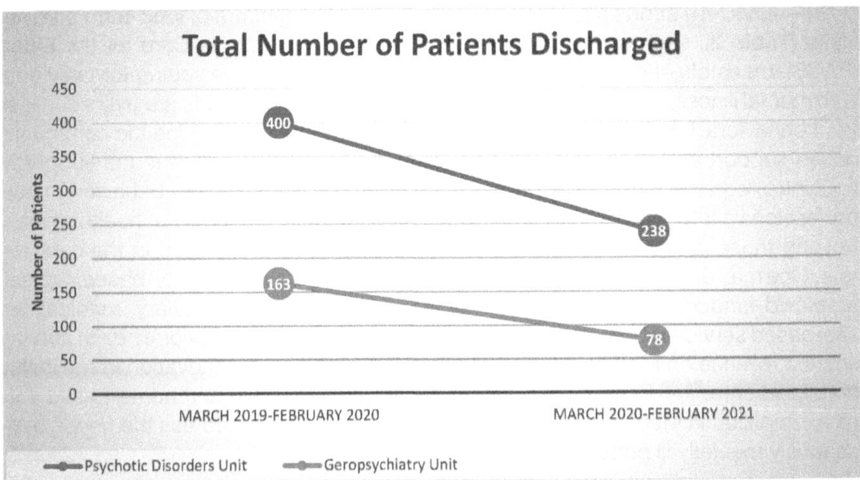

Fig. 5. Comparison of patient discharges before COVID-19 and during COVID-19. (*Data from* Millard H, Wilson C, Fortunati F, Li L. COVID-19 to 19 psychiatric patients: Impact of variability in testing on length of hospital stay and disposition back to congregate care settings. Psychiatry Res. 2020 Oct;292:113324. https://doi.org/10.1016/j.psychres.2020.113324. Epub 2020 Jul 24. PMID: 32736265; PMCID: PMC7380225.)

The COVID-19 pandemic turned up the volume on growing efforts to reinvent financing of long-term care, such as assisted living and skilled nursing facilities,[25] especially given the higher COVID-19 morbidity and mortality rate in long-term care facilities. Long-term care financial reform continues to challenge policymakers and families, as evidenced by the 2019 launch of the CMS value-based program for long-term care, focused on the skilled nursing level of care, the Skilled Nursing Value-Based Purchasing Program. The program rewards skilled nursing facilities for meeting quality of care goals, such as hospital readmissions.[26,27] Even modest long-term care finance reform proposals overlook the needs of long-term care residents with behavioral health conditions.

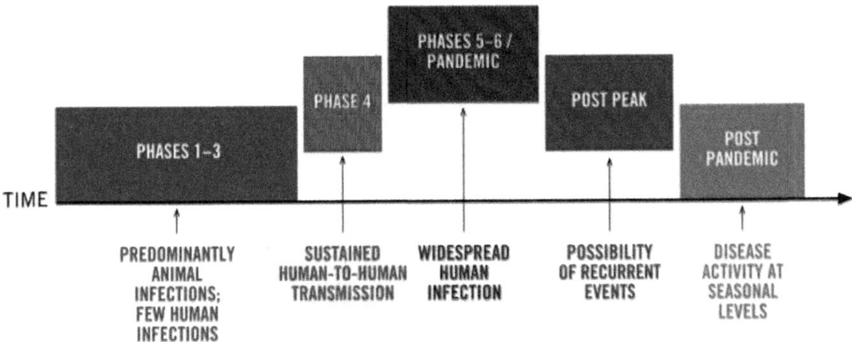

Fig. 6. Pandemic phases of preparedness. (*From* Pandemic Influenza Preparedness and Response: A WHO Guidance Document. Geneva: World Health Organization; 2009. 4, THE WHO PANDEMIC PHASES. Available from: https://www.ncbi.nlm.nih.gov/books/NBK143061/.)

Pre–COVID-19 efforts to achieve a more nuanced continuum of long-term care services (**Table 2**), such as the capitated Program for All-Inclusive Care for the Elderly (PACE), resemble efforts to promote care in the least restrictive setting for individuals with mental illness. Policymakers, facility owners, consumers, and caregivers can learn from behavioral health experiments in creating less restrictive therapeutic community-based support and services, such as assertive community treatment and supportive housing programs. The PACE program, for example, incorporates behavioral health professionals into the core staffing model, although direct behavioral health services beyond those provided by primary care providers, are not included in the capitated rate. One may even liken PACE to a collection of piecemeal community-based, typically Medicaid-funded, behavioral health services that incorporate ancillary, medical, and site-based services. Long-term care and community-based behavioral health services share a reliance on Medicaid for primary funding and, hence, innovation in noninstitutionalized care.[28,29] Perhaps a middle ground between PACE and home-based care, as exemplified in Medicaid innovations, is a starting point to address the needs of the seriously mentally ill population in long-term care facilities.

Preparing for the Next Pandemic

Although the COVID-19 pandemic is unprecedented in scale and virus transmissibility, a pandemic viral respiratory illness was not unexpected and remains an ongoing threat. The COVID-19 pandemic resulted in, as of June 24, 2021, 603,181 excess deaths in the United States and 3,902,187 in the world,[30] in addition to an increase in job loss, school disruption, social isolation, and child abuse. The unprecedented and rapid global research and dissemination of COVID-19 pathophysiology, epidemiology, clinical course, public health prevention, and immunotherapy represents a triumph; yet we learned that effective state, national and international leadership, communication and coordination are critical to improve the global response to the next pandemic.[31]

How can behavioral health leaders financially prepare their organizations and patients for the next pandemic? We categorize pandemic preparedness within 2 World Health Organization phases of a pandemic: phases 5 and 6 and after the peak.

Initial pandemic response

Pandemic declaration occurs when an epidemic affects multiple countries or continents and indicates geographic spread as opposed to disease severity. As we described, the pace of financial policy change was a key influence on the ability to maintain behavioral health services across the care continuum after the pandemic

Table 2
Care continuum

	Home-based Care	Community-based Care	Facility-based Care
LTC example	Home health, caregiver support	PACE program[a], senior centers, Kapuna Caregivers Program[a]	Skilled nursing facility
BH example	Assertive community treatment[a]	Psychosocial rehabilitation	Residential

[a] Value-based program.

Adapted from: National Conference of State Legislatures: Long-Term Services and Supports: FAQs: 2013. http://www.ncsl.org/research/health/long-term-services-and-supports-faqs.aspx.

declaration. In future pandemics, policymakers and payers can build from COVID-19 lessons learned to more quickly allow providers to transition to virtual care and ensure safe conditions for patients and providers in office-based or facility-centered care. Proactive strategies to obtain personal protective equipment access and implement social distancing strategies are critical to allow behavioral health providers time to safely transition, as indicated, to virtual care methods. Facility-based partners should be included in surge and initial pandemic planning to ensure the employment conditions of behavioral health workers and needs of behavioral health patients are well-represented.

Finally, the reliable and accurate communication of pandemic conditions, evolving disease burden, and health sector service use are critical to ensuring health security for patients and providers. Anticipatory guidance to obtain and interpret accurate, timely and relevant information to guide financial and operational policy for behavioral health services coverage, payment, and provision is as critical in the acute pandemic response phase and pathophysiology and treatment. For example, the Centers for Disease Control and Prevention outlines an entire health communication strategy at their website https://npin.cdc.gov/pages/health-communication-strategies.

CLINICS CARE POINTS

- Financing models shoud be evaluated for their resilience and abilty to maintain services during a crisis.
- Developing alternative payment models that are more flexible are necessary to address the need for a rapid response to a finanacial health care crisis.
- Develping and sustaining partnerships between governmnent agencies and behavioral health clinicians is essential for a rapid response to any crisis.

ACKNOWLEDGMENTS/CONTRIBUTING AUTHORS

Jacob Kannarkat, MD, Psychiatry Resident, Jackson Health System; Kenan Penaskovic, MD, Associate Professor and Associate Vice-Chair for Clinical Affairs, Psychiatry Physician Service Line Leader, Adult Psychiatry, University of North Carolina; and Robin Reed, MD, MPH, Medical Director, United Health Group and Associate Professor, University of Arkansas for Medical Sciences.

DISCLOSURE

The authors have nothing to disclose.

REFERENCES

1. Moreland A, Herlihy C, Tynan MA, et al. Timing of state and territorial COVID-19 stay-at-home orders and changes in population movement — United States, March 1–May 31, 2020. MMWR Morb Mortal Wkly Rep 2020;69:1198–203.
2. Adams K. A timeline of telehealth support from the federal government during the pandemic. Becker's Hospital Review. 2020. Available at: https://www.beckershospitalreview.com/telehealth/a-timeline-of-telehealth-support-from-the-federal-government-during-the-pandemic.html. Accessed January 20, 2021.
3. National Council Behavioral Health and analytics. Covid 19 economic impacts on behavioral health organizations. 2020. Available at: https://www.

thenationalcouncil.org/wp-content/uploads/2020/04/NCBH_COVID19_Survey_Findings_04152020.pdf?daf=375ateTbd56. Accessed January 10, 2021.
4. National Council Behavioral Health and and analytics. The financial viability of the nation's mental health and addiction treatment organizations is in jeopardy. 2020. Available at: https://www.thenationalcouncil.org/wp-content/uploads/2020/06/200616_NCBH_OnePager.pdf?daf=375ateTbd56. Accessed January 10, 2021.
5. National Council Behavioral Health and Member Consult. Member survey. 2020. Available at: https://www.thenationalcouncil.org/wp-content/uploads/2020/09/NCBH_Member_Survey_Sept_2020_CTD2.pdf?daf=375ateTbd56. Accessed January 10, 2021.
6. Hawkins M. Physicians and COVID-19, a survey examining how physicians are being affected by and are responding to the coronavirus pandemic. 2020. Available at: https://www.hasc.org/sites/main/files/file-attachments/mhacoronasurveyreport.pdf?1589491793. Accessed February 2021.
7. Doximity study finds physician compensation slowed in 2020. 2020. Available at: https://press.doximity.com/articles/doximity-study-finds-physician-compensation-slowed-in-2020. Accessed March 23, 2021.
8. Medscape psychiatrist compensation report 2021. Medscape. Available at: https://www.medscape.com/slideshow/2021-compensation-psychiatrist-6013867. Accessed June 6, 2021.
9. CMS. Medicaid & CHIP and the COVID-19-19 public health emergency: preliminary Medicaid & CHIP data snapshot, services through October 31, 2020. 2021. Available at: https://www.medicaid.gov/state-resource-center/downloads/COVID-19-19-medicaid-data-snapshot.pdf. Accessed May 15, 2021.
10. The high cost of compliance: assessing the regulatory burden on inpatient psychiatric facilities. National Association for Behavioral Healthcare; 2019. Available at: https://www.nabh.org/the-high-cost-of-compliance/. Accessed January 2021.
11. CMS. Medicare and Medicaid Programs, basic health program, and exchanges; additional policy and regulatory revisions in response to the COVID–19 public health emergency and delay of certain reporting requirements for the skilled nursing facility quality reporting program. 45 CFR Part 156. CMS; 2020. 27550-27629. CMS–5531–IFC. Available at: https://www.govinfo.gov/content/pkg/FR-2020-05-08/pdf/2020-09608.pdf. Accessed July 2021.
12. CMS. COVID-19 emergency declaration blanket waivers for health care providers. 2021. Available at: https://www.cms.gov/files/document/summary-covid-19-emergency-declaration-waivers.pdf. Accessed July 2021.
13. Zimmerman M, Benjamin I, Tirpak JW, et al. Patient satisfaction with partial hospital telehealth treatment during the COVID-19 pandemic: comparison to in-person treatment. Psychiatry Res 2021;301:113966.
14. Holland KM, Jones C, Vivolo-Kantor AM, et al. Trends in US emergency department visits for mental health, overdose, and violence outcomes before and during the COVID-19-19 pandemic. JAMA Psychiatry 2021;78(4):372–9.
15. Millard H, Wilson C, Fortunati F, et al. COVID-19-19 psychiatric patients: impact of variability in testing on length of hospital stay and disposition back to congregate care settings. Psychiatry Res 2020;292:113324.
16. World Health Organization. The impact of COVID-19 on mental, neurological and substance use services: results of a rapid assessment 2020. Available at: https://www.who.int/publications/i/item/978924012455. Accessed February 2021.
17. Hybels CF, Blazer DG. Epidemiology of late-life mental disorders. Clin Geriatr Med 2003;19(4):663–696, v.

18. National Coalition on Mental Health and Aging. Integrating older adult behavioral health into long-Term care rebalancing. 2017. Available at: http://www.ncmha.org/wp-content/uploads/2019/04/2017-NCMHA-Report-on-Integrating-Older-Adult-Behavioral-Health-into-Long-Term-Care-Rebalancing.pdf. Accessed February 2021.
19. Reeves WC, Strine TW, Pratt LA, et al. CDC report: mental illness surveillance among adults in the United States. MMWR Morb Mortal Wkly Rep 2011; 60(03):1–32.
20. Centers for Disease Control and Prevention. People with certain health conditions. 2021. Available at: https://www.cdc.gov/coronavirus/2019-ncov/need-extra-precautions/people-with-medical-conditions.html. Accessed February 2020.
21. Mechanic D, McAlpi D. Use of nursing homes in the care of persons with severe mental illness: 1985 to 1995. J Am Psychiatr Assoc 2000;51:354–8.
22. Center for Medicare and Medicaid Services. CMS OSCAR data current surveys: medical condition-mental status. 2013. Available at: http://www.ahcancal.org/research_data/oscar_data/NursingFacilityPatientCharacteristics/LTC%20STATS_HSNF_PATIENT _2013Q2_FINAL.pdf. Accessed February 2020.
23. Yi SH, See I, Kent AG, et al. Characterization of COVID-19 in assisted living facilities — 39 states, 2020. MMWR Morb Mortal Wkly Rep 2020;69:1730–5.
24. Shippee TP, Akosionu O, Ng W, et al. COVID-19 pandemic: exacerbating racial/ethnic disparities in long-term services and supports. J Aging Soc Policy 2020; 32(4–5):323–33.
25. Inzitari M, Risco E, Cesari M, et al. Nursing homes and long term care after COVID-19: a new ERA? J Nutr Health Aging 2020;24:1042–6.
26. Daras LC, Vadnais A, Pogue YZ, et al. Nearly one in five skilled nursing facilities awarded positive incentives under value-based purchasing. Health Aff (Millwood) 2021;40(1):146–55.
27. Weiner J, Coe NB, Hoffman AK, et al. Policy options for financing long-term care in the United States. University of Pennsylvania Leonard Davis Institute of Health Economics. Vol 23 No 3. 2020. Available at: https://ldi.upenn.edu/sites/default/files/pdf/LDI%20Issue%20Brief%202020%20Vol.%2023%20No.%203_6_0.pdf. Accessed February 2021.
28. Program for all-inclusive care for the elderly. CMS. Available at;. https://www.cms.gov/Medicare-Medicaid-Coordination/Medicare-and-Medicaid-Coordination/Medicare-Medicaid-Coordination-Office/PACE/PACE. Accessed February 2021.
29. Werner RM, Hoffman AK, Coe NB. Long-term care policy after Covid-19 — solving the nursing home crisis. N Engl J Med 2020;383:903–5.
30. COVID-19 Dashboard. Johns Hopkins University and Medicine; 2021. Available at: https://coronavirus.jhu.edu/map.html. Accessed June 24, 2021.
31. Preparing for the next pandemic. Nat Med 2021;27:357.

Mental Health Clinical Research Innovations during the COVID-19 Pandemic

The Future Is Now

Kelly B. Ahern, BS, Eric J. Lenze, MD*

KEYWORDS

• COVID-19 • Fluvoxamine • Remote • Trials • Decentralized

KEY POINTS

- The COVID-19 pandemic presented unprecedented challenges to clinical research.
- Telemedicine was frequently used to continue clinical care while prioritizing patient and provider safety.
- Using telemedicine technology, remote or decentralized clinical trials have risen to prominence during this era of "physical distancing."
- The feasibility of fully remote trials testing psychiatric medications was demonstrated by studies of the selective serotonin reuptake inhibitor fluvoxamine in COVID-19.
- Telemedicine and remote clinical trials are the future of psychiatric clinical research.

INTRODUCTION

The beginning of the COVID-19 pandemic brought most clinical research to a sudden halt. Enrollment in clinical trials per site plummeted by approximately 80% between April 2019 and April 2020.[1] When COVID-19 reached our institution, the Washington University School of Medicine, a multitude of restrictions were placed on clinical research. Research staff began working remotely, nonessential visits were canceled or postponed indefinitely, and most clinical trials became impossible to conduct without significantly modifying the study protocols. It soon became clear that the 2-week quarantine period would extend longer, with great uncertainty to this duration. Clinical researchers were faced with a daunting choice: cease research activity altogether or find new, innovative ways to move forward in these unprecedented times. In early 2021, more than 1 year since the pandemic first began, more than a thousand

Department of Psychiatry, Washington University School of Medicine, St Louis, MO, USA
* Corresponding author. Campus Box 8134, 660 S. Euclid, St Louis, MO 63110.
E-mail address: lenzee@wustl.edu

Psychiatr Clin N Am 45 (2022) 179–189
https://doi.org/10.1016/j.psc.2021.11.011

trials were listed as suspended on ClinicalTrials.gov, most owing to the COVID-19 pandemic.[2] However, the time from 2020 to 2021 was also a period of incredible adaptation and innovation in psychiatric clinical research. This article summarizes some of the key changes and assesses their future impact.

TELEMEDICINE

One of the innovative tools with the most significant potential for use in clinical research during the pandemic has been around for more than a century. Little-used in psychiatric research before 2020, telemedicine has become prominent, in research and practice, during the COVID-19 pandemic. The umbrella of what could be considered "telemedicine" is broad and encompasses many types of remote communication, ranging from telephone consultations to videoconferencing sessions.

Telemedicine, which is becoming increasingly commonplace in our clinical and research practices, has a fascinating history worth reviewing. Because of the fluidity of the definition of "telemedicine," the exact date of the genesis of telemedicine is unknown.[3] Technological advances in telecommunications in the twentieth century continued to evolve the landscape of telemedicine. Casualty lists and medical supplies orders were communicated via telegraph during the civil war and there are reports of telephone wires being used for medical communication as early as 1906.[3,4] Radio communication opened new avenues for telemedicine after World War II and was followed by the development of television several decades later.[3] The first predecessor to the modern virtual appointment (now over Skype, Zoom, or other major teleconferencing software) occurred in 1964 via interactive video linking the Nebraska Psychiatric Institute to the Norfolk State Hospital. State funding for telemedicine research projects in the 1960s and 1970s allowed for testing the feasibility and clinical efficacy of telemedicine with somewhat positive results.[3]

NASA and the developing space programs further expanded the capabilities of telemedicine. One such example occurred in 1975 with the Space Technology Applied to Rural Papago Advanced Health Care (STARPAHC) project, wherein television radio and remote telemetry were used to connect an Indian Health Service hospital to a mobile health unit in the Indian reservation.[5] Although the use of technology was more time consuming than in-person visits, the providers who participated felt that the STARPAHC program was successful in extending health care to the somewhat isolated population on the reservation. The development of modern internet in the 1990s, followed by subsequent widespread availability in the 2000s allowed for more widespread use of telemedicine.[5]

There are some advantages to telemedicine over the traditional model of face-to-face medical care. It allows physicians to treat patients in underserved areas who otherwise cannot attend in-person appointments owing to physical or logistical constraints. Additionally, virtual or telephone appointments can be more convenient for both parties and more cost effective in certain situations than traditional in-person appointments.[6,7] Although several arguments against telehealth cite a lack of interpersonal contact and a possible decreased quality of care, there is evidence to suggest that the accessibility that telehealth affords can lead to high levels of patient satisfaction.[6,7]

During the COVID-19 pandemic, telemedicine was used to provide health care in outpatient settings—especially in mental health—while decreasing risk of COVID-19 exposure and subsequent illness. The COVID-19 pandemic also saw the rapid and successful implementation of remote monitoring programs specifically for patients with COVID-19.[8,9]

TELEMEDICINE AND RESEARCH

Telemedicine has great potential in the world of fully remote or decentralized clinical trials, which are trials that do not require participant visits to clinical sites.[10] These trials rely on telephone communication, emails, texting, smartphone applications, video-conferencing, and many other technologies to deliver interventions and collect data. Although several significant challenges can affect these trials, the benefits they may deliver to current and future clinical trials merit their consideration.

In the prepandemic world, clinical research faced several significant hurdles to participant recruitment and engagement. In particular, rural populations have been historically difficult to engage in clinical trials. One potential driver of this phenomenon is the higher costs and travel time required to attend appointments at academic medical centers, which are often located in urban areas. A systematic review by Ross and colleagues[11] (1999) found that inconvenient travel and its associated expenses were a driver of trial refusal and participant attrition across many trials. Because of distance and a lack of exposure, rural populations may also be limited in their awareness and knowledge of clinical trials, which poses further obstacles to obtaining geographically diverse samples.[12,13] Telemedicine offers a workable solution to these problems, allowing investigators in a central location to easily reach and communicate regularly with participants, regardless of their geographic location.[14,15] Supporting this notion, a study by Sommer and colleagues[16] (2018) found that participants undergoing the decentralized model of their study had greater geographic diversity when compared with those who underwent the conventional (or in-clinic) arm. Additionally, the implementation of a decentralized study model also may increase convenience to those enrolled in the study by decreasing travel time.[15]

Coming to clinical trial visits poses burdens related to travel and potentially time off work, which may disproportionately affect individuals in minority groups that are historically underrepresented in clinical trials. One strategy to overcome this lack of diversity is to decrease participant burden, which decentralized trials can help accomplish.[17] In particular, the US Food and Drug Administration encourages the use of online recruitment strategies and electronic informed consent documents when needed to include underrepresented populations in research trials.[18]

Another important benefit of remote or decentralized clinical trials is the rate at which recruitment can occur.[16] As mentioned elsewhere in this article, studies do not require visits to a central site, so there are fewer geographic limitations on recruitment. With the help of online advertising, these studies can also quickly and efficiently reach and enroll many more people than an in-person study would, facilitating larger sample sizes and a greater impact of the study results. A wider study reach and faster recruitment can also be particularly advantageous when the study criteria are more specific or if the trial is recruiting patients with a rare condition.

There are also limitations of decentralized or remote clinical trials. First and foremost, it is important to consider that not all trials are well-suited to a remote or decentralized model. For example, more involved studies that require specialized medical tests and/or large or expensive equipment would be poor candidates for a decentralized model owing to the lack of acceptable remote alternatives. Second, privacy and data quality concerns accompany remote clinical trials.[15] By conducting a clinical trial remotely, the investigator relinquishes a great degree of control over the participant's physical environment and, subsequently, the trial participant's privacy. This lack of control, and its associated privacy concerns, lends itself better to some types of studies than others. For example, a simple online questionnaire can be completed discreetly on a mobile device in most settings. Conversely, neurocognitive or other performance testing is significantly more difficult to conduct remotely and the investigator is unable to tightly control trial participant's immediate environment, which may lead to privacy concerns. Third, assessments requiring a participant to remain undisturbed for a length of time are particularly difficult to coordinate remotely and may require flexibility in the study protocol if the assessment is interrupted. Fourth, if a medication or intervention is riskier, it is more difficult to monitor adverse events and intervene if necessary if a participant is local and the study is in-person; interventions that are high risk (ie, early phase/phase I in human pharmaceuticals or invasive devices) or high intensity (ie, infusions or implants) likely need in-person contact with the investigative team. Overall, it is crucial that investigators critically evaluate the experimental intervention and trial requirements to determine if a remote or decentralized trial is the best option.

Additionally, there are legal limitations on remote clinical trials, although the status of these restrictions may be in flux. One such limitation, prescription privileges, can vary across different states.[15] This legal obstacle can limit a certain investigator's ability to recruit and may necessitate the foundation of additional sites in each of the states from which participants are being recruited. This hurdle can be overcome by involving investigators licensed in different states, including investigators licensed in multiple states, or by partnering with licensed mobile health care provider services.[19] Beginning in March 2020, most US states relaxed their intersite prescribing and telemedicine laws in the wake of the pandemic. It is unclear at this time how many of these states will continue to allow intersite prescribing over the long term. It is also anticipated that the US Department of Health and Human Services may continue to relax intersite telemedicine restrictions, thereby overriding any state-level restrictions. For example, on December 3 it was reported that the US Department of Health and Human Services instituted a new policy allowing telemedicine services across state lines during the COVID-19 emergency. Further, the US federal government's push for more decentralized trials, outlined in the 2021 Senate Appropriation Committee funding bills for US Department of Health and Human Services (including the National Institutes of Health) and the US Food and Drug Administration, included specific language furthering the use of decentralized trials. This wording may accelerate legal changes allowing interstate prescribing.

It is also important to keep the population of interest in mind when deciding to conduct a clinical trial, particularly a fully remote clinical trial. The technological requirements that often accompany decentralized trials may pose a high hurdle and learning curve for participants less familiar with technology. Although at least 50% of every age group (including older adults) possessed a smartphone in 2017, older participants and those who are cognitively impaired may struggle more with a technology-driven study than an in-person one.[10,20] Additionally, high-speed internet, reliable phone service, and other elements of technical infrastructure are luxuries for some people, posing a significant barrier to making clinical trials more universally accessible. Per the 2018 US census, thousands of households in each state were estimated to lack internet access.[21] In 2019, the Federal Communications Commission reported that 21.3 million Americans had no internet connection or internet connections with speeds lower than 25 Mbps/3 Mbps at the end of 2017.[22] Although deployment of broadband internet has improved in rural and tribal lands, as of April 2020, 22.3% of rural Americans and 27.7% of those inhabiting tribal lands still lack internet with speeds of more than 25 Mbps/3 Mbps.[23] These inequities present a quandary to equitable participant recruitment and adequate sample diversity for trials relying on the internet.

Although there is no single solution for including Americans who lack the technological literacy or infrastructure to fully participate in remote or decentralized clinical trials, there are a few strategies that can be used to remediate the problem. Allowing various modalities for study assessments, including online questionnaires, phone questionnaires, and even carrier mail, may help to make study participation possible for those lacking reliable internet or phone lines. Depending on the nature of the study and the limitations of the participants, a hybrid in-person/remote approach may be more appropriate than a fully remote trial.[19]

Furthermore, even the safest interventions can still carry some degree of risk. In these cases, it is necessary to ensure that the trial participants are well-informed on what actions should be taken in the event of a health emergency. Such information can include a list of local approved providers, clear instructions on when to seek help, and how to inform the study team of any changes in medical care or study participation.[19]

Maintaining high levels of participant engagement from informed consent to study termination is critical to study success. Those of us who have read the Apple terms and conditions may already be familiar with a few of the significant difficulties of remote consent processes. For any study—whether remote, in-person, or hybrid—a thorough consent process is ethically desired and can decrease participant attrition in the future. The aforementioned systematic review by Ross and colleagues[11] (1999) found that participants across many studies desired more information about a trial than was provided to them by the trial team and called for a simpler, more readable consent form. For in-person clinical visits, it is much easier to keep the participant engaged. Those who consent participants should probe for questions and gauge participant understanding of the study. Although not necessarily the same as an in-person consent visit, ensuring that a study staff member is available to discuss the consent either by phone or email with the participant before enrollment can help to ensure a thorough consent process.

However, the hurdles to maintaining participant engagement in a remote clinical trial do not end with an interactive consent process. Trial participant attrition is a concern for in-person and fully remote trials alike, and thus it is important to maintain participant interest and engagement in the trial from consent to completion. Although extensive visits and procedures are objectively less convenient than answering a simple phone survey, they also require a high level of commitment to the study and the study mission. The ability to easily interact with study staff can also make a difference when it comes to improving recruitment outcomes and decreasing attrition. Corcoran and colleagues[24] (2015) found that social interaction from staff members helped to improve participant recruitment and retention rates. In contrast, Sommer and colleagues[16] (2018) compared decentralized and conventional/in-person clinical trial questionnaire administration and found that significantly more participants completed the decentralized assessments (89%) compared with the conventional or in-person assessment (60%).

INNOVATIONS IN REMOTE MONITORING

Remote monitoring has been a long-standing focus of our laboratory. Several of our studies have used ecological momentary assessment (EMA) technology, requiring participants to complete quick daily surveys on a mobile device. EMA is a type of assessment that prompts participants to evaluate their status in the moment (eg, “Right now I feel . . . ”), rather than retrospectively. Retrospective outcome measures, especially in mental health, which relies on subjective reporting, suffer from a variety of biases, particularly the peak-end rule. The peak-end rule refers to the human tendency to judge the entirety of a subjective experience by prototypical moments, most notably the moments where the experience was the most extreme and the final moment.[25,26] Using EMA helps to mitigate the peak-end rule by encouraging contemporaneous evaluations rather than asking the individual to retroactively evaluate a period of time. It has been successfully implemented in several of our laboratory's current and former studies (eg, Moore and colleagues,[27] 2016). EMA also aids in examining the variability of symptoms (such as depressed mood) over a defined span of time. For example, Rodebaugh and colleagues[28] (2021) successfully used EMA to track the rapid individualized changes in COVID-19 symptoms that occurred over 15 days after illness onset. Additionally, before the onset of the pandemic, we had begun to explore mHealth research and recently founded an mHealth Research Core at our university to increase uptake in such measurement advances.

ANATOMY OF A FULLY REMOTE CLINICAL TRIAL: THE STOP COVID TRIAL

Before the pandemic, telemedicine was already implemented to a degree in some of our multisite studies, such as the OPTIMUM study.[29] However, perhaps our most unique and timely application of novel strategies to conduct clinical research remotely occurred in our laboratory's STOP COVID trial, which was a placebo-controlled randomized controlled trial testing fluvoxamine for COVID-19. For that reason, it makes an excellent example of clinical research adaptations to the pandemic, including psychiatric researchers repurposing themselves to fight the pandemic itself.

STOP COVID was motivated by basic research showing that the antidepressant fluvoxamine demonstrated effectiveness in preventing sepsis in mouse models, and its need was spurred by the urgent need for an effective acute treatment for outpatients with mild COVID-19.[30,31] Although many early pandemic research studies focused on new drug development, we instead explored repurposing an existing US Food and Drug Administration–approved medication.

Just as the urgent nature of the pandemic required many physicians to step out of their traditional specialties and roles, this trial was different from our other trials.[32] For this trial, we reached beyond our own department and partnered with the division of infectious diseases to approach a largely nonpsychiatric problem with a psychiatric medication.

We recruited exclusively from the St. Louis metropolitan area owing to challenges in recruiting, and getting study supplies to, participants. In the past, we have largely used advertisements, word of mouth, and referrals for study recruitment, but the isolation of the pandemic made it difficult for us to reach eligible patients within our limited window of time without us first initiating the contact. For this particular study, we advertised locally with signs at testing sites, emails to local physicians, and the news media. The bulk of our participants were identified via electronic health records (EHR) from the local hospital system, then screened and recruited by study staff via telephone and email. Additionally, traditional and social media were used as strategies for remote trial recruitment.

Once contact was initiated, participants were rapidly screened through a short prescreen on our database. If the prospective trial participant passed the prescreen, they were then emailed a link to a consent form under their identifying number in our database. We were ultimately successful in recruiting and consenting 152 participants.

Once participants consented, we had to quickly enroll them to get study medication started within the first week of being actively symptomatic. This meant getting participants randomized and on treatment within hours of first contact by the study team. Similar to the remote monitoring program led by Agarwal and colleagues[33] (2021), staff members carried out a no-contact delivery of the study medication (or placebo) and required supplies to the participants' doorsteps. Participants were asked to complete brief online surveys twice daily for the first 15 days, followed by a short set of online surveys at the 30-day mark. These surveys requested the participants use their own supplies or provided study supplies to report their oxygen saturation, blood pressure, temperature, and pulse. They were also asked to report the presence and severity of their current dyspnea.

Our findings suggested that fluvoxamine, taken early in COVID infection, was effective in preventing clinical deterioration. In the placebo group, 6 of the 72 randomized patients (approximately 8%) met our criteria for clinical deterioration during the 15-day study. In contrast, no individuals in the fluvoxamine group (n = 80) deteriorated.

A key outcome of the STOP COVID trial was to demonstrate the feasibility of a fully remote clinical trial. The highly contagious nature of COVID-19 precluded any in-person interaction. We were working with an entirely remote study population with various levels of illness severity, technological literacy, and interest in our study. From a participant standpoint, we wanted the study to be high touch, but not high tech. We aimed to generate a simple, user-friendly interface for the participants to interact with.

We also tried to keep the study as simple and straightforward as possible. Cummings[8] (2021) discussed the difficulties that arise from complicating a participant's experience by adding additional measures to the primary outcome variable. In general, in-person clinical trial visits can easily fall prey to investigators' desires to screen patients extensively against a long list of inclusion and exclusion criteria or acquire as much data as possible. Although certainly burdensome for the participant, this is not always detrimental to in-person clinical trials. The Research on Electronic Monitoring of Overactive Bladder Treatment Experience (REMOTE) trial, the first published fully remote trial of a pharmaceutical drug, demonstrates the pitfalls of a complicated enrollment and participation process. Although their initial aim was to enroll and randomize 283 participants, the study only randomized 18 participants, in part owing to attrition during screening that resulted from a time-consuming multistep process involving online questionnaires, laboratory testing, and additional medical screening.[34]

Also worth consideration is that fluvoxamine is not without side effects. For these reasons, maintaining adherence and compliance were crucial to having a good outcome with the study. The side effects of a selective serotonin reuptake inhibitor tend to be at their worst during the first few days of treatment, so to increase participant comfort, staff members would call the participants for the first 2 days and help them to manage any side effects they may be experiencing. This gesture had the dual purpose of keeping participants engaged, as well as allowing them to feel well-supported in our study, thereby likely decreasing attrition rates. From a participant retention standpoint, we were successful: only 9 participants dropped out before taking their first dose of the medication and 27 failed to complete the 15-day assessment; only 13% of daily surveys were left uncompleted.

With only 1 week from symptom onset to enroll each individual, we needed to be strategic in how we recruited and consented participants. Owing to the urgent nature of starting treatment rapidly in acute COVID-19, we instituted a mandatory 7-day window from onset of symptoms to first dose of study medication. For analyses, we developed a modified intention-to-treat group comprising all those included in the analyses meeting 2 distinct criteria: (1) they met all study inclusion and exclusion criteria and (2) they took the first dose of the study medication within the 7-day window from symptom onset. This modified intention-to-treat group is often seen in infectious disease studies, but is uncommon in mental health.

Our primary outcome variable was respiratory decompensation (operationally defined as an oxygen saturation of <92% and a dyspnea rating of >3), so it was important that we ensure that our randomized and then lost to follow-up participants had not decompensated. The study was designed so that all participants were in the St. Louis area, allowing us to first check our own EHR for emergency visits or hospitalizations. However, this process was not a complete solution because our EHR access was limited only to those who visited our own hospital. For the participants who were lost to follow-up and were not part of our EHR, staff members called them to ensure that they had not visited a hospital, emergency room, or urgent care after they left our study. This addition to the study protocol helped us to obtain the most complete dataset possible.

After the success of our pilot/feasibility trial, we set out to complete a nationwide confirmatory trial (STOP COVID 2). Although we were the sole site for the pilot trial and had the intention of keeping it remote, the larger workload necessitated bringing other institutions onboard as satellite sites. We partnered with the Fred Hutchinson Cancer Research Center, Northwestern University, the University of Utah, McGill University, and University of Toronto to recruit, screen, and monitor our study participants. This trial commenced in December 2020, during a peak in cases in the United States. The Pfizer and Moderna vaccines had just been made available to certain populations, but were limited in availability to the public. However, beginning in 2021, vaccination rates increased rapidly, and the number of eligible patients with COVID-19 eventually plummeted. Although the swift vaccine uptake and steep reduction in COVID-19 cases was a victory against the pandemic that had cost many lives and kept people physically distant for more than a year, it severely limited our ability to recruit individuals into STOP COVID 2. We also noticed a decrease in participant engagement, with noticeably higher levels of enrolled participant attrition in April compared with the earlier months of the year. As a result, we stopped recruitment in May 2021. Results are pending at the time of this writing.

ADDITIONAL COVID-19 CLINICAL TRIAL ADAPTATIONS IN OUR LABORATORY

As a clinical laboratory focused on geriatric mental health, the majority of our other studies work with adults 60 years and older. Although some studies were stopped entirely, others were able to proceed with significant modifications to protect the health and safety of our participants while also maintaining data integrity. For a study relying on neuropsychological testing, a remote neuropsychological test battery that bore similarities to the in-person battery was developed. This test, which could be administered over teleconferencing software, allowed testing to be continued remotely for participants with a webcam and stable internet connection.

Toward the end of the pandemic, we began inviting participants back into our laboratory for physically distant visits. Following university policy, masks were worn at all times by all parties involved, and surfaces were sanitized thoroughly before and after each testing session. The participant was placed in an empty office with a computer while the testing was administered remotely by staff through videoconferencing software. This protocol allowed us to exercise a greater amount of control over our participants' surroundings and equipment during neuropsychological testing without compromising their safety. No known cases of COVID-19 have been linked to these physically distanced, in-person visits.

SUMMARY

Much as the STOP COVID study repurposed medication to treat COVID-19, the pandemic forced us to repurpose existing technology to solve one of our most pressing problems. Telemedicine has demonstrated clear strengths in the past, along with a few significant limitations that need to be overcome, but our STOP COVID studies have demonstrated that fully remote or decentralized clinical trials can be successful.

Looking Toward the Future

As the COVID-19 pandemic wanes, it is imperative that we look to the future and carry the lessons imparted to us by the pandemic forward. The COVID-19 pandemic has necessitated innovation in the area of remote clinical research. As our technology continues to improve, our capabilities and horizons continue to expand.

Sometimes the baseline tools to solve our most pressing problems already exist, and they just require creativity, courage, and good old-fashioned elbow grease to mold them into what we need them to be. Much like fluvoxamine itself in the STOP COVID study, remote and decentralized clinical research is an excellent tool that needed to be repurposed for the pandemic. The limitations that this pandemic has placed on in-person research have taught us the power and utilities of decentralized clinical research. Now, the onus is on us to figure out how we can take this lesson and use it to improve future clinical research.

CLINICS CARE POINTS

- Remote or decentralized clinical trials are an underused resource that can be used to reach out to difficult-to-recruit populations for greater sample diversity.
- Ensure that a decentralized model is the best fit for the topic of interest. Not all trials are well-suited for a decentralized model.
- When applied appropriately, a decentralized clinical trial design is a step forward in clinical trials, improving both efficiency and equitable access by patients.
- To promote equity and inclusion, make sure that study participation is straightforward and that you can provide necessary study materials to prospective participants if needed.
- Decrease attrition by frequently and consistently communicating with participants, ensuring that the study model is broad and not overly complicated, implementing an interactive informed consent procedure.

DISCLOSURE

Dr E.J. Lenze: Grant support (nonfederal): COVID Early Treatment Fund, Mercatus Center Emergent Ventures, the Skoll Foundation, the Taylor Family Institute for Innovative Psychiatric Research, the Center for Brain Research in Mood Disorders, the Patient-Centered Outcomes Research Institute, and the Barnes Jewish Foundation. Consulting fees: Janssen and Jazz Pharmaceuticals. Patent: Has applied for a patent for the use of fluvoxamine in the treatment of COVID-19. Ms K.B. Ahern has nothing to disclose.

REFERENCES

1. Xue JZ, Smietana K, Poda P, et al. Clinical trial recovery from COVID-19 disruption. Nat Rev Drug Discov 2020;19(10):662–3.
2. McDermott MM, Newman AB. Remote research and clinical trial integrity during and after the coronavirus pandemic. JAMA 2021;325(19):1935–6.

3. Zundel KM. Telemedicine: history, applications, and impact on librarianship. Bull Med Libr Assoc 1996;84(1):71–9.
4. Whitten P, Collins B. The diffusion of telemedicine: communicating an innovation. Sci Commun 1997;19(1):21–40.
5. Jagarapu J, Savani RC. A brief history of telemedicine and the evolution of teleneonatology. Semin Perinatol 2021;151416. https://doi.org/10.1016/j.semperi.2021.151416.
6. Wootton R. Telemedicine: a cautious welcome. BMJ 1996;313(7069):1375–7.
7. Wootton R. Recent advances: telemedicine. BMJ 2001;323(7312):557–60.
8. Annis T, Pleasants S, Hultman G, et al. Rapid implementation of a COVID-19 remote patient monitoring program. J Am Med Inform Assoc 2020;27(8):1326–30.
9. Gordon WJ, Henderson D, DeSharone A, et al. Remote Patient Monitoring Program for Hospital Discharged COVID-19 Patients. Appl Clin Inform 2020;11(5):792–801.
10. Cummings SR. Clinical Trials Without Clinical Sites. JAMA Intern Med 2021;181(5):680–4.
11. Ross S, Grant A, Counsell C, et al. Barriers to participation in randomised controlled trials: a systematic review. J Clin Epidemiol 1999;52(12):1143–56.
12. Sabesan S, Burgher B, Buettner P, et al. Attitudes, knowledge and barriers to participation in cancer clinical trials among rural and remote patients. Asia Pac J Clin Oncol 2011;7(1):27–33.
13. Ford JG, Howerton MW, Lai GY, et al. Barriers to recruiting underrepresented populations to cancer clinical trials: a systematic review. Cancer 2008;112(2):228–42.
14. Dorsey ER, Topol EJ. State of Telehealth. N Engl J Med 2016;375(2):154–61.
15. Apostolaros M, Babaian D, Corneli A, et al. Legal, regulatory, and practical issues to consider when adopting decentralized clinical trials: recommendations from the clinical trials transformation initiative. Ther Innov Regul Sci 2020;54(4):779–87.
16. Sommer C, Zuccolin D, Arnera V, et al. Building clinical trials around patients: evaluation and comparison of decentralized and conventional site models in patients with low back pain. Contemp Clin Trials Commun 2018;11:120–6.
17. Ortega RF, Yancy CW, Mehran R, et al. Overcoming lack of diversity in cardiovascular clinical trials: a new challenge and strategies for success. Circulation 2019;140(21):1690–2.
18. U.S. Department of Health and Human Services. Enhancing the diversity of clinical trial populations — eligibility criteria, enrollment practices, and trial designs guidance for industry. Silver Spring, MD: US Food and Drug Administration; 2020.
19. Clinical Trials Transformation Initiative. CTTI Recommendations: decentralized clinical trials 2018. Available at: https://ctti-clinicaltrials.org/wp-content/uploads/2021/06/CTTI_DCT_Recs.pdf. June 27, 2021.
20. Gitlow L. Technology use by older adults and barriers to using technology. Phys Occup Ther Geriatr 2014;32:3.
21. U.S. Census Bureau. American community survey 1-year estimates 2018. Available at: https://data.census.gov/cedsci/table?q=B28002&g=0100000US.04000.001&tid=ACSDT1Y2018.B28002&hidePreview=true. June 27, 2021.
22. Federal Communications Commission. 2019 Broadband deployment report. 2019. Available at: https://docs.fcc.gov/public/attachments/FCC-19-44A1.pdf. June 26, 2021.

23. Federal Communications Commission. 2020 Broadband deployment report. 2020. Available at: https://docs.fcc.gov/public/attachments/FCC-20-50A1.pdf. September 1, 2021.
24. Corcoran MP, Nelson ME, Sacheck JM, et al. Recruitment of mobility limited older adults into a facility-led exercise-nutrition study: the effect of social involvement. Gerontologist 2016;56(4):669–76.
25. Fredrickson BL, Kahneman D. Duration neglect in retrospective evaluations of affective episodes. J Pers Soc Psychol 1993;65(1):45–55.
26. Fredrickson BL. Extracting meaning from past affective experiences: the importance of peaks, ends, and specific emotions. Cogn Emot 2000;14(4):577–606.
27. Moore RC, Depp CA, Wetherell JL, et al. Ecological momentary assessment versus standard assessment instruments for measuring mindfulness, depressed mood, and anxiety among older adults. J Psychiatr Res 2016;75:116–23.
28. Rodebaugh TL, Frumkin MR, Reiersen AM, et al. Acute Symptoms of Mild to Moderate COVID-19 Are Highly Heterogeneous Across Individuals and Over Time. Open Forum Infect Dis 2021;8(3):ofab090.
29. Cristancho P, Lenard E, Lenze EJ, et al. Optimizing outcomes of treatment-resistant depression in older adults (OPTIMUM): study design and treatment characteristics of the first 396 participants randomized. Am J Geriatr Psychiatry 2019;27(10):1138–52.
30. Rosen DA, Seki SM, Fernández-Castañeda A, et al. Modulation of the sigma-1 receptor-IRE1 pathway is beneficial in preclinical models of inflammation and sepsis. Sci Transl Med 2019;11(478):eaau5266 [published correction appears in Sci Transl Med. 2019 Mar 27;11(485):].
31. Lenze EJ, Mattar C, Zorumski CF, et al. Fluvoxamine vs placebo and clinical deterioration in outpatients with symptomatic COVID-19: a randomized clinical trial. JAMA 2020;324(22):2292–300.
32. Nicol GE, Karp JF, Reiersen AM, et al. "What Were You Before the War?" Repurposing Psychiatry During the COVID-19 Pandemic. J Clin Psychiatry 2020;81(3): 20com13373.
33. Agarwal P, Mukerji G, Laur C, et al. Adoption, feasibility and safety of a family medicine-led remote monitoring program for patients with COVID-19: a descriptive study. CMAJ Open 2021;9(2):E324–30.
34. Orri M, Lipset CH, Jacobs BP, et al. Web-based trial to evaluate the efficacy and safety of tolterodine ER 4 mg in participants with overactive bladder: REMOTE trial. Contemp Clin Trials 2014;38(2):190–7.

Preparing for the Next Pandemic to Protect Public Mental Health

What Have We Learned from COVID-19?

Joshua C. Morganstein, MD

KEYWORDS

• Covid-19 • Pandemic • Preparedness • Mental health • Public health
• Interventions

KEY POINTS

- Public mental health practices and principles are critical in response to COVID-19 as well as in other pandemics and disasters.
- Distress reactions and health risk behaviors are early and common responses to COVID-19 in addition to psychiatric disorders.
- Risk and protective factors related to adverse psychological and behavioral health effects result from pre-event factors, aspects of impact, and recovery variables.
- Early interventions use an evidence-based framework to enhance well-being, reduce distress, and mitigate disorders.
- Adapting interventions from high-risk occupations provides a rapid and tailored response to enhance organizational sustainment.

INTRODUCTION

The COVID-19 pandemic is an unprecedented global disaster that has killed 5,203,000 people to date,[1] having an impact on nearly all sectors of society. The public's experience of the pandemic has been altered by the collision of multiple disasters: civil unrest, racial inequity, economic crises, political strife, and other events, such as hurricanes, floods, and mass violence. These events pull at the fault lines of communities and amplify distress, mistrust, and uncertainty, altering how these events are

Disclaimer (required for federal government employees): The views expressed are those of the authors and do not necessarily reflect the views of the Department of Defense, the Uniformed Services University, the Department of Health and Human Services, or the United States Public Health Service.

Center for the Study of Traumatic Stress, Department of Psychiatry, School of Medicine, Uniformed Services University, 6720B Rockledge Drive, Suite 550, Bethesda, MD 20817, USA
E-mail address: Joshua.morganstein@usuhs.edu

Psychiatr Clin N Am 45 (2022) 191–210
https://doi.org/10.1016/j.psc.2021.11.012
0193-953X/22/Published by Elsevier Inc.

experienced. Addressing public mental health needs involves an understanding of where risk is concentrated and how it changes over time to allow for more timely and tailored interventions that are altered to meet current and evolving needs. In disasters, certain populations bear a disproportionate burden of risk. For instance, in COVID-19, health care workers have experienced prolonged threats to health and safety for themselves and their families as well as exposure to death and dying.[2] People of color became sicker and died with greater frequency, with black and Hispanic citizens experiencing a 3-fold greater reduction in life expectancy than whites, directly resulting from the COVID-19 pandemic.[3]

Disasters cause an established range of adverse mental health effects, with pandemics creating unique impacts related to fear, uncertainty, and changing risk perceptions. Assessment and treatment of psychological disorders are aspects of managing public mental health during pandemics. Responses, such as distress reactions and health risk behaviors, also confer significant public mental health burden. The scope and magnitude of these events require a public mental health framework for interventions that focuses on disease prevention and wellness in addition to the treatment of disorders. Public health emergencies need coordinated and sustained public health approaches across various services and sectors of society.[4] These community-based approaches include public health education, communication, organizational sustainment, and leadership, all of which focus on fostering wellness, preventing disease, and promoting recovery.[5]

This article examines current findings from the pandemic and identifies gaps in the understanding of public mental health impact and mitigation strategies. Preparing for future pandemics requires examination of lessons learned and implementing relevant system changes, which require sustained commitment and collaboration from public and private sector entities.

SCOPE OF COVID-19 IMPACT ON MENTAL HEALTH

Disasters create adverse mental health effects, from distress to disorders, with various effects beginning early and others emerging over time,[6–9] some of which last for months or years and may result in prolonged or chronic functional impairment and disability. Pandemics produce unique psychological effects, related primarily to fear, and altered risk perception.[10] This perception of risk influences engagement in health behaviors required to control the outbreak, such as physical distancing, mask wearing, handwashing, and vaccinations.[10] During COVID-19, prolonged uncertainty, isolation and quarantine, concerns about shortages, and changing health recommendations exacerbated underlying concerns.

Psychological and Behavioral Effects of Disasters

Psychological and behavioral responses to disasters are depicted in **Fig. 1**. Psychiatric disorders often manifest after weeks or months with available evidence-based treatment. Other responses occur that often receive less clinical and media attention but cause significant public mental health burden. Distress reactions and risky health behaviors are well-established manifestations of disasters, including pandemics. In the severe acute respiratory syndrome (SARS) outbreak of 2007, approximately 40% of ICU nurses experienced significant insomnia,[11] which is associated with work errors, accidents, mental health disorders, exacerbation of cardiovascular and immune diseases, cognitive symptoms, and functional impairment. During COVID-19, for instance, insomnia has been studied largely in the context of sequelae from SARS coronavirus 2 infection, rather than as a distress reaction resulting from the

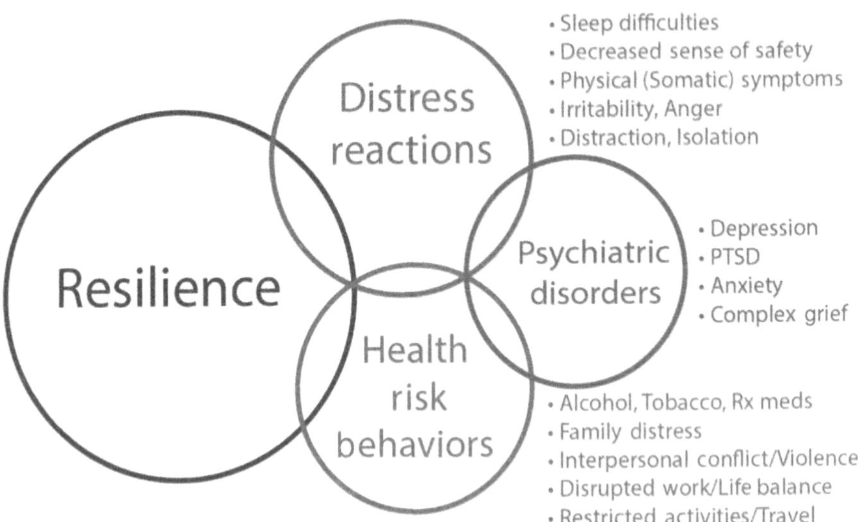

Fig. 1. Psychological and behavioral responses to pandemics and disasters.

experience of living through a pandemic, the latter having a far greater potential impact on public mental health.

Disasters, such as a hurricane, an earthquake, and a mass shooting, that are a single event and occur over a discrete period typically progress through well-established community phases. Initially, a honeymoon phase occurs when resources and support are brought to a community and individuals come together to connect and rebuild with the hope of being made whole again. Later, a disillusionment phase occurs when resources diminish, and mounting stressors reduce a sense of hope. Anniversary reactions remind individuals and communities of what has been lost. Finally is a reconstruction phase, when individuals find ways to make meaning of the event and move forward in the context of a new normal. COVID-19 disrupted these phases by limiting social connection and diminishing community cohesion, which made planning and allocation of community mental health resources more difficult.

The Unique Disaster of COVID-19

COVID-19 differs from other disasters by the very nature of the threat as well as its scope, magnitude, and duration. Even those with experience responding to disasters (eg, first responders, emergency workers, law enforcement, and health care workers) were ill-prepared for a novel infectious disease that has been hard to predict, caused significant illness, resulted in relatively high mortality, and presented significant risk to personal and family safety. Although risk mitigation is essential during COVID-19, risk cannot be eliminated. When the threat is a highly contagious respiratory virus, there is nowhere safety can be guaranteed. All members of society had to determine the extent to which loved ones, friends, and colleagues—traditionally a source of comfort, connection, and companionship—represented a threat to health and safety. These supportive resources often were less accessible due to required or voluntary physical distancing or quarantine after an exposure.

Health care workers played an essential role in preventing illness and death from COVID-19. Inadequate supplies, shifting policies and procedures, working outside their scope of care, and requirements to practice altered standards of care led to feelings of distress for some workers. Stigmatization by neighbors, friends, and family added to the burden of health care workers.[12] The extremes of COVID-19 caused mental health to become an increasingly significant threat to safety for health care workers around the world.[2]

Like most public health emergencies, the pandemic has pulled at the fault lines within society, further exposing divisions. These are predictable effects of disasters that have a broad impact on health, safety, security, and economics, particularly when they require sustained and changing behaviors to manage effectively. Community conflict over mask wearing, school closures, and vaccine acceptance were exacerbated by the emergence of more contagious and lethal viral variants, all of which served to fuel community anger and resentment and diminish social cohesion.

Psychological and Behavioral Health in COVID-19

Protecting health involves understanding psychological symptoms and behavioral effects of disasters. Symptoms of psychological disorders have received considerable attention, with studies demonstrating elevated rates of depression and anxiety during COVID-19 that persisted in communities around the world[13] and created considerable health burden, which benefited from evidence-based interventions. Beyond symptoms of disorders, insomnia, increased use of alcohol and tobacco, and family violence were responses to COVID-19, having an impact not only on individual health but also on the ability to sustain operations in occupational settings that were critical to maintaining community functioning.

Insomnia is a growing public health problem associated with worsening of underlying physical and mental health conditions,[14] diminished cognitive performance,[15] and impaired immune system. These create significant risks, particularly during a pandemic when decision making around family health behaviors and the ability to fight illness are critical to community health. COVID-19 had a negative impact on sleep around the world, with insomnia rates of 20% to 45% and health care workers reporting some of the highest overall rates,[16] where nurses and those working most closely with sick patients were at greatest risk.[17] Insomnia is both a risk factor for and an adverse clinical feature of numerous mental health conditions with elevated insomnia ratings in health care workers associated with higher rates of probable posttraumatic stress disorder (PTSD).[18] Nochaiwong and colleagues[13] reviewed the global prevalence of mental health symptoms from 32 countries and from approximately 400,000 participants and found a 27.6% prevalence of sleep disorders. Improved sleep can enhance the ability to solve problems, make decisions, and engage in behaviors needed to promote health during a pandemic and may be done through public health education about the benefits of re-establishing sleep and other daily routines, regular exposure to sunlight, calming behaviors that reduce arousal, and limiting exposure to disaster-related media. Access to self-directed cognitive behavioral therapy for insomnia using online and app-based programs and other technologies that foster calming and lower arousal may be useful as well, particularly when face-to-face health care is limited.

Alcohol often is used to manage sleep problems and distressing emotions, both of which are exacerbated during disasters. In March 2020, an online survey of US adults by the American Psychiatric Association revealed 8% of Americans already had begun increasing their consumption of alcohol.[19] Three months later, in June 2020, the Centers for Disease Control and Prevention found 13.3% of adults increased use of substances to manage pandemic-related distress.[20] Pollard and colleagues[21] quantified changes in alcohol use comparing the period during the pandemic with data from the year prior and observed 75% of adults reporting 1 additional drinking day per month, with 41% of women reporting increased binge drinking and a 39% increase on the Short Inventory of Problems scale related to use of alcohol. These findings have important public mental health implications. Even in the absence of alcohol use disorder, the increased use of alcohol within a community is associated with higher rates of accidents, violence, work and other errors, physical health ailments, and impaired decision making. The last can be particularly problematic when choices about pandemic behaviors have greater consequences for family health and safety. Home confinement, unemployment, work and family stresses, and the persistent availability of alcohol compounded these problems. Limiting access to alcohol as an intervention must be balanced against acute health consequences of abrupt discontinuation. Public health education, community support services, and timely and tailored resources to help mitigate the distress that often leads to increased alcohol use are important aspects of future interventions.

Grief is a near universal aspect of disasters, resulting from loss of possessions, health, perceptions of safety, and certainty about the future. Disenfranchised grief involves loss that is not acknowledged openly, validated socially, or mourned publicly in ways that promote healing, such as the inability to be at the bedside of dying loved or gather at a funeral service due to COVID-19–related health restrictions. Bereavement from the death of a loved one during disaster increases adverse mental health effects, with some estimates of 9 people experiencing bereavement for every COVID-19 death.[22] Hillis and colleagues[23] found more than 1.5 million children had a caregiver die from COVID-19, with the potential for this to increase greatly as more lethal viral variants became increasingly common. Evidence-based and actionable resources to support of children following the death of a caregiver were an important aspect of health education during COVID-19.[24]

Feeling safe during disasters is important to health, with decreased perceptions of safety associated with insomnia, increased substance use, depression, posttraumatic stress symptoms, and general psychological distress.[25] COVID-19 represents an amorphous and ongoing threat to safety, and further understanding the extent to which perceptions of safety influenced the onset of psychological and behavioral response is critical in developing effective interventions for future pandemics. The pandemic also created significant disruption to work-life balance, with virtual education and remote work commonplace. The presence of mental health symptoms and exposure to disasters both have been associated independently with occupational difficulties and impairment, including absenteeism and presenteeism.[26,27] Leveraging and adapting effective workplace health promotion programs that address unique changes required in the home-work environment during COVID-19 also can enhance pandemic preparedness.

Key Points

1. Responses to disasters include distress reactions, health risk behaviors, psychiatric disorders, and resilience. Understanding both the psychological and behavioral impacts of a pandemic on society provides the most robust understanding of community public mental health impacts.
2. Pandemics are characterized by fear and uncertainty that alter perceptions of risk, which directly influence engagement in recommended health behaviors. The ability to alter risk perception is essential to optimizing health behaviors required to control a pandemic.
3. Adverse responses to pandemics that negatively affect community functioning and occupational performance are important targets for interventions that protect health and sustain operations.

RETHINKING RISK AND RESILIENCE

Far more is known about what creates risk for illness than what protects health. Risk and protection in COVID-19 result from a dynamic interplay of biopsychosocial factors related to predisaster factors, impact characteristics, and post-disaster recovery variables. From an occupational and public health perspective, stressors, such as living through a pandemic, can be thought of like a toxin, such as lead or radon. To understand the impact, it is important to know aspects of the exposure, such as who, when, how much, the response over time, and which factors buffered against negative effects. Health surveillance during and after disasters is complex and challenging but critical to understanding where risk is concentrated and how it changes over time, which is essential to developing timely and tailored interventions. Certain populations are at increased risks during disasters and certain groups bear a disproportionate burden of risk. COVID-19 created unique, although often predictable, challenges.

Health care workers had unique and wide-ranging experiences throughout the pandemic, such as (1) being called heroes where communities clapped for them, (2) lacking basic personal protective equipment (PPE) to maintain personal safety, (3) being required to decide which patients lived or died due to constrained resources, (4) begin stigmatized by friends and neighbors, and, ultimately, (5) being vilified by patients and public officials who opposed health recommendations.[28] Health care workers represent a group with numerous risk and protective factors that evolved throughout the pandemic (**Table 1**). Although the transition to recovery is far less clear during COVID-19, the factors listed provide an understanding of how risk and protection evolve throughout a pandemic life cycle.

Risks Created by COVID-19 Response

Health behaviors to control the spread of COVID-19 reduced the risk of illness and death from infections but created other health risks associated with increased mental health burden. Immediately after implementation of physical distancing and restrictions of movement, ambulatory health care visits dropped by approximately 60%,[29] creating risk for missed diagnoses, lack of preventive services, and decreased interventions for poorly controlled medical conditions. For instance, in the first 3 months of the pandemic, screening for breast cancer and for cervical cancer decreased by 87% and 84%, respectively, with significant reductions persisting more than 6 months into the pandemic and the greatest decrease observed geographically in the Department of Health and Human Services Region 2 (including New York), for cervical cancer screening among women who identified as Asian and Pacific Islander (92%) and for breast cancer screening in women who identified as American Indian/Alaskan Native (98%).[30] Santoli and colleagues[31] observed that, when compared with the same time frame in 2019, 3,000,000 fewer childhood vaccinations were given during the first month after lockdowns (March 2020) in the United States. Although it will be years before the full impact of these changes in health care engagement are fully quantified, they increase the likelihood that diseases are missed or are found at more advanced stages, morbidity is higher from poorly controlled illnesses, and preventable infectious illnesses become more prevalent. Increasing health care disease burden is associated with higher rates of mental health symptoms and disorders. Delays in care and missed preventive services during COVID-19 have significant implications for public mental health.

Individuals with serious and persistent mental illness (SPMI) experienced risk early in the pandemic when health care organizations were determining which services to deem essential, allowing patients to continue accessing them when health care

Table 1
Risk and protective factors for health care workers during COVID-19

Time	Risk Factors	Protective Factors
Pre-event period	• Active health problems, mental health, substance use • Need for access to self/family health care • Limited/poor coping skills • Limited social supports • Financial difficulties • Lack of training • Poor team cohesion • Resistance to help-seeking	• Positive health status • Availability/use of health resources • Limited exposure to adverse environmental health factors • History of positive adaptation to stress or stress resistance • Hopeful outlook • Creative coping skills/strategies • Screening and identification of health risk status • Reducing stigma for non-frontline personnel • Adequate training and preparation
Event/impact period	• Requirement to use crisis (altered) standards of care • Inadequate PPE • Moral distress/injury • High exposure to infection • Exposure to death, dying, and human remains • Required work outside specialty training • Weakened community fabric • Punitive or unsupportive work environment • Toxic leadership • Lack of empathy • Poor communication • Death of loved ones	• Short duration, minimal disruption to work/personal life • Community fabric intact • Adequate PPE • Exposure risks and sacrifices shared equitably • Clear communication about evolving infection control and safety policies and procedures • Supportive and accessible leaders • Help-seeking organizational culture • Regular monitoring of health and behavioral health status through multiple means • Early identification and intervention with health and behavioral health issues • Accessible supports, interventions, and referral options • Monitor impact of organizational status and change on well-being of all personnel
Recovery period	• Illness stigma from neighbors/family/friends • Disjointed community response • Isolation from social support systems • Inability to grieve • Job loss • Extended virtual/home school requirements • Lack of access to childcare	• Strong workplace and personal support • Range of supports and interventions • Options and opportunities for personnel interactions • Family friendly personnel policies and strategies • Adaptation to changing patterns of needs, demands

(*continued on next page*)

Table 1
(*continued*)

Time	Risk Factors	Protective Factors
	• Fatigue; inability to reset or recover • Diminished health • Vaccination concerns and barriers	• Work culture continues to encourage interventions and support • Rest and reset options provided and encouraged • Health issues addressed • Leadership remains engaged and communicating regularly with personnel

services were being restricted to control spread of infection. Electroconvulsive therapy to manage psychosis and suicidal thinking and long-acting injectable medications to sustain abstinence from substance abuse and dependence often were the subject of debate regarding their "essential" nature. Public health education by psychiatrists and collaboration between health care disciplines elaborated the life-saving role these interventions play in the lives of individuals with SPMI.[32,33] Care for persons with SPMI will be improved in future pandemics when health care systems identify these as essential health care services in disaster planning and preparations and ensure that discussions about resource allocation include psychiatrists and other mental health professionals.

Concerns emerged early in the pandemic for increased child maltreatment and neglect as well as other forms of family violence. Heightened family stress related to shifts to virtual school and remote work, limited access to health care and other helping services, loss of employment, and continued access to alcohol created an environment in which violence is more likely to occur and less apt to be identified. Some studies revealed a reduction in rates of emergency department visits for interpersonal violence as well as child abuse and neglect early in the pandemic.[34] This did not necessarily indicate these events were less common, however, only that presentation to emergency health care settings (where the risk for COVID-19 infection was perceived to be high) decreased over a given period of time. By contrast, law enforcement calls for domestic violence increased significantly during the early months of lockdowns and restrictions of movement, with many of these perceived to be related to pandemic stressors.[35,36] These findings, along with increased calls to domestic violence hotlines around the world, serve as a reminder that people chose to present distress during COVID-19 to places perceived as most safe. Anticipating these shifts, adequately staffing helping resources, rapidly transitioning to remote support services, and community health education campaigns to inform the public about available resources and lower barriers to help-seeking are important aspects of preparing for future pandemics.

Inequitable Distribution of Risk

In disasters, risk is not distributed equitably. Lower socioeconomic status is one of the most consistent global predictors of adverse outcomes following disasters, resulting from factors, such as reduced preparedness and insufficient systems of care. Unsurprisingly, inequities in risk have been observed in COVID-19. During April 2020 and May 2020, Hispanic respondents reported high rates of depression (40.3%) and suicidal thoughts (22.9%) and increased use or initiation of substances (36.9%), remarkably higher than those of white counterparts, and endorsed high rates of worry about having enough food and stable housing.[37] In the state of Maryland during the first 5 months of the pandemic, suicide mortality for white citizens decreased by approximately 40% but increased approximately 5% for black citizens.[38] Systemic racism, inequities in health care treatment and delivery, and overt harm to people of color fueled feelings of hesitancy and lower rates of vaccination in these communities during the pandemic.[39] Around the world, vaccination rates of developed nations in Asia, North America, and Europe eclipsed vaccination rates in African nations.[40] These findings highlight the importance of engaging with marginalized communities before, during, and after disasters like COVID-19; partnering with community leaders; acknowledging current and historic inequities; and seeking culturally sensitive and collaborative approaches to enhance preparedness and strengthen community resilience.

Changing Risks Over Time

In COVID-19 and other disasters, much of risk comes from evolving health behaviors. Understanding how risk changes over time, what new risks emerge, and where risk is concentrated is essential to protect health. Research found that from March 2020 to November 2020 adherence diminished significantly in nearly all health behaviors recommended to control the spread of the pandemic, with mask wearing remaining the one behavior done with greater frequency.[41] Pew Research tracked trends in willingness to accept the COVID-19 vaccine, observing that althoughb more individuals expressed willingness after the vaccines were first released, hesitancy and refusal persisted, particularly among certain demographics, including those with lower education and less knowledge about the vaccines.[42]

Misinformation created one of the most significant and evolving threats to public health during COVID-19, prompting a report from the US Surgeon General[43] as well as information campaigns from the United Kingdom and the World Health Organization.[44] A significant area of misinformation occurred around vaccines. In July of 2021, a national survey of adults in the United States found that, among those who indicated they were "definitely not" getting vaccinated, a vast majority believed the health risk related to vaccines was higher than the health risk of contracting COVID-19.[45] The prominence of social media and the proliferation of Internet-connected digital devices facilitated global spread of misinformation. Senior government officials and media pundits around the world fueled divisions and misinformation by delivering conflicting messages about the threat of COVID-19, casting blame on its origins in favor of engaging in behaviors to contain spread, suggesting unapproved and untested treatments, undermining the utility of health behaviors intended to prevent the spread of the infection, and minimizing the need for vaccinations. Misinformation will be a predictable aspect of future pandemics and effectively countering it will require early and robust communication using principles of behavioral sciences to develop messages shared by trusted and credible messengers that address the broad range of concerns across different communities.[46]

Reconsidering Assumptions About Risk

Media messages about concerns for severe and prolonged mental health outcomes transmitted the direst projections from health care providers.[47] Historically, mental health difficulties have persisted for long periods of time in certain populations after disasters, and this is important for planning for future events. But, once a new disaster, such as COVID-19, occurs, historical lessons become more speculative. Health surveillance over time is needed to understand community impact during and after COVID-19.

Suicide has been an ongoing focus of global public mental health concern. Loss of employment, social isolation, and family and work stress contribute to suicide.

Research in previous disasters revealed mixed results with respect to the impact of disasters on suicide rates, with infectious disease outbreaks typically showing no association.[48] Temporal changes have been observed with risk changing over time, where suicidal behavior diminished during the time frame typically corresponding to the honeymoon phase of community response but increased in the time frame corresponding to the disillusionment phase.[49] Concerns emerged early in the pandemic about suicide as an adverse outcome. Media attention following the suicide of Dr Lorna Breen, a prominent emergency physician in New York, further heightened fears of suicide in frontline health care workers. Recent global data on suicide and suicidal behaviors have demonstrated mixed findings, with certain demographics and other factors associated with increased risk and others with reduced risk. For instance, studies identified younger age[50] and female gender[51] as risk factors for suicidal ideation and related behaviors during COVID-19. Other studies suggest, however, that overall suicide rates have not increased and, in some cases, have modestly decreased during the pandemic. An understanding of how COVID-19 has had an impact on suicidal thoughts and behaviors during various community phases of the pandemic and steps to help mitigate and intervene require an understanding of the factors that predispose to suicidality during the pandemic as well as interventions that are accessible and adaptable within various social and occupational communities.

Older adults have been found to be at risk for adverse mental health outcomes in disasters, predominantly due to diseases of aging, such as cognitive impairment, diminished vision and hearing, mobility limitations, and increased reliance on systems of care.[52] Increasing age also is associated, however, with increased stress tolerance and resilience to adversities, including disasters. During COVID-19, many studies found older participants reported lower rates of depression, anxiety, sleep disruption, and suicidal thoughts.[53] A literature review by Parlapani and colleagues[54] of studies examining the impact of COVID-19 revealed that older age largely buffered against many of the adverse effects of the pandemic. Factors impacting the experience of older adults during the pandemic include having a fixed income, lower likelihood of job loss concerns, less work-life imbalance due to lack of young children at home requiring childcare and oversight for virtual schooling, and the ability to experience feelings of self-efficacy from serving as a source of support to children and grandchildren dealing with these very challenges. The experience of older adults likely is nuanced and impacted by socioeconomic, cultural, and other regional factors.

Key Points

1. The impact of pandemics and behaviors required to effectively manage the spread of infection will mitigate certain health risks, while exacerbating or creating other risks. Addressing evolving risk protects health and reduces morbidity.
2. Risk is not distributed equitably in disasters, and understanding which populations are at risk during pandemics, as well as how those risks change over time, allows for effective planning and preparation as well as enhanced response.
3. Risk should be evaluated broadly, with ongoing health surveillance among different communities and sectors of society informing where risk is concentrated to provide timely and tailored interventions.

INTERVENTION TO PROTECT MENTAL HEALTH

Public mental health interventions are essential to sustain community well-being and functioning in disasters, such as COVID-19, including public health education, risk and crisis communication, and leadership.[6,55] Approaches should extend beyond treatment of disorders and emphasize wellness and protective health behaviors. Adapting interventions from occupations with experience in prolonged high-stress environments allowed for a more timely and efficient response to support community health and enhance operational sustainment.[56] Effective interventions to sustain organizations, such as health care systems, include actions by individuals, organizations, and leaders (**Box 1**).

Interventions should foster the 5 essential elements that are protective during disasters, including a sense of safety, calming, social connectedness, self-efficacy and community efficacy, and hope.[57] These elements form what has been called Psychological First Aid (PFA), an evidence-based framework for enhancing well-being and resilience for individuals and communities. Early efforts were made to adapt these elements to address unique aspects of the pandemic.[58] Health care system intervention frameworks that incorporated principles of PFA were better able to address distress and health risk behaviors through interventions other than clinical care. This is particularly important to lower barriers to care because health care workers may perceive mental illness as stigmatizing, whereas interventions that focus on distress and transient impairment may be more accessible. These approaches also enabled organizations to recognize and promote nonclinical, evidence-based interventions to reduce distress.[59] Organizational efforts to acquire protective equipment and establish protocols enable a sense of safety among workers. Enhancement of respite areas within hospitals and promotion of self-help interventions, such as mindfulness and meditation, promote calming. After action reviews and shift huddles create opportunities to reinforce self-efficacy and collective efficacy, promote connectedness among health care teams, and dispel misconceptions or distortions of thought that otherwise might lead to feelings of blame and guilt.

Health education is critical to fostering the principles of PFA for individuals and communities during COVID-19 and other disasters. The Center for the Study of Traumatic Stress developed COVID-19 health education resources that address the unique risks and exposures of various communities, including responder and emergency personnel, health care workers, patients, families, and community leaders.[60] These brief, easy-to-read, just-in-time resources explain complex topics in a way that is easy to understand and address the critical question, "What do I do?" to protect individual, family, and community health during public health emergencies and other disasters. In collaboration with partners around the world, many of these resources have been translated into different languages to support global health throughout the pandemic. Online training in community-based PFA is available through the National Child Traumatic Stress Network that prepares individuals to support community health following disasters.[61] PFA training for supervisors and leaders also is available from the National Association of County and City Healthcare Organizations. Based on the principles of PFA, the Massachusetts Medical Society created training to enhance sustainment of health care workers during COVID-19, through self-care and other actions.[62]

Mobile apps can provide information and access to location-based resources tailored to individual risks and needs. The Heroes Health app provides location-based well-being resources and a weekly self-assessment for health care workers and allows user-approved information to be shared with health care organizations to facilitate the delivery of timely and tailored interventions that address evolving risks for workers.[63] The COVID Coach app provides information about coping during the pandemic, tools for self-care, and trackers to observe trends over time in mood and other measures of well-being.[64] Resources that support interventions in future pandemics should leverage technology, such as wearables, to assess and optimize

Box 1
Actions to promote organizational sustainment during COVID-19

Individual
Self-care: sleep, nutrition, hydration, and exercise help with decision making.
Media use: limiting exposure to disaster-related and other negative media lowers distress.
Self-monitoring: taking our own pulse through self-checks and feedback from others
Self-advocacy: speaking up when things do not seem right improves efficacy.
Social connections: reaching out and connecting with others reminds us we are not alone.

Organizational
Communication: timely, regular, updated, and accurate messages build trust.
Training: thorough and realistic training to prepare workers lowers uncertainty.
Education: understand normal psychological and behavioral responses to stress.
Practical supports: food, parking, lodging, and childcare meet essential needs.
Camaraderie: connections among personnel (colleagues, managers, and others)
Equipment: adequate supplies of protective equipment to feel safer
Peer support: peer buddies and other support systems to sustain well-being
Growth mindset: team learning and growing together through difficulties

Leadership
Modeling self-care: gives permission to all personnel to do the same
Effective communication: using effective strategies enhances health behaviors.
Grief leadership: acknowledging grief and honoring losses make meaning of the event.

physiologic measures of distress, including heart rate and sleep quality. The ability to crowdsource information from wearables and other mobile devices could provide significant insights into community psychological responses and health behaviors that identify evolving public mental health hot spots to which resources can be more efficiently directed in future pandemics.

Adapting Interventions

During the pandemic, considerable work was done adapting interventions used in occupations that routinely conduct prolonged operations in unsafe, high-stress environments, such as the military, for use in health care systems and other settings to support well-being and enhance sustainment for workers. Public-private partnership facilitated adaptation of interventions through the rapid transfer of information, resource sharing, and proliferation of lessons learned across sectors.

In New York City, a collaboration of public and private partners created Healing, Education, Resilience & Opportunity for New York's Frontline Workforce (HERO-NY).[65] This interdisciplinary group developed training materials to help workers and supervisors manage the stresses of multiple pandemic waves. HERO-NY applied a tiered approach that reinforced principles of self-care, buddy aid, and help-seeking. The University of Minnesota Medical School promoted a battle buddy system, adapted from the US Army, using periodic check-in meetings with a designated peer as a means of reinforcing safety, social connectedness, and efficacy during pandemic surges.[66] Buddy systems and other formal, rather than ad hoc, peer support can be helpful in organizations where personnel have more difficulty asking for help, such as health care workers, military personnel, first responders, and other emergency workers.

Principles of the military's Stress Continuum model (**Fig. 2**) shaped approaches to interventions aimed at worker sustainment. This framework emphasizes that

- Workers' experience generally occurs on a continuum of expectable responses and does not require clinical care or medicalizing.

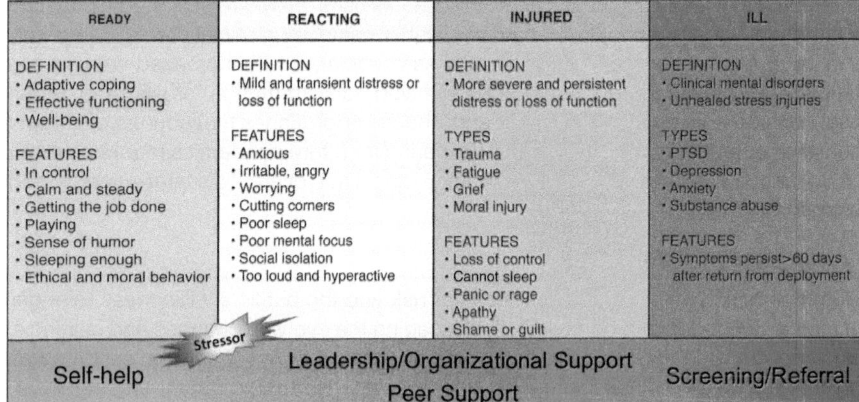

Fig. 2. Stress continuum model. (*Adapted from* Nash WP. US Marine Corps and Navy combat and operational stress continuum model: a tool for leaders. In: Ritchie EC, ed. Combat and Operational Behavioral Health. Fort Detrick, MD: Borden Institute; 2011.)

- Communities in which individuals live and work greatly influence their well-being and serve as the main source of support and sustainment.
- Support systems should focus primarily on identifying reactions on the continuum and providing interventions to facilitate adaptation and wellness.

Interventions that incorporated a stress continuum allowed health care system leaders and wellness experts to think beyond a model that limits responses to illness and individual treatment to also recognize a range of distress responses and health risk behaviors that may or may not ultimately result in lasting illness. The Mount Sinai Center for Stress, Resilience, and Personal Growth incorporated a stress continuum approach as part of facilitating peer support and guiding health care workers to optimal helping resources.[67] In the United Kingdom, hospitals created Supported Wellbeing Centres, providing employees with rest facilities and trained peer supporters.[68] These approaches incorporated aspects of embedded mental health, which utilizes mental health providers as members of a care team without providing direct care to colleagues. Instead, their presence fosters connections, facilitates communication, encourages help-seeking, and lowers stigma. Deploying support staff in an embedded mental health model can enhance access to interventions for stressed workers.[69]

Media Exposure

Some studies have revealed that use of media in disasters may increase compliance with recommended health behaviors and reduce distress. Disaster-related media exposure, however, also is associated with disrupted sleep, increased use of alcohol and tobacco, elevated symptoms of depression and posttraumatic stress, and higher general psychological distress.[70] Bendau and colleagues[71] found that German citizens with increased exposure to COVID-19 media indicated greater symptoms of depression and anxiety and similar associations were found in other countries.[72] Increasing use of social media and use of a greater number of sources of media were associated with higher rates of general psychological distress.[73] Engaging with the media to create messages that inform the public while avoiding sensationalized and distress-related messaging is an important aspect of public health education.

Infectious disease outbreaks create additional risks related to how media consumption has an impact on health behaviors. Higher reliance on social media as a primary source of information about COVID-19 was associated with increased vaccine hesitancy.[74] As health recommendations evolved, disinformation proliferated rapidly, with considerable effort given to evidence-based approaches that counter disinformation and protect community health.[75] Preparing for future pandemics requires the public to use trusted sources of information and limit overall disaster-related media exposure.

Communication and Messaging

Communication influences perceptions of risk and the public's willingness to engage in recommended health behaviors.[76] Messaging the evolving changes and helping society manage ongoing uncertainty requires trusted principles of risk and crisis communication,[77] which include being first and accurate with information, sharing what is known and unknown, committing to finding answers, and then following up, letting the public know when further information will be shared and avoiding efforts to mislead or provide excessive reassurance. The conflicting messages from community leaders and elected officials as well as deliberate efforts to spread misinformation made obtaining accurate health information difficult for the public during COVID-19.

Clinicians, public health professionals, community leaders, and the media play an important role in creating messages to the public that lower distress and enhance community cohesion. Using a word like "concern" rather than "anxiety" helps normalize the public's experiences. Using language that is understandable is increasingly important because society has a growing mistrust of scientific information with medical jargon, fostering disengagement.[78] A mistrust in science has been associated with increased interest, adoption, and spread of misinformation during COVID-19.[79] Although efforts have been made to draw attention to the importance of communication with the public during COVID-19,[80] virtually no literature has been published to inform understanding of how communication and messaging have had an impact on engagement in health behaviors and public mental health during the pandemic. Research on the effects of communication and messaging during COVID-19 is essential to develop lessons learned to inform the development of interventions more precisely for specific communities. Consistent application of the principles of communication and messaging during disasters, by scientists, elected officials, and community leaders, will be critical to optimize health behaviors in future pandemics.

Leadership in Crisis

Leadership during crisis plays an essential role in community recovery. The actions and words of leaders play a vital role in the overall well-being of organizations and communities after crisis events and can even facilitate growth following exposure to trauma.[81] Leaders exist at many levels within organizations and communities. During times of crisis, individuals also rise and exert leadership influence regardless of their formal position or established authority. In addition to effective communication, leaders model behavior for members of their communities. Decisions by leaders to support health professionals and encourage health behaviors, such as wearing masks, physical distancing, and vaccinations set a tone that often is modeled by community members aligned with those leaders. There have been efforts to bring attention to principles and practices for leaders to support communities during COVID-19, emphasizing important crisis leadership actions, such as communication, collaboration, and connection.[82] Nevertheless, little research exists on the impact of leadership behaviors on community well-being during the current pandemic.

Grief leadership is a critical aspect of leading during a crisis that is associated with improved community well-being and recovery.[83] Grief leadership involves ongoing communication that acknowledges losses through community-conceived and implemented rituals, efforts to help make meaning of the event, and, ultimately, helping communities look hopefully to the future. Efforts by community leaders to address loss within their communities, collaborate with community members in developing rituals and symbolic acts to recognize and honor aspects of loss, and foster a sense of hope moving forward even through uncertain times can aid in recovery of communities around the world.

Key Points

1. The 5 essential elements of PFA (safety, calming, self-efficacy and community efficacy, social connectedness, and hope) form the foundation for interventions in COVID-19 and other disasters.
2. Effective interventions incorporate a stress continuum that extends beyond illness and addresses distress and health risk behaviors while incorporating actions that involve the individual, peers, organizational practices, and leadership support.
3. Risk and crisis communication principles should inform messaging through media and other means to reduce community distress, inform risk perceptions, and optimize engagement in pandemic-related health behaviors.

SUMMARY

The COVID-19 pandemic has brought unprecedented uncertainty to the global society. The evolving impact on public mental health is only beginning to be understood and includes numerous responses beyond psychiatric illness, such as distress reactions, health risk behaviors, resilience, and growth. Recognition of this continuum of response allows for more effective interventions. Risk for adverse outcomes during this pandemic is not distributed equitably, will change over time, and may emerge in unexpected communities. Ongoing health surveillance will inform understanding of who is at risk and when, temporal responses, and factors that buffer against this far-reaching disaster event. Continued research to better understand the unique aspects of risk created by this global event is critical to future preparedness efforts. Public mental health interventions in COVID-19, as with all disasters and future pandemics, must consider the full range of responses beyond medical illness, rapidly adapt established interventions to address current needs, and be developed within an evidence-based framework that includes established principles of PFA, communication and messaging, and leadership behaviors. Additional studies are essential to better inform understanding of how adapted interventions have an impact on outcomes to prepare the global society more effectively for future pandemics.

DISCLOSURE AND DISCLAIMER STATEMENT

The author has nothing to disclose.

REFERENCES

1. Alcantara C, Shin Y, Shapiro L, et al. Mapping the worldwide spread of the coronavirus. The Washington Post. Available at: https://www.washingtonpost.com/graphics/2020/world/mapping-spread-new-coronavirus/?no_nav=true&p9w22b2p=b2p22p9w00098. Accessed November 30, 2021.

2. National Academies of Sciences E, Medicine. Rapid expert consultation on understanding causes of health care worker deaths due to the COVID-19 pandemic (December 10, 2020). Washington, DC: The National Academies Press; 2020. p. 10.
3. Arias E, Tejada-Vera B, Ahmad F, et al. Provisional life expectancy estimates for 2020. Hyattsville, MD: Vital Statistics Rapid Release; 2021.
4. DeSalvo K, Hughes B, Bassett M, et al. Public health COVID-19 impact assessment: lessons learned and compelling needs. NAM Perspect 2021;1–29. https://doi.org/10.31478/202104c.
5. National Academies of Sciences E, Medicine. Evidence-based practice for public health emergency preparedness and response. Washington, DC: The National Academies Press; 2020. p. 500.
6. Ursano RJ, Fullerton CS, Weisaeth L, et al. Textbook of disaster psychiatry. Cambridge, UK: Cambridge University Press; 2017.
7. National Academies of Sciences E, Medicine. Long-Term Health Monitoring of Populations Following a Nuclear or Radiological Incident in the United States: Proceedings of a Workshop. 2019;
8. Hansel TC, Osofsky JD, Osofsky HJ, et al. The effect of long-term relocation on child and adolescent survivors of Hurricane Katrina. J Trauma Stress 2013; 26(5):613–20.
9. van der Velden PG, Wong A, Boshuizen HC, et al. Persistent mental health disturbances during the 10 years after a disaster: Four-wave longitudinal comparative study. Psychiatry Clin Neurosci 2013;67(2):110–8.
10. Morganstein JC, Fullerton CS, Ursano RJ, et al. Pandemics: health care emergencies. Textbook of disaster psychiatry. 2017:270-284.
11. Su T-P, Lien T-C, Yang C-Y, et al. Prevalence of psychiatric morbidity and psychological adaptation of the nurses in a structured SARS caring unit during outbreak: a prospective and periodic assessment study in Taiwan. J Psychiatr Res 2007; 41(1–2):119–30.
12. Ramaci T, Barattucci M, Ledda C, et al. Social stigma during COVID-19 and its impact on HCWs outcomes. Sustainability 2020;12(9):3834.
13. Nochaiwong S, Ruengorn C, Thavorn K, et al. Global prevalence of mental health issues among the general population during the coronavirus disease-2019 pandemic: a systematic review and meta-analysis. Sci Rep 2021;11(1):1–18.
14. Fernandez-Mendoza J, Vgontzas AN. Insomnia and its impact on physical and mental health. Curr Psychiatry Rep 2013;15(12):418.
15. Hajak G, Petukhova M, Lakoma MD, et al. Days-out-of-role associated with insomnia and comorbid conditions in the America Insomnia Survey. Biol Psychiatry 2011;70(11):1063–73.
16. Cénat JM, Blais-Rochette C, Kokou-Kpolou CK, et al. Prevalence of symptoms of depression, anxiety, insomnia, posttraumatic stress disorder, and psychological distress among populations affected by the COVID-19 pandemic: A systematic review and meta-analysis. Psychiatry Res 2021;295:113599.
17. Lai J, Ma S, Wang Y, et al. Factors associated with mental health outcomes among health care workers exposed to coronavirus disease 2019. JAMA Netw open 2020;3(3):e203976.
18. Zhang H, Shi Y, Jing P, et al. Posttraumatic stress disorder symptoms in healthcare workers after the peak of the COVID-19 outbreak: a survey of a large tertiary care hospital in Wuhan. Psychiatry Res 2020;294:113541.
19. Connors E. New Poll: COVID-19 Impacting Mental Well-Being: Americans Feeling Anxious, Especially for Loved Ones; Older Adults are Less Anxious. American

Psychiatric Association. Accessed August 31, 2021. Available at: https://www.psychiatry.org/newsroom/news-releases/new-poll-covid-19-impacting-mental-well-being-americans-feeling-anxious-especially-for-loved-ones-older-adults-are-less-anxious.

20. Czeisler MÉ, Lane RI, Petrosky E, et al. Mental health, substance use, and suicidal ideation during the COVID-19 pandemic—United States, June 24–30, 2020. MMWR Morb Mortal Wkly Rep 2020;69(32):1049.
21. Pollard MS, Tucker JS, Green HD. Changes in adult alcohol use and consequences during the COVID-19 pandemic in the US. JAMA Netw open 2020;3(9):e2022942.
22. Verdery AM, Smith-Greenaway E, Margolis R, et al. Tracking the reach of COVID-19 kin loss with a bereavement multiplier applied to the United States. Proc Natl Acad Sci 2020;117(30):17695–701.
23. Hillis SD, Unwin HJT, Chen Y, et al. Global minimum estimates of children affected by COVID-19-associated orphanhood and deaths of caregivers: a modelling study. Lancet 2021;398(10298):391–402.
24. Center for the Study of Traumatic Stress. Caring for Children After Parental Death: Guidelines for Primary Care Providers.
25. Morganstein JC, Ursano RJ. Ecological disasters and mental health: causes, consequences, and interventions. Front Psychiatry 2020;11:1.
26. Lerner D, Adler DA, Rogers WH, et al. A randomized clinical trial of a telephone depression intervention to reduce employee presenteeism and absenteeism. Psychiatr Serv 2015;66(6):570–7.
27. Qin X, Jiang Y. The impact of natural disaster on absenteeism, job satisfaction, and job performance of survival employees: An empirical study of the survivors in Wenchuan earthquake. Front Business Res China 2011;5(2):219–42.
28. Shigemura J, Ursano RJ, Morganstein JC, et al. Public responses to the novel 2019 coronavirus (2019-nCoV) in Japan: Mental health consequences and target populations. Psychiatry Clin Neurosci 2020;74(4):281.
29. Mehrotra A, Chernew ME, Linetsky D, et al. The Impact of the COVID-19 Pandemic on Outpatient Visits: A Rebound Emerges. Accessed August 31, 2021. Available at: https://www.commonwealthfund.org/publications/2020/apr/impact-covid-19-outpatient-visits.
30. DeGroff A, Miller J, Sharma K, et al. COVID-19 impact on screening test volume through the National Breast and Cervical Cancer early detection program, January–June 2020, in the United States. Prev Med 2021;151:106559.
31. Santoli JM. Effects of the COVID-19 pandemic on routine pediatric vaccine ordering and administration—United States, 2020. MMWR Morb Mortal Wkly Rep 2020;69:591–3.
32. APA Committee on the Psychiatric Dimensions of Disaster and COVID-19. Electroconvulsive Therapy as an Essential Procedure 2020.
33. APA Committee on the Psychiatric Dimensions of Disaster and COVID-19. Use of Long-Acting Injectables as a Clinically Necessary Treatment 2020.
34. Holland KM, Jones C, Vivolo-Kantor AM, et al. Trends in US emergency department visits for mental health, overdose, and violence outcomes before and during the COVID-19 pandemic. JAMA Psychiatry 2021;78(4):372–9.
35. Allen-Ebrahimian B. China's domestic violence epidemic. Axios 2020;10:w26823.
36. Hsu L-C, Henke A. COVID-19, staying at home, and domestic violence. Rev Econ Household 2021;19(1):145–55.
37. McKnight-Eily LR, Okoro CA, Strine TW, et al. Racial and ethnic disparities in the prevalence of stress and worry, mental health conditions, and increased

substance use among adults during the COVID-19 pandemic—United States, April and May 2020. MMWR Morb Mortal Wkly Rep 2021;70(5):162.

38. Bray MJC, Daneshvari NO, Radhakrishnan I, et al. Racial differences in statewide suicide mortality trends in Maryland during the coronavirus disease 2019 (COVID-19) pandemic. JAMA Psychiatry 2021;78(4):444–7.
39. Thompson HS, Manning M, Mitchell J, et al. Factors Associated With Racial/Ethnic Group–based medical mistrust and perspectives on COVID-19 vaccine trial participation and vaccine uptake in the US. JAMA Netw Open 2021;4(5):e2111629.
40. Abdi Latif Dahir, Holder J. Africa's Covid Crisis Deepens, but Vaccines Are Still Far Off. The New York Times. Accessed August 31, 2021. Available at: https://www.nytimes.com/interactive/2021/07/16/world/africa/africa-vaccination-rollout.html?action=click&module=Spotlight&pgtype=Homepage.
41. Crane MA, Shermock KM, Omer SB, et al. Change in reported adherence to non-pharmaceutical interventions during the COVID-19 pandemic, April-November 2020. JAMA 2021;325(9):883–5.
42. L Hamel, A Kirzinger, L Lopes, et al. KFF COVID-19 Vaccine Monitor: January 2021. 2021.
43. Murthy VH. Confronting Health Misinformation - The U.S. Surgeon General's Advisory on Building a Healthy Information Environment. 2021.
44. World Health Organization. Fighting misinformation in the time of COVID-19, one click at a time. Accessed August 31, 2021. Available at: https://www.who.int/news-room/feature-stories/detail/fighting-misinformation-in-the-time-of-covid-19-one-click-at-a-time.
45. Kirzinger A, Sparks G, Hamel L, et al. KFF COVID-19 Vaccine Monitor: July 2021. Accessed August 31, 2021. Available at: https://www.kff.org/coronavirus-covid-19/poll-finding/kff-covid-19-vaccine-monitor-july-2021/.
46. Bursztyn L, Rao A, Roth CP, Yanagizawa-Drott DH. Misinformation during a pandemic. 2020.
47. Roxby P. Psychiatrists fear 'tsunami' of mental illness after lockdown. Accessed August 31, 2021. Available at: https://www.bbc.com/news/health-52676981.
48. Leaune E, Samuel M, Oh H, et al. Suicidal behaviors and ideation during emerging viral disease outbreaks before the COVID-19 pandemic: a systematic rapid review. Prev Med 2020;106264. https://doi.org/10.1016/j.ypmed.2020.106264.
49. Kessler RC, Galea S, Gruber MJ, et al. Trends in mental illness and suicidality after Hurricane Katrina. Mol Psychiatry 2008;13(4):374–84.
50. O'Connor RC, Wetherall K, Cleare S, et al. Mental health and well-being during the COVID-19 pandemic: longitudinal analyses of adults in the UK COVID-19 Mental Health & Wellbeing study. Br J Psychiatry 2021;218(6):326–33.
51. Nomura S, Kawashima T, Yoneoka D, et al. Trends in suicide in Japan by gender during the COVID-19 pandemic, up to September 2020. Psychiatry Res 2021;295:113622.
52. Sakauye KM, Streim JE, Kennedy GJ, et al. AAGP position statement: disaster preparedness for older Americans: critical issues for the preservation of mental health. Am J Geriatr Psychiatry 2009;17(11):916–24.
53. Czeisler MÉ, Lane RI, Wiley JF, et al. Follow-up survey of US adult reports of mental health, substance use, and suicidal ideation during the COVID-19 pandemic, September 2020. JAMA Netw open 2021;4(2):e2037665.

54. Parlapani E, Holeva V, Nikopoulou VA, et al. A review on the COVID-19-related psychological impact on older adults: vulnerable or not? Aging Clin Exp Res 2021;33(6):1729–43.
55. Morganstein JC, Herberman Mash H, Vance MC, et al. Public Mental Health Interventions Following Disasters. In: Friedman MJ, Schnurr PP, Keane TM, editors. Handbook of PTSD. 3rd edition. Guilford Press; 2021. p. 570–88. Science and Practice.
56. Morganstein JC, Flynn BW. Enhancing Psychological Sustainment & Promoting Resilience in Healthcare Workers During COVID-19 & Beyond: Adapting Crisis Interventions from High-Risk Occupations. J Occup Environ Med 2021;63(6):482.
57. Hobfoll SE, Watson P, Bell CC, et al. Five essential elements of immediate and mid–term mass trauma intervention: Empirical evidence. Psychiatry Interpersonal Biol Process 2007;70(4):283–315.
58. Sulaiman AH, Ahmad Sabki Z, Jaafa MJ, et al. Development of a remote psychological first aid protocol for healthcare workers following the COVID-19 pandemic in a university teaching hospital. Malaysia: Multidisciplinary Digital Publishing Institute; 2020. p. 228.
59. Brooks SK, Dunn R, Amlôt R, et al. A systematic, thematic review of social and occupational factors associated with psychological outcomes in healthcare employees during an infectious disease outbreak. J Occup Environ Med 2018; 60(3):248–57.
60. Center for the Study of Traumatic Stress. COVID-19 PANDEMIC RESPONSE RESOURCES. Accessed August 31, 2021. Available at: https://www.cstsonline.org/resources/resource-master-list/coronavirus-and-emerging-infectious-disease-outbreaks-response.
61. The National Child Traumatic Stress Network. Accessed August 31, 2021. Available at: https://learn.nctsn.org/enrol/index.php?id=38.
62. NACCHO. Building Workforce Resilience through the Practice of Psychological First Aid – A Course for Supervisors and Leaders. Accessed August 31, 2021. Available at: https://www.massmed.org/Continuing-Education-and-Events/Online-CME/Courses/Psychological-First-Aid/Psychological-First-Aid–Healthy-Recovery-Now-and-in-the-Aftermath-of-the-COVID-19-Public-Health-Crisis/.
63. Heroes Health Initiative. Accessed August 31, 2021. Available at: https://heroeshealth.unc.edu/.
64. U.S. Department of Veteran Affairs. PTSD: National Center for PTSD, Mobile Apps: COVID Coach. Accessed August 31, 2021. Available at: https://www.ptsd.va.gov/appvid/mobile/COVID_coach_app.asp.
65. Burke A. Healing, Education, Resilience & Opportunity for New York's Frontline Workforce (HERO-NY). Accessed August 31, 2021. Available at: https://www.gnyha.org/program/hero-ny/.
66. Albott CS, Wozniak JR, McGlinch BP, et al. Battle Buddies: Rapid Deployment of a Psychological Resilience Intervention for Health Care Workers During the COVID-19 Pandemic. Anesth Analg 2020;131(1):43–54.
67. DePierro J, Katz CL, Marin D, et al. Mount Sinai's Center for Stress, Resilience and Personal Growth as a model for responding to the impact of COVID-19 on health care workers. Psychiatry Res 2020;293:113426.
68. Blake H, Yildirim M, Wood B, et al. COVID-Well: evaluation of the implementation of supported wellbeing centres for hospital employees during the COVID-19 pandemic. Int J Environ Res Public Health 2020;17(24):9401.

69. Malik M, Peirce J, Wert MV, et al. Psychological first aid well-being support rounds for frontline healthcare workers during COVID-19. Front Psychiatry 2021;12:766.
70. Pfefferbaum B, Newman E, Nelson SD, et al. Disaster media coverage and psychological outcomes: descriptive findings in the extant research. Curr Psychiatry Rep 2014;16(9):464.
71. Bendau A, Petzold MB, Pyrkosch L, et al. Associations between COVID-19 related media consumption and symptoms of anxiety, depression and COVID-19 related fear in the general population in Germany. Eur Arch Psychiatry Clin Neurosci 2021;271(2):283–91.
72. Gao J, Zheng P, Jia Y, et al. Mental health problems and social media exposure during COVID-19 outbreak. PLoS One 2020;15(4):e0231924.
73. Riehm KE, Holingue C, Kalb LG, et al. Associations between media exposure and mental distress among US adults at the beginning of the COVID-19 pandemic. Am J Prev Med 2020;59(5):630–8.
74. Allington D, McAndrew S, Moxham-Hall V, et al. Coronavirus conspiracy suspicions, general vaccine attitudes, trust and coronavirus information source as predictors of vaccine hesitancy among UK residents during the COVID-19 pandemic. Psychol Med 2021;1–12. https://doi.org/10.1017/S0033291721001434.
75. National Academy of Sciences Engineering and Medicine. Building COVID-19 Vaccine Confidence. Accessed August 31, 2021. Available at: https://www.nap.edu/resource/26068/interactive/.
76. World Health O. Communicating risk in public health emergencies: a WHO guideline for emergency risk communication (ERC) policy and practice. Geneva: World Health Organization; 2017.
77. Reynolds B. Crisis and emergency risk communication (Manual). 2014th edition. Atlanta, GA: CDC; 2014.
78. Shulman HC, Dixon GN, Bullock OM, et al. The effects of jargon on processing fluency, self-perceptions, and scientific engagement. J Lang Social Psychol 2020;39(5–6):579–97.
79. Agley J, Xiao Y. Misinformation about COVID-19: evidence for differential latent profiles and a strong association with trust in science. BMC Public Health 2021;21(1):1–12.
80. APA Committee on Psychiatric Dimensions of Disaster. Communicating With The Public During The COVID-19 Pandemic. 2021.
81. Wood MD, Walker T, Adler AB, et al. Post-traumatic growth leadership: mitigating stress in a high-risk occupation. Occup Health Sci 2020;4:1–20.
82. McKinsey, Company. Leadership in a crisis: How leaders can support their organizations during the COVID-19 crisis and recovery. Accessed August 31, 2021. Available at: https://www.mckinsey.com/business-functions/organization/our-insights/leadership-in-a-crisis.
83. Wright KS, Sparacino L, Bartone P, et al. The human response to the Gander military air disaster: A summary report. 1987.

Sheppard Pratt

Lessons Learned During COVID Across a System of Care

Harsh K. Trivedi, MD, MBA

KEYWORDS

• COVID • System of care • Lessons learned • Behavioral health

KEY POINTS

- Across the nation, each organization and every leadership team has become battle-tested during the COVID-19 pandemic.
- There is a greater need for behavioral health services due to burnout, as well as generalized trauma due to racial injustices and COVID.
- Key leadership and operational lessons learned during COVID are presented for a health system with 387 care sites, across 160 programs, serving 70,000 patients.
- General preparedness, maintaining access to care, staffing plan strategies, supporting our employees, and moving forward beyond the pandemic are presented.

INTRODUCTION

Across the nation, each organization and every leadership team has become battle-tested during the coronavirus disease 2019 (COVID-19) pandemic. Health care has been impacted in every community, and the mental health toll of the pandemic continues to worsen each day. At Sheppard Pratt, we have offered several webinars, resource tools, and technical assistance to our colleagues across the nation throughout the pandemic. The lessons highlighted in this article form key learnings made possible through discussions from within the organization and reflections of many colleagues nationwide.

THE IMPENDING TIDAL WAVE

In early 2020, coronavirus was not a household name and certainly not a worldwide pandemic. Instead, our nation was grappling with all-time high rates of suicide, including an alarming trend among young people. Drug overdose deaths soared, and people lacked access to psychiatric services.

Sheppard Pratt, 6501 N. Charles St, Baltimore, MD 21204, USA
E-mail address: htrivedi@sheppardpratt.org
Twitter: @HarshTrivediMD (H.K.T.)

Psychiatr Clin N Am 45 (2022) 211–225
https://doi.org/10.1016/j.psc.2021.11.015
psych.theclinics.com
0193-953X/22/

As COVID-19 cases continue to surge and are well nearly 45 million in the United States at the time of this writing, an even larger crisis is barreling toward us like a tidal wave—the impending behavioral health surge created by COVID-19 (**Fig. 1**).

In the aforementioned depiction, within that first wave, those that have psychiatric comorbidity were staying at home trying to manage their condition or illness so they would not end up in an emergency room. As we moved into the second wave, we saw an impact on non-COVID conditions and how people were having negative health outcomes as a result.

Then there is the third wave—interrupted care for chronic conditions, including mental health. The fourth wave is pending. After nearly 2 years of uncertainty, fear, social isolation, stress, and anxiety, we are seeing the beginnings of this wave: psychiatric trauma, mental illness, and burnout.

In a 2020 Centers for Disease Control and Prevention report, 10% of respondents reported having seriously considered suicide in the prior 30 days.[2] Only 4% of respondents in a relatively similar study considered taking their own lives in 2018[3]—and in that year, 48,000 died of suicide.[4] Suicide rates, which were already alarmingly high prepandemic, are expected to increase. In addition, the CDC report indicated that almost 41% of respondents reported at least one mental health concern, and experiences of distress such as depressive and anxiety symptoms were reported as 3 to 4 times greater than prepandemic periods.[2] The Maryland Opioid Operational Command Center reported an overall 9.1% jump in drug-related overdose deaths in the first half of 2020 compared with the same period in 2019,[5] which it attributed to the COVID-19 pandemic.

We envision a greater need for behavioral health services due to the burnout of health care providers and the broader community, as well as the generalized trauma many have seen and experienced due to racial injustices and COVID.

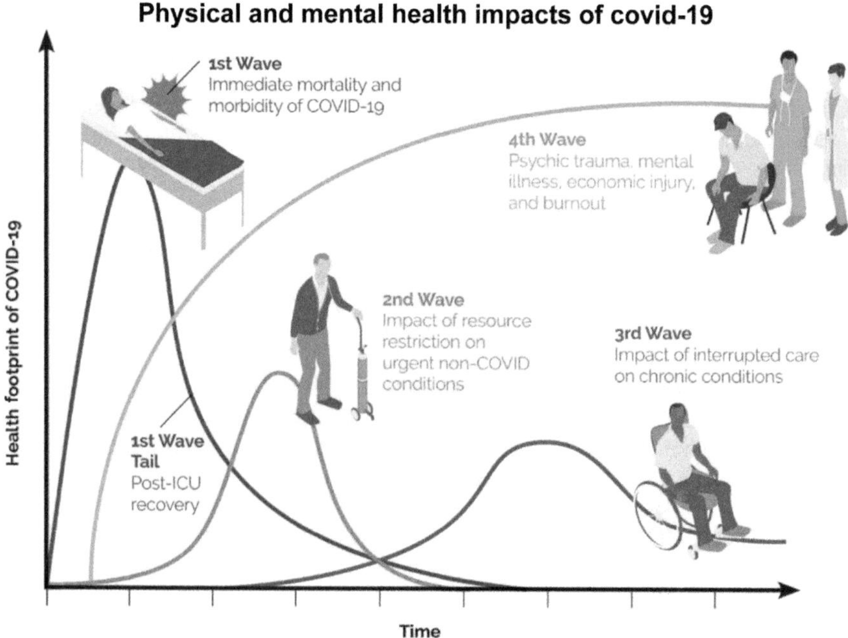

Fig. 1. Physical and mental health impacts of COVID-19.[1] (*Adapted with permission from* Victor Tseng, MD.)

PROVIDING A SYSTEM OF CARE

What helps to make Sheppard Pratt unique is also what has been most challenging in planning a response to COVID-19. Since its founding in 1853, Sheppard Pratt has been innovating the field through research, best practice implementation, and a focus on improving the quality of mental health care on a global level. As the nation's largest private, nonprofit provider of mental health, substance use, developmental disability, special education, and social services in the country, there were challenges in our response. Challenges ranged from managing COVID protocols across 387 sites of care to maintaining access for patients across the nation and the globe. As a safety-net provider, we had to ensure solutions worked for people with serious mental illness and who have significant barriers to accessing care, such as homelessness and lack of broadband access. We serve more than 70,000 individuals in more than 160 programs, including inpatient and outpatient treatment, housing, education, job training, and rehabilitation services, among many others. With such a broad and diverse system of care—including heterogeneity in types of programs and levels of care—the first lessons became quite clear, quite fast (**Fig. 2**).

In a Rapidly Changing Environment, Use Organizational Culture as a Strength

From the beginning, what we believed to be true and the directives coming from local, state, and federal authorities were rapidly evolving. In order for an organization to be nimble enough to keep up with the breakneck pace of change, there had to be an acknowledgment that a strictly top-down approach was not feasible. Rather, the importance of empowering local leaders and frontline staff to problem solve and share what works became energizing to teams across our organization.

Information Is a Liberator, Be Transparent and Message Often

During times of significant and rapid change, one of the greatest problems can be information gaps. Increasing anxiety combined with a lack of transparency leaves ample room for conjecture or detrimental misinformation to take hold. Updates should be

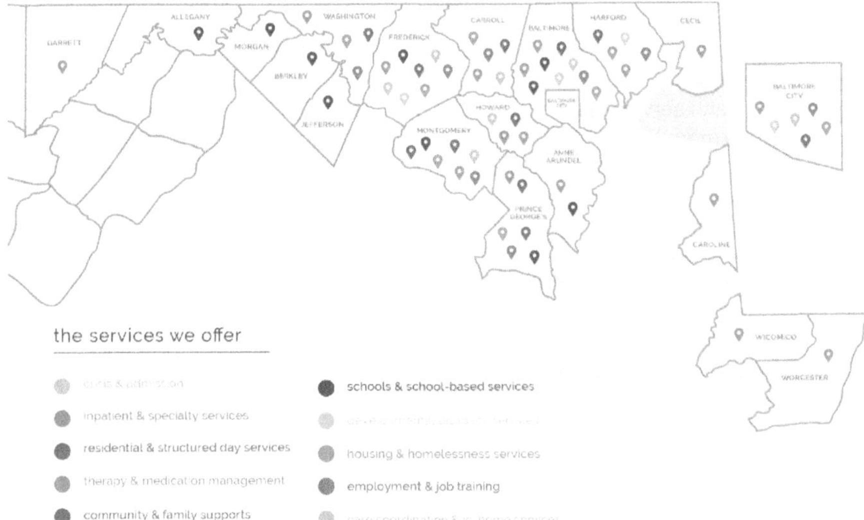

Fig. 2. Location overview of Sheppard Pratt programs and services.

provided at regularly scheduled intervals and there should be transparency about what we know and what is uncertain. Multiple formats should be used to communicate to align with reaching various internal audiences and external stakeholders.

The Role of a Leader Is to Set the Tone and Unite the Team in Purpose

From the onset of the pandemic, we had regular conversations with leaders across the organization. These virtual calls allowed nearly 300 leaders to hear directly from members of the executive team on a regular basis. Beyond data and updates, careful effort was placed to help leaders set the tone for a robust and organized response. We had discussions that framed the response to COVID as being a marathon and not a sprint. We discussed the importance of a leader in helping to smooth the bumps, rather than feeding into the uncertainty. The message was consistent from the beginning—we will get through this together, supporting one another, helping each other through difficult days at work and at home, and providing the care we would expect for our own loved ones throughout. We routinely refocused on our mission and why we each come to work.

MAINTAINING ACCESS TO LIFE-SAVING CARE

As behavioral health needs are increasing across the nation, we are seeing an alarming trend of decreasing behavioral health services across many communities. The number of state-funded psychiatric beds per capita has decreased by 97% between 1955 and 2016,[6] with the per capita psychiatric inpatient bed count approximately 70% lower than the average among developed nations.[6]

Many hospitals and health systems were decreasing bed capacity before COVID-19, and as COVID continued, more had to reduce bed capacity due to COVID-19 concerns as well as close units temporarily to accommodate patients with medical/respiratory COVID-19. In June 2020, the University of Washington Medicine shut down its 14-bed psychiatric unit amid financial shortfalls.[7] Providence Behavioral Health also ended its inpatient services in June 2020 reducing the number of psychiatric beds for children and adolescents in the western part of Massachusetts to zero.[8] Heywood Healthcare in Massachusetts also closed its adult mental health unit in April 2020 as a result of the financial effects of COVID-19 and was uncertain if it would be able to reopen.[9]

In contrast, Sheppard Pratt recognized the importance of remaining open and providing access for those who need care and services at a time when the need for behavioral health services is greater than ever. Sheppard Pratt has more than 160 programs across more than 380 sites of service in Maryland and West Virginia. It was critical to support the patients, clients, and students we serve so they had timely access to quality care and services (**Fig. 3**).

Sheppard Pratt rapidly adapted its care and services across the continuum of care to meet the wide-ranging demands. We have been able to keep all 19 of our hospital inpatient units open and operating during the pandemic. In addition, we reimagined our community-based and school-based programs to ensure our clients and students were able to get the support and help they needed.

Part of the process early on in COVID was forming good partnerships with health departments at the county and state level in an effort to maintain our services. Substantial education and partnership was required so as not to accept the status quo of psychiatric care being automatically deemed congregate care. Rather, officials were engaged to understand that every emergency room across our state would come to a standstill if Sheppard Pratt was unable to maintain the flow of psychiatric patients in acute crisis.

Crisis & Admission
- Psychiatric urgent care/Virtual Psychiatric Urgent Care
- Assessment and intake services
- Therapy referral services
- Mobile crisis services

Inpatient & Specialty Services
- Child, adolescent, adult, geriatric services
- Intellectual disabilities, neuropsychiatry
- OCD and anxiety, psychotic disorders, trauma, eating disorders, sports psychiatry, autism, direct-to-employer services

Residential & Structured Day Services
- Day hospitals
- Crisis residential services
- Psychiatric rehabilitation services
- Residential treatment services

Therapy & Medication Management
- Addiction services
- Outpatient and in-home/in-community behavioral health services
- Integrated primary and behavioral health care services
- Telepsychiatry services
- Neurostimulation

Community & Family Supports
- Head start program
- Domestic violence shelter
- Early intervention parenting support
- Supervised visitation, monitored exchange
- Substance use and recovery support services
- Child development center, family counseling and education services

Schools & School-Based Services
- Nonpublic special education
- School-based mental health and substance use support services
- Residential treatment centers

Developmental Disability Services
- Neuropsychiatry services
- Inpatient and outpatient intellectual disabilities and autism care
- Schools and school-based programs

Housing & Homelessness Services
- Homeless outreach services
- Housing counselor services
- Veterans service center

Employment & Job Training
- Business services
- Employment support
- Vocational services
- Project SEARCH

Care Coordination & In-Home Services
- Assertive community treatment services
- Behavioral health home services
- In-home counseling services

Fig. 3. Overview of Sheppard Pratt programs and services.

Maintaining Care in Our Hospitals

We developed a personalized patient care approach in our hospitals during COVID that differed from patient to patient. We looked closely at managing our therapeutic environments to maintain social distancing—from rearranging and eliminating furniture to changing the size of our therapy groups (**Fig. 4**).

For example, on our child unit wherein the children are very active and often cling together, how could we maintain a therapeutic environment and keep them safe from an infection control perspective? We gave visual cues to help our patients see what it means to be socially distanced. This was helpful with many of our specialty units (**Fig. 5**).

Patients were also encouraged to wear a mask to practice infection control prevention measures. When patients were noncompliant with wearing personal protective equipment (PPE), we took an individualized approach with successful interventions for all patients. We ensured staff maintained social distancing. There were also alternative activities provided that were therapeutic and interactive, but could be

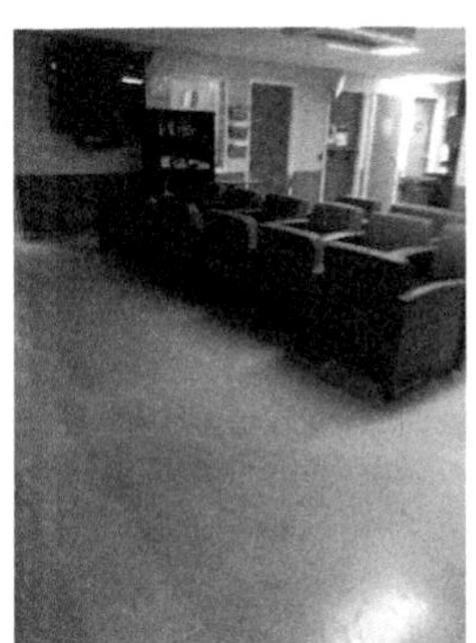
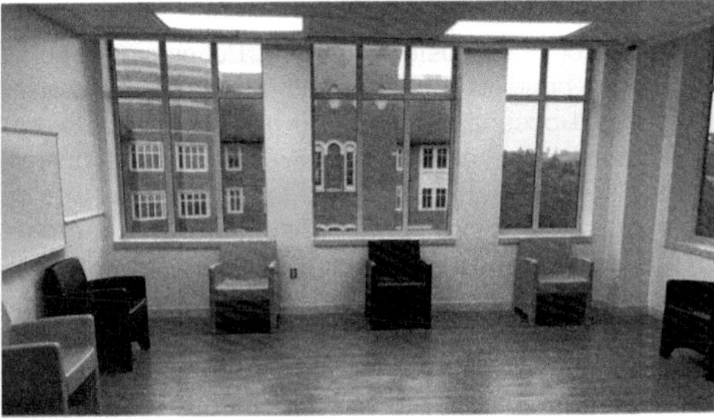

Fig. 4. Managing therapeutic environments to maintain social distancing.

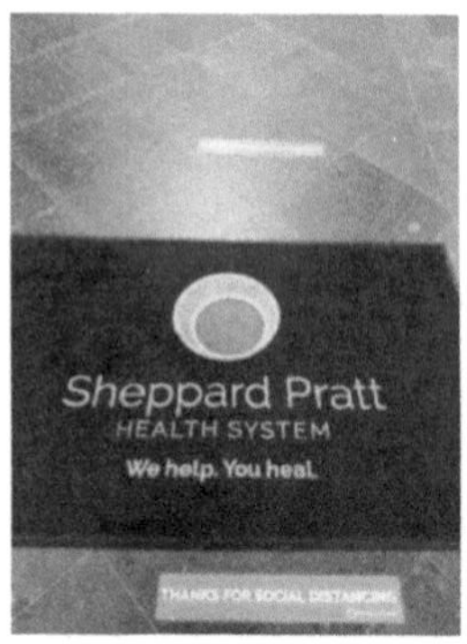

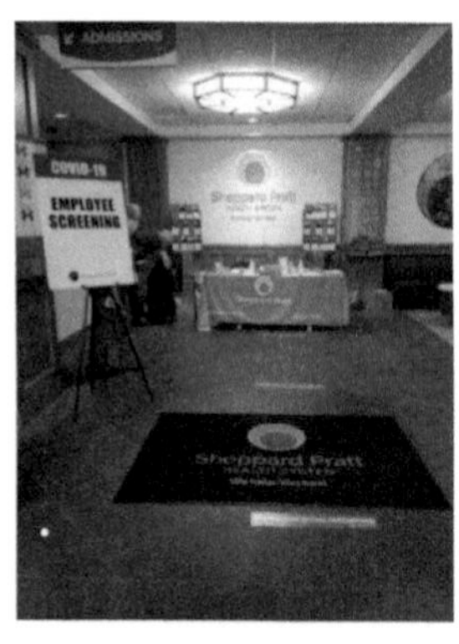

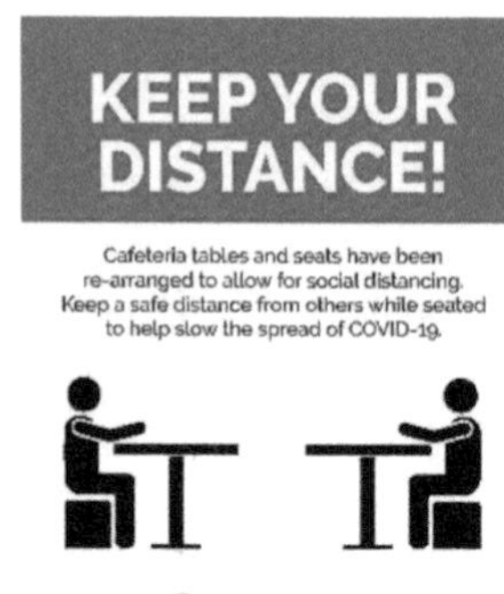

Fig. 5. Examples of social distancing signage and graphics.

accomplished at a distance. In addition, we had PPE code kits so that staff assisting for medical or psychiatric emergencies had everything they needed at a moment's notice to feel protected and safe. We also reduced the areas from which staff could respond to minimize interactions and potential spread should anyone become COVID positive (**Fig. 6**).

Our partial hospitalization programs also had to get creative when it came to programming as our day programs went virtual. We made sure patients had access to zoom rooms. We have provided a mix of individual sessions while also using interactive sessions to get them up and moving, like yoga or helping them walk through guided meditation or mindfulness.

In any given year, Sheppard Pratt cares for patients from 42 states and 19 foreign countries. Many of our hospital programs are renown in their expertise, and people travel from outside of the region to receive this specialized care. In the early months of COVID, when there were hotspots, we wanted to ensure the safety of our patients and employees. We focused our specialty program admissions on areas within driving distance, tested upon arrival, and had a mandatory quarantine period.

For our regular hospital admissions from emergency department (ED) referrals, the ED tested for COVID before approval. Patients were subsequently room restricted for the first 72 hours of their stay with clinical services delivered in the room. We also limited dual occupancy rooms to ensure that we were not placing someone who had quarantined already with a new patient in the quarantine period.

Our Care Connect team, similar to a call center, was critical during this time. Team members act as navigators for Sheppard Pratt's programs; they triaged calls and responded to e-mail inquiries to connect people to the program that fits their needs—from level of care, to therapeutic interventions, to insurance, and location. Our national outreach team was similarly working with referring providers to help them with the referral process to get patients the specialty care they needed and make the admissions process as smooth as possible, including managing travel logistics.

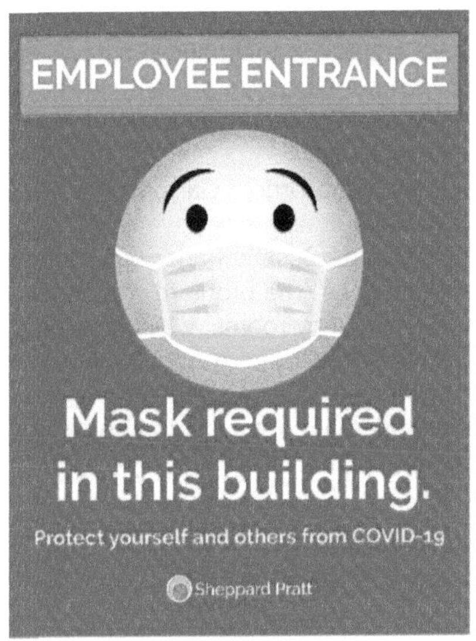

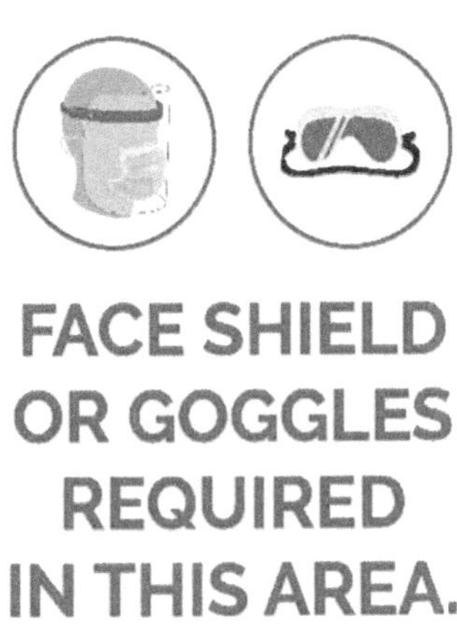

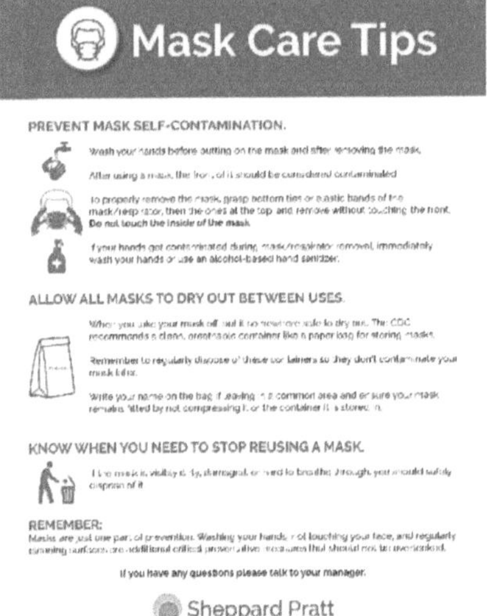

Fig. 6. Examples of PPE signage utilized across the health system.

Maintaining Care in the Community

Much of our outpatient care was converted to telehealth, providing virtual access to thousands of patients, including more than 500,000 virtual visits that were conducted from April through just the first half of 2021. For our most vulnerable, staff members were redeployed to conduct home visits across 200 supportive housing locations to help manage food and shelter, providing more than 250,000 meals to the community. And for those who need long-acting injections, we created mobile nursing teams to provide in-home medication administration and injections. We worked closely to help people learn to manage their own care, especially some of our more vulnerable populations with developmental disabilities. We ensured people had thermometers, and we taught them how to check their own temperature. We are certain that we kept thousands of people with serious mental illness alive and safe during this most uncertain time (**Figs. 7** and **8**).

In April 2020, we also launched our Virtual Psychiatric Urgent Care, which was an extension of our in-person services for those seeking emergency psychiatric care; it provides those in crisis with an online mental health assessment and then connects them to the most appropriate level of care and services. The program was meant to decrease the volume of psychiatric patients in emergency rooms, which are integral when hospitals are taking care of patients with COVID-19. From April 2020 through June 2021, our virtual crisis clinic provided more than 3500 crisis evaluations and urgent follow-up appointments for medication management or psychotherapy.

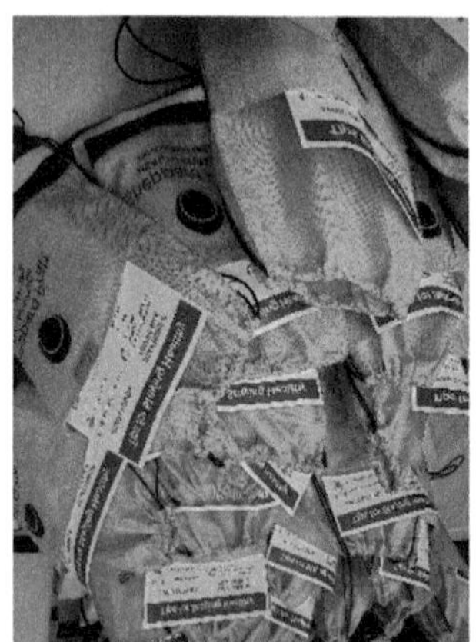

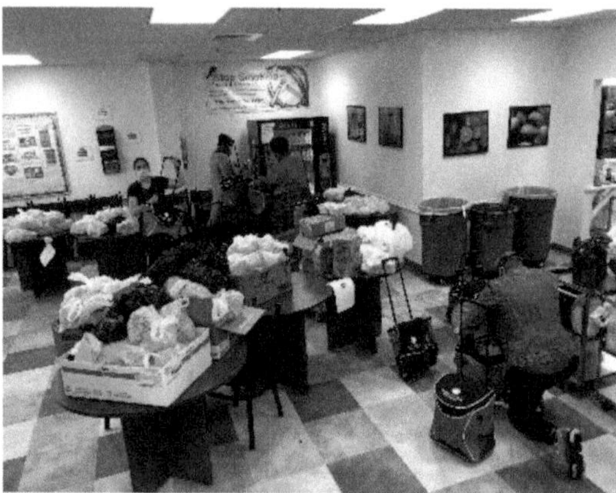

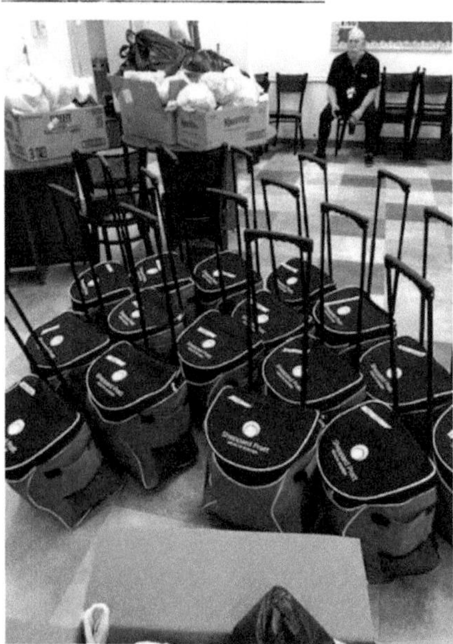

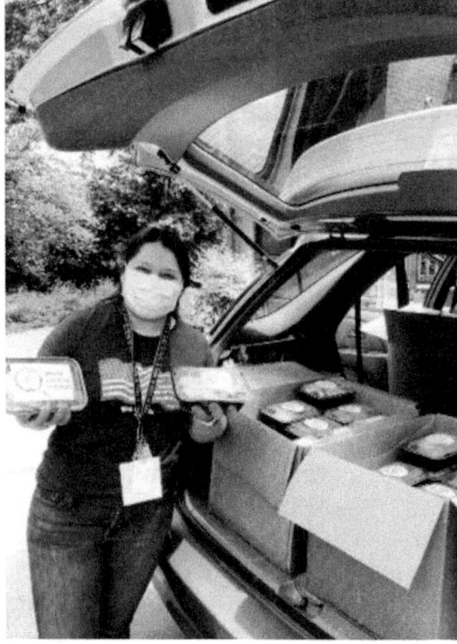

Fig. 7. Adapting services to maintain care in the community.

Staying Healthy During Coronavirus

It is important to know if I am sick. Some signs I might be sick are:

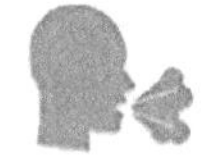

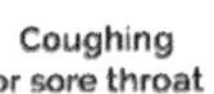

Feeling very tired

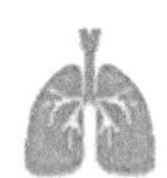

Feeling out of breath

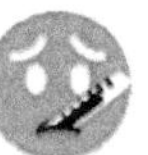

Fever

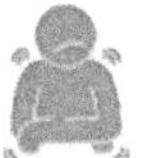

Chills and body aches

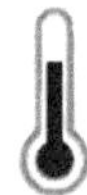

A fever means my body temperature is over 100.4 degrees. If I have a fever my skin might feel hot. I might shiver or have chills.

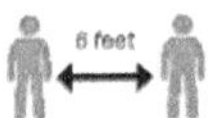

If I might be sick, I need to stay away from other people so that I do not spread germs.

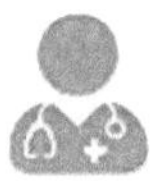

It is important to tell someone so that I can get help to get better. I might need to call my doctor.

There are ways I can try to stay healthy. I stay healthy by:

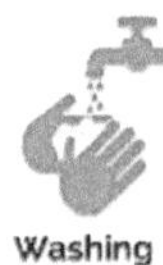

Washing my hands

Exercising

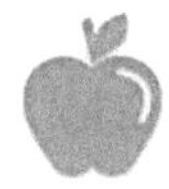

Healthy eating

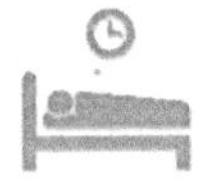

Getting enough sleep

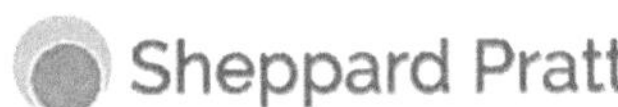

Fig. 8. Social story example.

Telehealth can be a game changer and equalizer when it comes to access. For many, transportation can be a barrier to accessing quality care. Following the virtual evaluation, if in-person care was needed, our transportation team picked up the patient and brought them to the program for further evaluation and treatment. This innovative virtual program was awarded the Innovation in Health Care award by a local business publication. Our chief of medical staff and medical director of outpatient services received the health care outcomes award from our local business journal for his work with our Virtual Psychiatric Urgent Care.

We developed and launched other programs to support our community. The Retreat, our premier program for mood disorders and substance use, began offering a virtual program in light of the COVID-19 pandemic.

The continued uncertainty surrounding COVID-19 has caused many people to evaluate the impact of anxiety, obsessive-compulsive disorder (OCD), and related disorders on their daily lives. Sheppard Pratt launched the Center for OCD and Anxiety during the pandemic in response to increased community need to help more people get the specialized and compassionate care they need. We also added confidential access to crisis care for health care workers that are on the frontlines of this pandemic, including internal counseling appointments and resiliency training.

Our schools and school-based programs continued to support students and families in Maryland and the surrounding area. We operate 12 nonpublic special education schools throughout the state that support more than 700 students with autism spectrum disorders, behavioral disabilities, and intellectual disabilities.

During COVID, our schools pivoted to develop continuation of learning plans for when schools were not in session and established a comprehensive task force to review metrics and develop safe reopening strategies. Our teams had to think creatively about how to deliver not only education but also mental health services in new and innovative ways, whereas both our schools and public schools remained closed during the COVID pandemic. Last fall and winter, clinicians made therapy kits that included some basic materials such as journals, crayons, color pencils, and fidget toys. These resources served as materials to be used during the telehealth sessions and also for the children to have some materials when they felt anxious or upset.

Throughout all the transitions, changes, and uncertainties, bottom-up solution-finding was encouraged. Employees were empowered to suggest solutions that could help the organization and those we serve thrive.

STAFFING PLAN STRATEGIES

Within our hospitals, we created almost 19 different subpockets so our units became sites where we did not look to do transfers from unit to unit. These are things that naturally occur when we are in non-COVID times, but are especially important to limit during the current environment.

We also used a modified provider staffing schedule of 7 days on/7 days off, with one provider on a unit at a time and another provider that is supporting off-unit via telehealth. Normally, we could have anywhere from 2 to 3, maybe even four doctors or nurse practitioners providing care on our inpatient setting. We limited it to just one doctor or nurse practitioner on the unit at any given time. During their 7 days on, it was one person physically on the unit that could be seeing up to 20 patients, maybe even up to 22 patients if our largest unit was filled. We did a similar staffing schedule with nurse leaders.

From an infection control standpoint, but also from a burnout standpoint, we saw the impact COVID was having and how it was wearing our employees down. Having an alternate schedule gave some reprieve. With our other frontline staff, we were also trying to compress their schedules so that they are on 3 or 4 days at a time and not on/off/on to get a much-needed reprieve as well as limit their exposure.

In addition, we worked to limit our float pool. Before our first patient with COVID-19, we tried to find a home base for our float pool so that we had extra people in service lines and areas to limit floating. We have also been very attentive to when staff get sick and how we support them. We set up a screening process early on in the pandemic, which includes screening before entering our hospitals and throughout the day on our units. And we pay really close attention to how people are feeling. We send people home, and we encourage them not to come to work if they have any symptoms.

SUPPORTING OUR EMPLOYEES

From the onset, in addition to ensuring we provide the best care and services to those we serve, our focus has also been on our 5000 employees. We know how critical they are to the success of the organization and providing the high-quality, compassionate care that we are known for.

As we adapted to the changing circumstances of COVID-19, it was critical that employees had timely and accurate information. Our executive leadership team began hosting daily calls with more than 200 leaders in our organization to share important information about COVID, share success stories, as well as support our leaders so they could in turn support their team. These calls have moved to a biweekly update, but still continue today. In addition, to better communicate with all employees, we launched an internal communications platform that was accessible via desktop and mobile to not only provide information about COVID-19 and resources but also keep employees energized and motivated about the work they were doing each day (**Fig. 9**).

Early on during the pandemic when an executive order to shut down schools in Maryland was issued—including our own special education schools—it became clear that our employees would need support while working and handling duties as caregivers. We quickly created day camps staffed by our school-based employees at 5 locations across the state to provide a free, safe space for children of our employees (**Fig. 10**).

We also provided telehealth counseling resources for our staff, offered free therapy groups for employees led by one of our providers, as well as provided our leaders access to coaching resources to help them lead and to support their staff. Employees and their loved ones also had access to a wealth of mental health, wellness, and self-care resources that we developed and housed on our Web site including blogs on reducing anxiety and sharing mindfulness tips, links to free at-home fitness options, and resources for parents about coping with online learning and managing during a lockdown. We regularly encouraged employees to access these free resources and to also use our Employee Assistance Program.

As leaders, we needed to role model vulnerability and healthy behaviors. It is the role of leadership to carry organizational anxiety and work actively to reduce barriers. Our

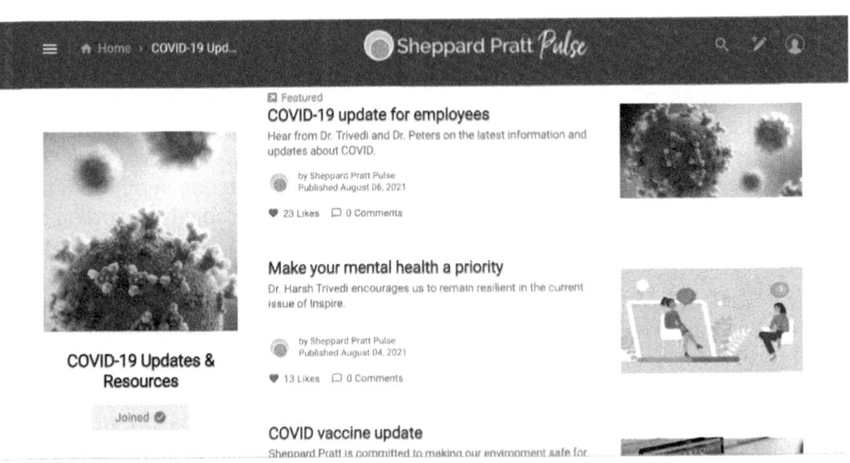

Fig. 9. Internal communication platform with COVID-19 updates and resources.

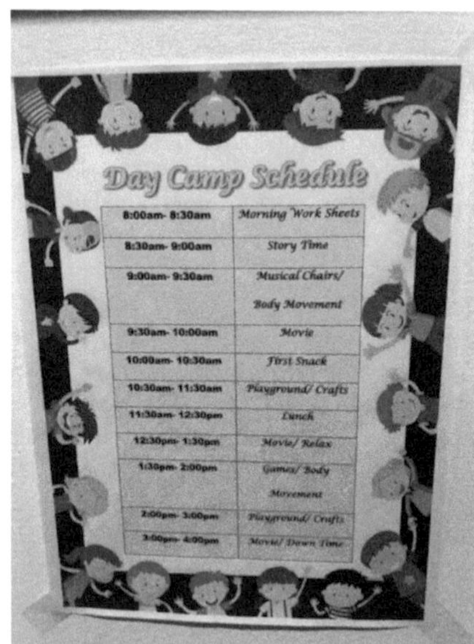

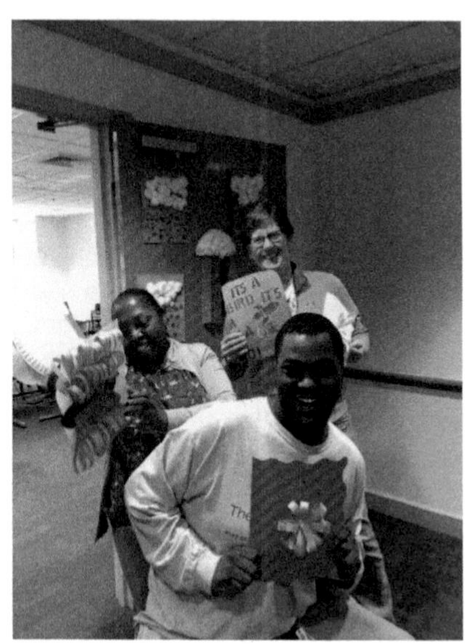

Fig. 10. Sheppard Pratt day camps were created early in the pandemic to support children of our employees.

leadership team prioritized making it "okay to not be okay." We encouraged employees to embrace uncertainty and know that this was a marathon not a sprint. Employees were also encouraged to stop and share how hard the journey has been and support one another to the finish line. And where possible, encourage people to take time off to recharge, find ways for people to disconnect from work, and place an importance on family and community.

GENERAL PREPAREDNESS AND RESPONSE

Following the state of emergency declared by the Governor of Maryland in March 2020, Sheppard Pratt initiated a Code Yellow (Disaster/Emergency code) to ensure we were on standby notice and ready to activate our emergency preparedness plan as needed given the potential surge of patients to hospitals.

Although a surge did not mean our hospitals would receive patients with potential or confirmed cases of COVID-19, it did mean that we needed to think about our discharge plans for patients so that we can continue to receive psychiatric patients (who are not medically at risk) from other area hospitals. This proactive thinking allowed area hospitals to have greater capacity to care for those in our communities with the virus. We maintained ongoing dialogue with area hospitals regarding our admissions so that we could be a resource and quickly move psychiatric patients to our facilities.

All throughout COVID, we were fortunate to stay ahead of PPE needs by empowering our supply chain team to use their expertise and ensure adequate PPE supply. Our operational excellence team developed new programs for supply control and sourcing materials to sites across the state, something practically unheard of within psychiatric hospitals. To ensure we had sufficient supplies of PPE at each location, we developed a new process for requesting and tracking daily consumption of supplies to manage our organizational supply chain most efficiently.

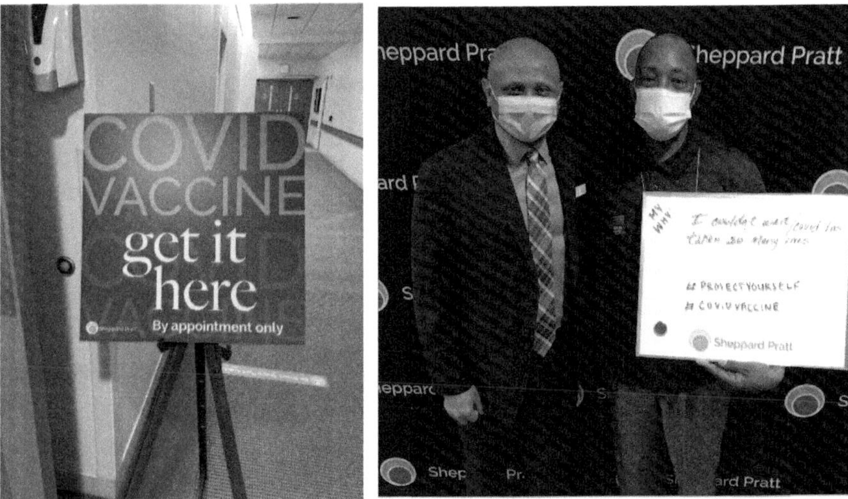

Fig. 11. Hosted vaccine clinics to vaccinate employees as well as some of the most vulnerable in our communities.

We identified designated PPE requestors to submit daily consumption tracking of PPE and new requests for PPE-related supplies. All PPE-related requests went through these designated requestors for processing. By following this process, we maintained an efficient and centralized critical supply distribution process.

It was also seen as an imperative for Sheppard Pratt to lead the way and secure COVID-19 vaccine access for our broader mental health community. Beginning in late December 2020, we hosted vaccine clinics daily at our conference center in Baltimore County as well as through pop-up clinics throughout the state to help vaccinate employees, including our psychiatry residents/fellows, as well as vaccinating some of the most vulnerable in our group homes (**Fig. 11**).

We also contacted the Maryland Psychiatric Society as well as local providers to offer access to our vaccine clinic to ensure psychiatrists and other mental health practitioners were vaccinated.

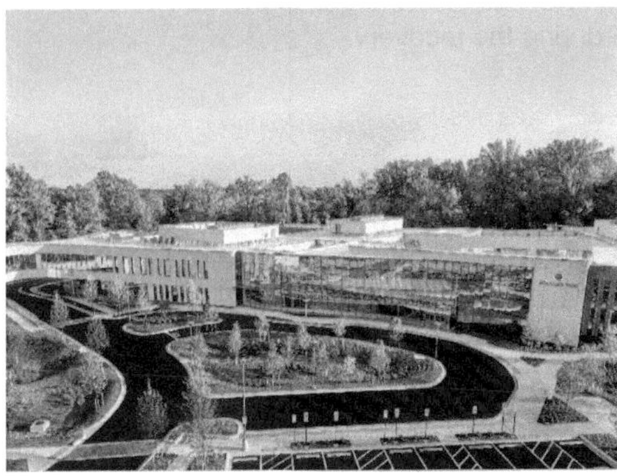

Fig. 12. The new Sheppard Pratt - Baltimore/Washington Campus

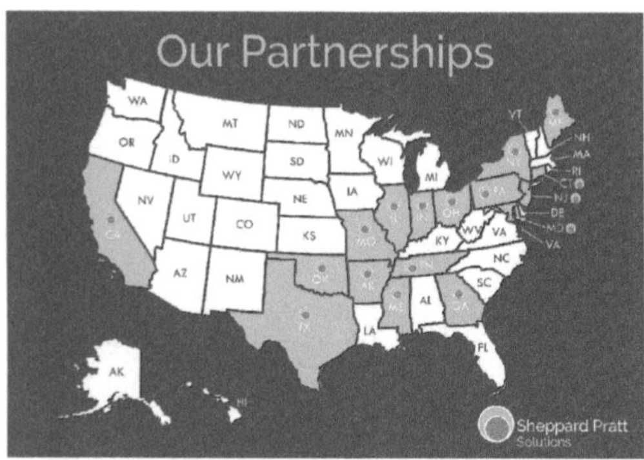

Fig. 13. Sheppard Pratt Solutions partnerships to meet the behavioral health demand in communities nationwide as of November 2021.

MOVING FORWARD

The last 2 years have shown that mental health services are needed now, more than ever. Beyond managing our COVID response, Sheppard Pratt doubled down on innovation and developing the next set of resources our nation would need. From opening a brand new psychiatric hospital in the Baltimore-Washington corridor, to opening additional crisis beds, to beginning a replication of Vermont's statewide hub-and-spoke model for opioid treatment, to penning the next Textbook on Hospital Psychiatry for the field, we have mobilized all of our care teams and dedicated care providers to do more. We do not plan to give up the organizational agility that we have gained during COVID because there is so much more that we all need to do (**Fig. 12**).

We have also seen the need for solutions to meet the increased demand for behavioral health services locally, regionally, and nationally. Recently, we launched Sheppard Pratt Solutions, a new division that uses the extensive expertise of our mental health professionals to provide consulting, management services, and development-based partnerships to help health care organizations nationwide establish and improve delivery of hospital and community-based behavioral health services in their community (**Fig. 13**).

Now begins the hard work for all of us to work together and find the path forward.

As the need for more behavioral and mental health treatment options increases and as psychiatric bed capacity remains almost full, it is critical to have access to care and services. Sheppard Pratt has been integral to the COVID response, and all of us will be ever more integral during the recovery.

DISCLOSURE

The author has nothing to disclose.

REFERENCES

1. Adapted from: https://twitter.com/VectorSting, Accessed October 22, 2021.
2. Czeisler MÉ, Lane RI, Petrosky E, et al. Mental health, substance use, and suicidal ideation during the COVID-19 pandemic — United States, June 24–30, 2020. Available at: https://www.cdc.gov/mmwr/volumes/69/wr/pdfs/mm6932a1-H.pdf. [Accessed 14 August 2020].

3. Substance Abuse and Mental Health Services Administration. Key substance use and mental health indicators in the United States: results from the 2018 National Survey on Drug Use and Health (HHS Publication No. PEP19-5068, NSDUH Series H-54). Rockville (MD): Center for Behavioral Health Statistics and Quality,Substance Abuse and Mental Health Services Administration; 2019. Available at: https://www.samhsa.gov/data/.
4. Data Brief 355. Mortality in the United States, 2018. (PDF). CDC.
5. Oxenden MK. Drug- and alcohol-related deaths across Maryland jump more than 9% due to the coronavirus, officials say. Baltimore Sun 2020. Available at: https://www.baltimoresun.com/health/bs-hs-opioid-report-first-half-of-year-20200922-2khvu37zhngf7dsiqivulv6ctu-story.html.
6. National Association for Behavioral Healthcare. The high cost of compliance: assessing the regulatory burden on inpatient psychiatric facilities. Washington, DC: National Association for Behavioral Healthcare; 2020. p. 7. Available at: https://www.nabh.org/wp-content/uploads/2019/03/The-High-Cost-of-Compliance.pdf.
7. Bush E. UW Medicine shuts down psychiatric unit amid financial shortfall. Seattle Times. 2020. Available at: https://www.seattletimes.com/seattle-news/health/uw-medicine-shuts-down-psychiatric-unit-amid-financial-shortfall/. Accessed October 22, 2021.
8. Barry S. 'This is a scary, ugly system': Families say loss of Providence Behavioral Health Hospital beds endangers kids. MassLive.com. 2020. Available at: https://www.masslive.com/coronavirus/2020/05/this-is-a-scary-ugly-system-families-say-loss-of-providence-behavioral-health-hospital-beds-endangers-kids.html. Accessed October 22, 2021.
9. Durling D. Heywood healthcare closes mental health unit in cost-saving move. Massachusettes: The Gardner News; 2020. Available at: https://www.thegardnernews.com/news/20200417/heywood-healthcare-closes-mental-health-unit-in-cost-saving-move.

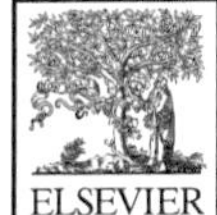
ELSEVIER

9780323848589